D1738589

PSYCHIATRY INSIDE OUT: SELECTED WRITINGS OF FRANCO BASAGLIA

EUROPEAN PERSPECTIVES

A series of the Columbia University Press

Psychiatry Inside Out: Selected Writings of Franco Basaglia

edited by Nancy Scheper-Hughes and Anne M. Lovell

Foreword by Robert Coles

Translated from the Italian
by Anne M. Lovell and Teresa Shtob

Columbia University Press   New York   1987

Library of Congress Cataloging-in-Publication Data

Basaglia, Franco.
  Psychiatry inside out.

  (European perspectives)
  Selected and translated from Scritti.
  Bibliography: p.
  1. Psychiatry.   2. Psychology, Pathological.
3. Psychotherapy.   I. Scheper-Huges, Nancy.
II. Lovell, Anne.   III. Title.   IV. Series.
RC458.B362513   1987   616.89   86-23287
ISBN 0-231-05718-0

Columbia University Press
New York Guildford, Surrey
Copyright © 1987 Columbia University Press
All rights reserved

Printed in the United States of America

This book is
Smyth-sewn.

Book design by J.S. Roberts

Contents

Foreword Robert Coles   vii

Preface Franca Ongaro Basaglia   xi

Acknowledgments   xxvii

Editors' Note   xxix

Introduction The Utopia of Reality: Franco Basaglia
and the Practice of a Democratic Psychiatry

Anne M. Lovell and Nancy Scheper-Hughes   1

Part One DESTROYING THE MENTAL HOSPITAL:
WRITINGS FROM GORIZIA

Introduction—Nancy Scheper-Hughes   53
1. Institutions of Violence   59
2. The Problem of the Incident   87

Part Two DEVIANCE, "TOLERANCE,"
AND MARGINALITY: WRITINGS
FROM ITALY AND AMERICA

Introduction—Naomar de Almeida-Filho
and Nancy Scheper-Hughes   95
3. The Disease and Its Double and the Deviant Majority:
Critical Propositions on the Problem of Deviance   101
4. Letter from America: The Artificial Patient   127

Part Three PRACTICING KNOWLEDGE:
REFLECTIONS ON THE ROLE OF INTELLECTUALS

Introduction—Anne M. Lovell   137
5. Peacetime Crimes: Technicians of Practical Knowledge   143
A Conversation with Jean-Paul Sartre   169

A Dialogue with R.D. Laing   194
Science and the Criminalization of Need   202

Part Four ON THE NATURE OF MADNESS

Introduction—Anne M. Lovell   227
6. Madness/Delirium   231

Part Five ANTI-INSTITUTIONAL POLITICS
AND REFORM: ON PSYCHIATRY AND LAW

Introduction—Anne M. Lovell   267
7. Problems of Law and Psychiatry: The Italian Experience 271
Appendix: Law N. 180   292
8. Critical Psychiatry After the Law 180   299

Notes   305

Foreword

Robert Coles

As I read this book I kept thinking of one of the "psychotic" patients I met when a resident in psychiatry at the Massachusetts General Hospital in Boston. She was, by her own telling, sad and worried and fearful. She was also plagued by "ghosts," as she called them. The more I talked with her, the more I was convinced that she was "delusional," that she was having "hallucinations," both auditory and visual. I concluded that she was "schizophrenic," and prepared to fill out a "pink paper"—that name we young psychiatrists-in-training used for the commitment form then in common use throughout the Commonwealth of Massachusetts. I became brisk, efficient, determined; I was working in the emergency room of the hospital, after all, and there were others to see—"alcoholics," men and women with various psychological difficulties (anxieties, fears), whom I would evaluate, and usually refer to the outpatient service. But this woman was really "sick," I concluded, and she needed to be hospitalized as soon as possible. Why? I knew the answer, of course: she was "delusional"—and on and on. I was, then, in a circle of sorts—the likes of which I fear I did not understand and was trained not to question. Yet the woman challenged me, and to this day, I can remember her unnerving question: "Why are you in such a hurry to lock me up?" Her voice had a wry, detached tone. I think I would have found the question easier to answer had she been more excited, truculent, or fearful. As I prepared, nevertheless, to answer her and to mobilize my self-important psychological pieties, she did an end-run around me. She spoke again and offered a calm, shrewd interpretation: "I'm sure you'll feel better when the ambulance comes to take me away. I'm glad I can help you this way!"

I was jolted by that second sentence, especially by the

matter-of-fact remark from a person I'd just declared to be insane! As I sat there I could recall the relief to which she'd been referring—that mix of satisfaction at wielding power (I'm not helpless, after all!) and relief that a disturbed person is out of the way (Who can understand what "they" have to say, anyway, at least at my level of training!). As I left the room I gave her one final glance before the police arrived, and hoped, I now realized for an outburst which would have made things right in my mind—relieved me of some growing sense that I was as sick in my own way as this patient, and indeed, that we both were part of some larger social, cultural, and political craziness.

Readers of this book will soon enough begin to understand what was happening to that woman and to me—both of us victims. I might have sat there, gotten to know her, tried to be of help to her; instead, I was sure that she needed confinement. A few years later, of course, people like me wouldn't be so quick, if not reflexic with our judgments, because the laws and some of our attitudes would have changed: we'd be all in favor of deinstitutionalization. Yet, such "progress" hasn't really addressed the fundamental matter, it has only shifted the locale of a particular kind of human struggle: that of men and women whose minds don't quite work the way many of our minds work. Now our streets are full of so-called homeless people who once lived on the back wards of mental hospitals—and still, we haven't significantly tried to work with such people, to *be* with them in such a way that their ideas and hopes come across to us, even as we might come across to them.

The point is *not* to romanticize what it is that causes some people, say, to hallucinate, and to feel terrified by voices, thoughts, and concerns within their minds. The point is not, either, to deny their pain, even their oft-stated right to feel not only "different" but "sick" in certain respects. The point is what we do with our labels, our diagnoses, our clinical determinations—what it is that happens in our minds that keeps us from putting ourselves alongside, existentially, another human being? What keeps us from approaching that person with an openness to their lives, and with a desire to learn from them as well as, perhaps, to be of assistance to them? What keeps us from offering them what thoughts and comfort we can muster that might, we hope be useful—a helping hand extended, rather than the ruling hand exercising its legally-sanctioned prerogatives? As in so many other matters of this life, the issue, finally, is one of sharing as opposed to controlling and dominance. Let us all allow Franco Basaglia to share his wise and important ideas and experiences with us, and thereby give us, (one hopes and prays) a bit of understanding not only with respect to the way he dealt with various challenges in Italy, but how we might meet our own challenges as they present themselves to us, day by day, here in America.

Preface

Franca Ongaro Basaglia

At the beginning of the sixties, the problem of psychiatric care in Italy appeared analagous to that of every other country. Its generalized response was the asylum as a closed and totalizing structure, whose birth had confirmed the incurability of mental illness and had protected a civil society that defended itself against the real and presumed danger posed by the sick, by segregating them for life. The Italian situation was certainly backwards (poorer, culturally more archaic, its contradictions harsher and social conflicts more in evidence, hence, its institutions more violent), with respect to other European countries. But essentially our asylums and the prevailing psychiatry were no different from the French and British ones, where since the end of the [Second World] war a movement among the general public and a series of technical actions had inaugurated discussions and denunciations of the problem, without, however, modifying the logic of the asylum in any concrete way.

During the sixties Italy had about 100,000 inpatients, whose fates were marked by the confinement that official psychiatry accepted as the only measure capable of controlling and containing illness. Fifteen years later, in 1978, the number of patients had been halved and a law—the Law 180—promulgated that prohibited the construction of new asylums, imposed the gradual phasing and emptying out of the old ones, and dictated norms for instituting community-based sociomedical structures to cope with the problem of mental disturbances without falling back on confinement.

Translated by Anne M. Lovell.

How is it possible that over a fifteen-year period, a culture as deeply rooted as that, based on the segregation, dangerousness, and identification of what is different, could have yielded to a new way of seeing and confronting problems? What forces were at play so that this new culture could impose itself as a law of the state? What elements made this operation possible and what is the status today of a reform that calls into question the roots of traditional psychiatry, its decision-making parameters, its tools, and even the entire logic of welfare that shapes our culture?

This brief preface to the American translation of selections from Franco Basaglia's writings hopes to respond to these queries, by reconstructing the general outline of an undertaking—a practical and theoretical itinerary—that over the course of a few years upset the very way psychiatry was practiced.

In 1961, Franco Basaglia, a young psychiatrist, intolerant of academic life, a scholar of phenomenology during a period when organicist theories were reigning, left the University of Padua, where he had worked for fourteen years, to direct a small provincial psychiatric hospital with 650 patients: the asylum of Gorizia, near the Yugoslavian border. The impact of this experience was severe. Although he had graduated in medicine with a specialty in mental and nervous disorders and was a tenured professor of psychiatry with fourteen years of clinical experience behind him, Basaglia had never seen an asylum. It was at that time possible, in other words, to prepare for twenty years of psychiatry without ever coming into contact with the reality to which it belonged. He was upset by that encounter; it was certainly the first emotional reaction from which stemmed his refusal of the reality of the asylum and its logic. He would either succeed in changing everything, or else he could never accept the position of warden.

With a small group of doctors, who would grow with time, he accepted the directorship, attempting, as a first step, to erase all traces of violence. Restraints, strait-jackets, wire-mesh fencing, grating, bars, gates, keys, all that had been locked, imprisoned, and segregated were gradually eliminated and replaced by the force and cohesion of the community. First of all, one had to restore dignity to the patient, whatever his or her illness, through the gradual recovery of freedom and responsibility lost at the moment of confinement, but also through the reconstruction of a hospital life that would be acceptable or at least tolerable. This meant restoring a sense of dignity to the profession of the psychiatrist as well as of the nurse, and thus going beyond pure custody of the inmate.

At a London conference in 1964, Basaglia presented a paper, based on three years of his experience, which was to form the first outline of the eventual foundations for his work. It was a lucid analysis of the asylum and its destructive power over its inmates; the identity forced upon patients in an institution that segregates and annihilates them; the predominance of the institutional system's values and rules over the value of those it is meant to protect and treat; the role of the psychiatrist as delegate appointed by society to contain and control the excesses of illness, and hence of social disturbances; the "risk" of inmate's freedom as the only guarantee of minimal reciprocity between them and whoever is in charge of them; the need for the psychiatrist to transcend an objectifying relationship with the patient, which assumes conquering one's own subjectivity and freedom; the aggression of the sick (which transcends the illness itself), as the first reaction with which psychiatrists must contend, a sign of the patients' conquest of themselves and of their right to a human life; the necessity of distinguishing between damage produced by the illness and that produced by segregation; the danger implicit in the new "good" organization of the hospital, whenever it is maintained as a closed world without relationships to the outside, and whenever the sick person's freedom is reduced to the doctor's largess rather than being the fruit of a conquest; and the destruction of the asylum as an "urgently needed if not simply obvious fact."

This was the first document that marked the passage from a phenomenological stance that he had held during the years of university work to what would subsequently become an anti-institutional struggle. The violent encounter with the violence of the institution, with the ultimate reality of psychiatry (the reality of confinement), ignored by a university that would not deal with it, wrecked the illusion that it is possible to search for subjectivity in a world where neither subjects nor bodies exist.

What in fact is the body of the inmate if it is not the body of internment? Where can one trace, in this total invasion and expropriation by the institution, the distance between the "I" and

the "self", the interval between the "I" and the body necessary for
the subject, if these bodies are possessed by the institution, if they
are the very body of the institution? How and where can one enable the subject to emerge in that humiliated humanity, in those
tortured bodies, in those truncated lives?

This inquiry proceeded in the thickness constituted by
the layers that surround illness and condition its expression. If
the sick have taken on the institution as their own body, the an-
nihilated human being encountered in the institution is above all
the product of the institution. But what role has illness played in
the process of totally destroying the individual? If it is true that
the asylum contains the various forms of mental illness that psychiatry has been limited to classifying and subdividing, what is
the significance of the fact that the asylum offers a univocal response—internment—to every form of disturbance? Beyond any
attempt to understand illness, the destruction of the reality and
the logic of the asylum becomes the first step that can guarantee
an approach to the patient as a problem to be deciphered, while
at the same time guaranteeing the survival of a professional responsibility that has been implicitly negated by the institution.

The wards were gradually unlocked and opened, furnished in part with what was already there, but with the attempt
to create a favorable and family-like environment. Every patient
was eventually able to use a small cupboard to keep his or her
things. Normal clothes were acquired for men and women, as the
old, grey, oversized shirts were completely eliminated. A cafe-bar
was opened, run by the patients, and it became a meeting place
where the entire hospital would gather. A beauty parlor was
equipped where some patients learned the trade, and women
were stimulated to look after themselves, to care for their physical
appearance, instead of letting themselves go. The men no longer
had their heads shaven, because it was important for them to
reacquire their image, their body, their dignity. All of these things
are simple and banal, but they help the patients to assume a respect heretofore nonexistent.

For a long time, running the hospital along a smooth
course had been the only goal, one reached at the expense of the
life of the individual patient. Now the subject for whom the hospital existed became the sick person; everything had to yield to his

or her needs. Thus the situation had been overturned in practice: here was a hospital at the service of the sick and not vice-versa, as usually happens. Together with the patients, the problems of the community were confronted: bad food which needed to be improved, the lack of toilets and showers, an outing to be organized, a party to plan, work for pay, and the refusal of ergotherapy [work therapy]. And then there were the problems of cohabitation: an aggressive patient who did not respect others or the rules of the community, the overbearing alcoholic, or the psychopath who betrayed the group's expectations. The ward meetings and the general assembly for the whole hospital were the occasions for discussion; voices no one had ever listened to found an audience. Those who had not spoken for years began to regain confidence in themselves, in others. And the once-lost hope for a different life, at home, with family, in the world, surfaced.

The violence and the dangerousness were reduced as the restrictions and threats disappeared, as the subjective possibilities of life and self-expression grew. Certainly, now the doctors could not stay on the wards for a few minutes only to close themselves in their silent studies, dedicating themselves to private practice; they had to stay with patients all day. Nurses could no longer calmly play cards. When the patients were tied to their beds it had been possible to pass the time away, but if they were free, someone had to be present for every occurrence, every necessity that might emerge. New needs—for relationships, movement, and autonomy—were being born.

In the climate of enthusiasm, of work and lives experienced in common, many young people had rushed in as volunteers. Even for them this was an opportunity, an experience rich in meaning. In the hospital, they "lived" the life of patients and with their presence they broke the hospital's monotony, bringing with them new activities and initiatives, movement, life, and their youth. One of them might play the guitar, another teach how to write or add; someone else might organize a gymnastics course for rehabilitation; still another accompany the older and more regressed people on walks in the park or to town, the movie, the store, or to a relative's home. Some assumed the task of spending an entire day, many days, with a patient who was going through a crisis. All this accomplished more than psychiatry had ever done. The young volunteers knew little or nothing about mental illness, the various forms of pathology, and therapies. But their practical actions, their availability—even emotional—for people who had always been rejected gave unexpected results.

In 1968 the asylum disappeared, leaving some traces in the most regressed patients, who were nevertheless protected by the collectivity. In place of the asylum was a completely open therapeutic community, where patients could gradually reappropriate all of which they had been deprived. The number of patients was reduced to less than half, because as they became re-habilitated, they were returned—wherever possible—to their homes. For those who did not have a family, home, work, other solutions had to be found: apartments for discharged patients; en-titlements for those who would not work or find work; outpatient centers that could follow ex-patients in their daily lives, with their difficulty of reentering and living in society but who, together, could face new problems without being committed. For this it was necessary to rally the support of local administrations that had always looked upon this experience with vexation, attacking and provoking attacks on every occasion with accusations, summonses, indictments, and trials.

The determining element in this struggle against the asy-lum was the identification of the political character of the entire undertaking. The fact of having understood that the asylum did not contain madness, but rather poverty and misery that, not be-ing able to resist harshness and suffering, can be expressed through madness, clearly demonstrated that the asylum, and therefore the psychiatry practiced within it, had an explicitly class character. The discourse about the nonneutrality of science that characterized those years found a practical confirmation in the Gorizia experience. Psychiatrists, working in a traditional asy-lum, performed a precise task, controlling and containing the ele-ment of disturbance belonging to the poorest strata of the popula-tion. This concerned not only a psychiatric, medical, or scientific problem to be discussed only among co-workers. If well-off mid-dle-class people can be treated differently, the fact that the entire population can be treated or only the most disenfranchised are set aside for confinement in the asylum was a problem of choice, of political will. Psychiatrists could not have continued this battle alone: they had to join with popular struggles, and act so that these themes—the asylum, segregation, the violence to which the sick were subjected, in that they were deprived of economic and cultural resources—might become the legacy of a struggle for health in the factories, the workplaces, homes, and hospitals. In 1968 the struggle against authoritarianism, hierarchy, the rigidity of roles, the nonneutrality of science had found in the struggle against the asylum a parallel anti-institutional practice against which to measure itself. The years that followed the end of the student movement signaled the qualitative leap of the anti-institutional movement.

Some aspects of the battle, premonitions of future developments, allow the struggle against the asylum and against every form of segregation and marginality to survive, even during the present ebb. There was a call for self-preservation in the political battle through strong ties to one's specific sector where one had to continue to act on its contradictions; and the need to involve political and union forces in a struggle that otherwise viewed nurses and inmates, who belonged to the same class, as enemies.

It was this extremely politically intelligent operation that allowed the field of action to broaden, on the one hand overcoming the risk of simply absorbing the movement into the general logic of the institutional political struggle, that would have reduced the specificity of the contradictions on which we worked and, on the other hand, the implicit risk of an isolated, separate struggle of enlightened technicians who were confronting the problem of mental illness and its archaic institutions in a different way, as a result limiting it to proposing a new technique to replace the old, with the reality left unaltered.

In 1974, at the first conference of democratic psychiatry—the movement which brought together psychiatrists, nurses, health workers, and local administrators fighting to abolish the asylum—in the presence of political and union forces, a proposal for creating liaisons was articulated. Identified with a struggle for the healthy and the sick, it would single out the processes through which the criminalization of illness and deviance are scientifically carried out; the processes through which the needs expressed therein are translated into crimes to be punished, to justify the criminality of the punishment.

In 1972 Gorizia was abandoned, with the mass resignation of the doctors, because of the barriers the local administration had created against proceeding beyond the walls of the open asylum. From then on the experience was broadened. In Perugia, at the same time as in Goriza, work was underway to prevent hospitalizations. Subsequently, the work continued in Arezzo, Ferrara, Parma (where Basaglia worked from 1969 to 1971), Reggio Emilia, Trieste, then Venice, Turin, Genoa, and Naples. The Gorizians had been dispersed, setting off the process of gradual dismantling of the asylum already carried out at Gorizia, but with different methods, which moved, as the next step, towards its total elimination.

In 1977, Trieste, where Basaglia had moved to in 1971, announced that the hospital would close, even though about 250 people out of the original 1,200 were still housed in the hospital, in small apartments carved out of the wards, but under conditions of total freedom and autonomy in relation to the organization of health care.

In those years the problem of psychiatry had become common knowledge: daily newspaper articles, radio broadcasts, television interviews, discussions, debates, publications, books, all involved people with a problem that was theirs and could not be delegated only to psychiatrists. This was the most difficult step, because it is convenient for everyone to think that if people with problems prevent us from living [as we wish], there must be a place where they can be relegated and entrusted to someone else. But the mere fact that this place does not exist or is no longer accessible can force us to confront these problems in a different way, to find ways of overcoming them that are not automatic and obvious or determined by the reassuring existence of a safety valve: the asylum.

As long as we are used to knowing that for every problem there is a ready answer (orphanages for abandoned children, special schools for retarded children, nursing homes for the elderly, and hospitals for the sick), it will be difficult to create a different culture that breaks with the process of delegating problems to others. Abandoned children need a family, not an institution; retarded children need to stay with others, to be stimulated, even if they cannot keep up with the rest of the class; old people need to continue participating in collective life and to imagine themselves useful in some way, not to be holed up in a ghetto waiting to die; the sick do well in hospitals during the acute phase of their illness, but then they heal faster at home, with their family, with their loved ones.

Our culture however, has tended to resolve things by creating an institution for every phenomenon, for every problem, where all phenomena and problems of the same type can be concentrated. Rather than being surmounted, they are confirmed. Children have continued to be abandoned, old people left isolated and alone, the mentally ill labelled chronics and each placed in the institution hypothesized for their recovery. While this might have appeared at one time as a useful and humanitarian service, in fact it served to rid us of our problems, making whoever has an illness or abnormality pay for it. Like the asylum, all care-giving institutions have functioned to relieve the healthy of the problem represented by the ill, the weak, the impaired, while the latter were punished for their condition. But this operation concerns only the weak, the impaired, the sick from the disadvantaged class, and as such has always had an explicit class meaning.

In Italy, the struggle against the asylum was essentially a struggle against this asylum logic, founded on the expropriation and annihilation of those who are helped, hence a struggle against social marginalization achieved under the guise of treatment, therapy, protection, and rehabilitation.

The political character of this battle and the links made with the labor movement and social forces engaged in changing society are what produced the new law on psychiatric care. But it must also be emphasized that the reform could be made possible only in that the experiences underway, from the beginning of the sixties on, had compelled all political forces to measure themselves against the standard of a theoretical-practical exchange that acted directly on "things," beyond preconceived notions.

The reform law enacted in 1978 [Law 180] provided for the following:

—a freeze on new admissions to the asylum (to avoid contagion, no new patients can come into contact with it); a deadline for imposing the freeze, which allowed alternatives to confinement to be established, where there was a will.

—a gradual phasing out of the asylum, through the gradual rehabilitation and resocialization of its inpatients and the creation of new outpatient structures (houses, apartments, supervised facilities, day and night hospitals, and cooperatives for work and social reintegration) for those who could not return to families.

—the establishment in general hospitals of "diagnosis and treatment units" [*servizi di diagnosi e cura,* or S.D.C.s] for compulsory treatment and crisis intervention; (these placed the mentally ill person on the same level as any other sick person).

—the creation of outpatient services of a sociomedical nature, where the problem of psychic disturbances could be confronted in all the elements that comprise it, whether biological, psychological, or social.

—the organization of new structures whose modalities were to be required from and implemented by the regional districts, thus falling under their competency. The provision, however, lacked specific funding.

—assignment to the ministry of health the task of overall coordination and direction.

These are the essential lines of a reform that, having fractured the old relationship between psychiatry and justice, tends at the same time to remove the exclusive management of the problem of mental disturbances from the hands of the doctor. Instead, it involves the community in changing the cultural attitudes toward every form of diversity. Given that what is done socially and culturally with biological and psychological factors conditions people's destinies, the emphasis is placed not so much on the institution as on new services—on the creation, through the services themselves, of a new more participatory mode, a joint way of experiencing relationships. The Law 180, in fact, is a reform that presupposes not only a change in services, but also the beginning of a radical change in social relations.

Where the law has been implemented, there now exist, in the place of asylums, community mental health centers open twenty-four hours a day, where illness is handled by taking charge of all problems that are biological, psychological, and social in nature and present in the psychic disturbance. A different approach to illness allows for a brief stay in a hospital ward (the diagnostic and treatment unit) during the crisis. When necessary, a subsequent stay is possible in a community mental health center that is a social center and meeting place, as well as a facility for treatment and rehabilitation. Or a supervised home that has the same goals can be used. Both cases avoid the serious consequences provoked by confinement.

By preventing a hospitalization, we participate in changing the very way illness is expressed (and this can be seen clearly in places where the reform has been implemented). For the moment the crisis is experienced without the anguish that accompanied it when it was only repressed and restrained, it can be expressed as a life experience capable of being communicated, and not just as an illness; hence it is a less anguishing and more understandable experience. Community mental health centers with several in-patient beds are not strict medical centers, but rather places to stay, be treated, congregate, and resocialize. As for example in Trieste, they tend to confront the problem without relegating, and hence forgetting it, in places intended for the most difficult cases. This is a measure that has revealed its capacity for hindering the process of chronicity implicit and inevitable in confinement.

Nevertheless, even if some cases exist in which all of this has been implemented with positive results, six years after its enactment the reform has not been applied evenly throughout the country, and discussions are already underway to modify it. The absence of funding allocated specifically for psychiatric care could be the tell-tale sign of the real political unwillingness to implement a difficult reform, one that twists the foundation of our culture. In fact, not only must a therapeutic technique that is anachronistic and has now been surpassed be questioned, but so must the function of traditional, asylum psychiatry. Science and its institutions as a system for control and containment of marginal strata, and as a cover for problems that often have little to do with illness, must also be questioned.

Working within the relationship between the dominant rationality in our culture (the rationality of efficiency and productive norms) and the material and psychological poverty that characterizes asylum inmates, it has finally been possible to carry out both a scientific and a political action that made obvious not only the backwardness of the institution, but also its discriminating function in the social game, a function usually covered by the alibi of treatment, protection, and rehabilitation.

The knowledge of this deep tie, between a rationality that marginalizes and excludes whatever does not resemble it and a segregated misery, has allowed the nucleus of the problem to be touched, avoiding the simple recourse to new therapeutic techniques that, in a phase of theoretical and institutional renewal, would have continued to confirm the role of the sick person, the illness, the psychiatrist, the institution, and in this way preserve the function of the social game.

The uniqueness of the Italian situation consists of having forced this submerged core to rise as an essentially political discourse. This is what has yielded the bond between technicians and politicians that brought about the reform law.

The reform has thus been possible in Italy to the extent that the struggle of the technicians, who called into question their own power and role and the traditional referents, could move beyond the alignments and alliances of the parties, causing all of the political forces at play to be measured against the weight of practical experiences that had already produced a change in the institutional reality, but also in the scientific ideology. By breaking with the asylum and its logic, and by rehabilitating the inpatients, the fragility of a scientific judgment that had confirmed the incurability of illness had been demonstrated in practice. And the use made of this judgment to mask social problems to which responses other than treatment and therapy can be given was covered, as were the role of psychiatry and the psychiatrist in this operation.

The conflict engendered by the Law 180 thus goes deeper than simply changing the organization of a branch of medicine, because it begins from the revelation that psychiatric problems are not of a strictly medical nature. It is against this conflict that we must measure ourselves in Italy today, at a time when there is an attempt to force every source of social conflict into the stream of technical responses most adaptable to covering them up. The ex-patient "tramp" who wanders the streets, unemployed and homeless, stirs our pity, but it is easier to be affected by that aspect of his illness that requires treatment and institutions, rather than to see the true nature of his needs.

An analysis of what has happened in these last six years can further clarify the present situation. From the moment the law was enacted, we have been witnessing a strengthening and spreading of the experiences that brought about the reform (in Trieste, Arezzo, Perugia, Ferrara, Pordenone, Genoa, Reggio Emilia, Venice, Turin, Modena, Livorno, Bari and Potenza the work is in keeping with the reform, even if at different levels of implementation), with a diversion of both financial and personal resources from asylums into community services. Many regions have launched programs, more or less in accordance with the law's precepts, often with lesser variations, which are still in the process of being implemented or are still on paper. Many local administrators have struggled against the regions in an attempt to institute outpatient services, often succeeding only in part; others, because of incapability or an explicit will not to do anything, have let time slide while waiting for the law to be revoked or modified.

As for mental health workers, there exists beside those who belong to the movement that brought about the reform, a considerable number who declare themselves still unwilling to be involved with a commitment that forces a not negligible cultural and behavioral change. We have witnessed doctors or paraprofessionals, who, while perhaps verbally in favor of the necessity to abolish the asylum, have declared, faced with a sick person in the midst of a crisis, that mental illness does not exist, that it is not within their competency; thus they have unloaded the burden onto the patient's family. At the beginning, especially, we verified the phenomenon of discharging en masse, or transferring to other agencies or institutions, people who had been hospitalized for twenty, thirty years, without minimal rehabilitation or recovery, and without any concern for their destiny.

Where community structures have not been established, the beds in the diagnosis and treatment units of general hospitals (a maximum of fifteen), being the only available service, have obviously turned out to be insufficient. This has created more than a few difficulties for patients' families, who have organized together, and justifiably so, refusing to bear unaided the burden of having a mentally disturbed person in the home. In the absence of other services and without the knowledge of any solutions other than the asylum, they have easily been manipulated into requesting it as the only response that might lift an unbearable weight. Moreover it is significant that in places where the law has been or is in the process of being implemented, family members are becoming involved in a positive way in the struggle to implement it, and are at our sides in this battle.

Several university psychiatric clinics have become connnected to the National Health Service, directly administering their services, while part of the academic world—that during the years of struggle kept themselves out of the fray—is now regaining a power that is certainly not out of keeping with the recent proposals to modify the law, and which tends implicitly to reconfirm the complete autonomy of their own world.

This, then, is the overview of the last few years: the only univocal position has been that of the Minister of Health, who from the law's enactment until the present, has been totally abscondent. No direction or coordination, no incentive or sanction has been given to the more passive and immobile regions and local administration. No funding has been provided for a reform that the Minister has allowed to drift.

We now find ourselves working on filling in these gaps; we can count on the cultural and practical changes acquired from the experiences underway, and, on the changed relationship between citizen and institutions that this has provoked. This involves a range of areas, such as the integration of handicapped children into normal schools, the practical critique of orphanages, nursing homes for the elderly, and prisons—and the consensus that underlies these movements.

The data speak for themselves: the number of hospitalized patients in public institutions and accredited ones receiving public funds went from 96,000 in 1968 to 54,480 in 1978, when the law was enacted, then fell to 44,450 at the end of 1979. From then on we witnessed noticeable slowing down of the rate of discharges (3,000–4,000 a year). In other words, before enactment of the law and under the thrust of a struggle that shook the country in the seventies, psychiatric hospitals were gradually discharging patients, unaccompanied by the polemics that would be pro-

voked at the beginning of the reform, and without the additional
weight produced by forms of resistence, from boycotts to manipulation by the law's detractors. Now we are also witnessing a gradual increase in compulsory treatment (*trattamenti sanitari
obbligatori*) that, in the first year of the reform, had fallen by 60%
nationwide. This means that, in the absence of alternative responses, and with the motivation for struggle weakening, the old
repressive techniques are proposed again intact.

        Another factor is yet at play. The novelty of the Italian
psychiatric reform consisted essentially in recognizing that, with
regard to mental disturbances, the medical intervention had to
play only a part—and not a predominant one—in a phenomenon that involves individuals in all the elements which make up
their biological, affective, and social lives. The establishment of
services that are more sociomedical than medical, such as community mental health centers that try to take charge of the problem in its totality (which means homelessness, unemployment,
solitude, old age, etc.), however, collides with the old medical
culture that continues to see and defend the centrality of the hospital and of medical interventions. Although the health reform
legislation was passed not long after the psychiatric reform,
breaking a medical model that often responds in terms of treatment and therapy to social problems that require another type of
response would require a radical questioning of our medical culture, one that cannot happen in a few months or even a few
years. The Italian psychiatric reform departing from a state of crisis into which psychiatry spilled over, has in some ways antici-
pated the crisis of medicine. The resistence to the application of
the law should also be understood as medicine's defense against
any increasingly urgent attack on the old way of understanding
medicine and its ability to translate into natural phenomena
even that which is an explicit social product.

Acknowledgments

The research for this book and translations from the Italian were supported by grants from: Mrs. Patricia Kind; the Department of Social and Administrative Medicine; and a Scholarly Publications and Artistic Exhibitions Award, both from the University of North Carolina, Chapel Hill. A University of California Humanities Research Fellowship and a Richard Carley Hunt Memorial Fellowship from the Wenner-Gren Foundation for Anthropological Research provided leave time during the fall of 1985 for one of us (NS-H) when the final stages of this project was completed.

Without the encouragement of Franca Ongaro Basaglia and the inspiration of Dr. Naomar Almeida-Filho of the School of Medicine, Salvador, Bahia, Brazil, this project would never have been initiated. Charles Webel's early support of the proposal to Columbia University Press was also crucial, for which we are deeply appreciative.

Many friends and colleagues read various drafts of the translations and the introduction, or listened patiently to our ideas in the process of putting together this volume, and they often provided suggestions, criticism, or emotional and intellectual support. In particular, we wish to acknowledge: Hans Baer, Susan Makiesky Barrow, Phil Brown, Yannick Durand, Sue E. Estroff, T.M.S. Evens, Kent Gerrard, Maria Grazia Giannichedda, Wolf Heydebrand, Michael Hughes, Peter Johnson, Sandra Karp, Judith Kempf, John Lovell, Diana Mauri, Lee Schlessinger, Merrill Singer, Michael Taussig, the late Anthony E. Thomas, Glenn Wilson, and Allan Young. Friends in Europe who provided useful discussion include Jean-Marie Alliaume, Robert Castel, Ronald Frankenberg, and Michel Legrand.

Grace Buzalkjo provided expert editorial assistance. The

manuscript was typed and prepared, with much patience, by Detra Allen, Susan Craddock, Jennifer Jones, Mattie Jones, Pam Owens, and Barbara Quigley.

Finally, our editor at Columbia University Press, Maureen MacGrogan, remained a steady support and a guide through the many dark and trying moments in the gestation and difficult delivery of this manuscript. Her faith in us and in the project encouraged us to forge on, and we are happy that her efforts, too, have been rewarded.

Part of this book's earnings will go to support the Berkeley Catholic Worker Movement on behalf of the homeless, especially those who struggle to remain free of institutional confinement. And part of the earnings will be contributed to the New York Coalition for the homeless.

The selections in this anthology have been taken from two volumes of Franco Basaglia's collected writings, *Scritti I* (1981), and *Scritti II* (1982), both edited by Franca Ongaro Basaglia and published by Einaudi (Turin). The selections originally appeared as follows:

1 and 2 *L'institutione negata.* Franco Basaglia, ed. Turin: Einaudi, 1968.

3 *La maggioranza deviante.* Franco Basaglia and Franca Ongaro Basaglia, eds. Turin: Einaudi, 1971.

4 In *Libri Nuovi.* Turin: Einaudi, 1969. Translation reprinted by permission of *Radical Therapist.*

5 *Crimini di pace.* Franco Basaglia and Franca Ongaro Basaglia, eds. Turin: Einaudi, 1975.

6 In *Enciclopedia Einaudi,* vol 5. Turin, 1979.

7 Paper presented to the International Congress of Law and Psychiatry. Oxford, 1979. Translation reprinted by permission of Pergamon Press.

8 *Il giardino dei gelsi.* E. Venturini, ed. Turin: Einaudi, 1979.

Nancy Scheper-Hughes,   Anne M. Lovell,
Berkeley   New York City

Editors' Note

The editors have occassionally taken the liberty to edit from the original verbatim translation repetitive phrases and to render the translation into a more colloquial and readable English in keeping with Basaglia's style.

NANCY SCHEPER-HUGHES is professor of anthropology at the University of California, Berkeley. She is the author of *Saints, Scholars, and Schizophrenics: Mental Illness in Rural Ireland* (University of California Press, 1979, 1982), for which she received the Margaret Mead Award. She has also published widely on the plight of the chronically mentally ill in the United States, and on mother love and child death in Northeast Brazil, for which she was awarded a Guggenheim Fellowship in 1986.

ANNE M. LOVELL is a research fellow at the French National Institute of Health and Medical Research (INSERM) and is affiliated with the New York State Psychiatric Institute. As a Fulbright scholar, she worked and studied with Franco Basaglia. She is coauthor, with Robert Castel and Francoise Castel, of *The Psychiatric Society* (Columbia University Press, 1982) and has published articles on Italian psychiatry as well as on homelessness.

Introduction The Utopia of Reality: Franco Basaglia and the Practice of a Democratic Psychiatry

Anne M. Lovell and Nancy Scheper-Hughes

It was as if history had hesitated, as if there had been an oscillation between two antagonistic models of care. The first was the totalitarian utopia of the Ancien Régime: cleaning up the mass of deviants, first neutralizing and isolating them, then disciplining them within the institution with a range of correctional techniques based on activity manuals, religious exercises, and moral regulations. The second strategy of care was already a utopia one might call capillary. It aims to fix the risk of deviance in the place from which it emerges, to avoid a dangerous drift from public order.[1]

The history of psychiatry is replete with the myth making that perpetuates such utopian visions. Social historians and sociologists have traced the shifts between the utopian proposals of the eighteenth-, nineteenth-, and twentieth-century psychiatries: some see these utopian ideals as alternating in cycles of reform;[2] others see them as revolutions occurring in a linear sequence;[3] for still others, they represent epistemological breaks in the way Western society has perceived and responded to madness.[4]

Witness, for example, the retelling of the Philippe Pinel story. These are the harsh words uttered by the president of the Paris commune in response to the young psychiatrist's proposal to unshackle the lunatics of Bicetre: "A plague upon you if you are deceiving us, and if among these madmen you are hiding enemies of the people. . ."[5] And Pinel's response: "Citizen, I am of the conviction that these lunatics are so intractable only because they have been deprived of air and liberty."[6] Pinel's act was first recorded as a liberation of the insane from archaic forms of treatment/torture, a liberation that was in keeping with the revolutionary philanthropy that followed the French Revolution of 1789. That history has since been retold by Foucault, not as a phase in the gradual evolution of more benevolent or enlightened models of psychiatric care, but rather as an abrupt rupture, marking the transformation from a corporal discipline that would inscribe society's norms on the body of the mental patient, to a "moralizing sadism" that sought to inscribe those norms on her very soul. The regime of moral treatment, often attributed to Pinel, then, transformed the mental asylum into a new kind of court of law in which the madman was continually judged guilty of the crime of unreason.

Similar utopias appeared elsewhere, with William Tuke's Quaker retreat in Victorian England that enclosed patients within a carefully regulated, moralistic, family-like milieu, designed to resocialize deviants into more conventional and useful citizens. The nineteenth-century American reformer, Thomas Kirkbridge, designed an asylum within an idyllic setting that would allow a hospital superintendent to rule "like a benevolent despot over a hospital kingdom in which every fixture and every inmate was part of his domain."[7] And the utopian vision offered by the so-called lunatic colony of Geel, Belgium—where the severely and chronically psychotic and mentally retarded have boarded with ordinary families since at least the seventeenth century—appears and reappears in the annals of psychiatry, with alternate interpretations posited as to whether Geelians have by and large helped or exploited their vulnerable boarders, or whether these boarders have been abandoned by the medical profession. French, British, and American physicians and psychiatrists have argued the merits of this particular ideal of community care for at least two centuries.[8]

Whether the aim has been the perfect asylum, the well-run community or the territorial system, utopian visions have been borrowed and adapted continually, in accordance with the shifting goals of the social and historical context. Yet, their application always falls short of the ideal aspired to, and in the end custodialism or a new, more subtle form of domination, and an emergent professionalism is revealed or rediscovered.

The itinerary of the Italian psychiatrist, Franco Basaglia (1924-1980), however, marks an epistemological break, and hence a new chapter in the contemporary history of European psychiatry. In the 1960s, at the historical moment when the pendulum in Western countries was swinging toward the capillary utopias of the community model, Basaglia gave a new meaning to utopia. The earlier proposals were utopias in the sense that they generated ideologies, each with a preconceived future that would reinforce and improve upon existing patterns of management and control over excluded groups.

The alternative Basaglia proposed was what he called a *practical* utopia, creating new ways of responding to the needs of psychiatric patients, the handicapped, and the mentally retarded.[9] Rather than using blueprints for reform—and the innovations of the sixties produced a plethora of these from therapeutic communities to prevention to comprehensive health planning— Basaglia's changes were forged out of the specific context in which he worked. His work was utopian precisely because he was willing to open up new possibilities that broke sharply with the existing order, with Western conceptions of how psychiatry should be practiced and illness defined, and with the social, economic, and political purposes served by the psychiatric system. In his practical utopia, Basaglia wedded psychiatry to a political praxis—a collective effort for change that verified new ideas by putting them to work and by constructing further theories from what was learned through action. Basaglia's political dimension, so unique in psychiatry, corresponded to a whole generation of Italian intellectuals and activists who emerged beginning in the 1960s. As a psychiatrist, his actions extended far beyond psychiatry and its institutions, into the arena of political and social life.

As an individual—and this explained in part his enormous following and his effectiveness—Basaglia was brilliant, charismatic, direct, and never condescending. Whether talking to factory workers outside Venice, to students at the University of Paris, or to psychiatrists in São Paulo, he eschewed rules, models, and recipes, in keeping with his critique of ideological utopias. Rather, he provided a critical way of seeing, of spurning surface interpretations and easy solutions, and of experiencing the conditions of one's life. Although he recognized that a sprawling city in a developing country of Latin America or a psychiatric hospital in Franco's Spain were not analogous to the asylums of Gorizia or Trieste, he empathized without restraint and he stimulated and energized others, spurring them on to analyze their particular situations with their own cultural tools.

A close colleague captured some of these qualities in a description of his first meeting with Basaglia: "I found myself before a person who expressed a large, cultural openness but who could tie this general vision to everyday life, translating it into coherent behaviors and practical initiatives that—even if seemingly insignificant—were a stimulus to other people's participation in social change."[10] Thus, in his clinical work (as well as in his political praxis), Basaglia presented no famous case histories, and no specific therapeutic techniques or practices. Innovations, of course, require new conceptual schemes and reference points, but Basaglia's apprehension that these might freeze into ideological utopias was reminiscent of Sartre's observation that ideologies are liberating only while they are in the making, and oppressive once they are established.[11]

In contrast to what critics later referred to as the "Basaglian method," Basaglia himself saw his work as part of a dialectical process. For example, he explained that his excerpts on the events and radical changes at the asylum at Gorizia, some of which appear in this volume, were "not intended to be a description of technique, or of a system that is more efficient or more positive than any other. The reality of today will differ from the reality of tomorrow, and in trying to freeze it, it either becomes distorted or irrelevant. The excerpts are only conceptualizations of our practice that gradually developed as the original concentration camp environment gave way to more human relationships."[12]

The corpus of Basaglia's writings, published after his death and running to more than one thousand pages, is of a theoretical, sometimes philosophical, and often rhetorical nature, with only tantalizing and passing references to his own revolutionizing actions in the psychiatric institutions of Gorizia, Parma, Trieste, and later in the region of Rome.[13] A good third of the collected works concerns the applications of phenomenology to psychiatry. However, in the present volume we have limited ourselves to selections that constitute his critical reflections on the destruction of the institution, and his astute analyses of psychiatry, society, intellectuals, and social movements. In this introduction we provide some background on the early intellectual influences on Basaglia as well as the key concepts, many unfamiliar to an American audience, which pervade his work. The actual history of the anti-institutional movement he led is not to be found in Basaglia's own writings. It must be reconstructed from numerous books and articles, Italian and otherwise, and from the newspaper clippings and journalistic writings that captured the debates and controversies surrounding those crucial years from roughly 1964 to his death in 1980. Through these, the meaning of his practical utopia—or, as we prefer, his utopia of reality—can be derived.

From Phenomenology to Psychiatric Praxis

Before [Basaglia's arrival] those who were here prayed to be the next to die. When someone died the bells used to chime and everyone would say: "Oh God, if only they chimed for me; I'm so tired of this life in here." How many of us died who could have been alive and healthy! But humiliated and deprived of any way out, some would refuse to eat. Then the food would be forced down their nose with a tube. There was nothing else to do, because we were locked up inside here with no hope of ever leaving. Like scorched plants with leaves withered from the drought, this is how we were.[14]

In these words, a patient at the Gorizia psychiatric hospital in northeastern Italy, on the Yugoslav border, described the conditions there in the years before Franco Basaglia assumed its directorship. But he might have been describing any of the nearly one hundred provincial (public) psychiatric hospitals in Italy at the time. Basaglia was revolted by what he observed at Gorizia as the traditional regime of institutional care; his intellectual orientations and his medical training had not prepared him for his first confrontation with the reality of the asylum.

The first time he entered a mental hospital, Basaglia later recalled, he was struck by a terrible odor—an odor redolent of death and defecation—and one not unlike the fetid odor of the prison cell where Basaglia had experienced his first institutional encounter when, as a medical student active in the Italian resistance, he was arrested and held prisoner during the German occupation. This formative experience provided Basaglia with the materials for his evocative equation of asylum, prison, and concentration camp,[15] and incited him with the single-minded passion to destroy, once and for all, the imprisoning institution itself.

Basaglia's subsequent transformation of the asylum at Gorizia shared intellectual roots with the Saint-Alban group in France, who had provided health care for their companions in the French Resistance. Under the leadership of Francois Tosquelles, a psychiatrist and a Spanish Civil War hero, the group went on to humanize the mental hospital by uniting insights from Marxism and Freudian psychoanalysis. The Saint-Alban experience culminated in the movement known as French institutional psychotherapy, which interpreted the dynamics of the psychiatric hospital as the manifestations of a kind of collective unconscious, but which also took into account the social origins of psychological suffering. Institutional psychotherapy became the predominant alternative psychiatry in France, but it fell short in its ability to draw connections between the sources of oppression *inside* and *outside* the asylum, a task that Basaglia and his co-workers in Italy would accomplish later. Nor did institutional psychotherapy either challenge or change the fact of the mental hospital and its controlling functions. Nonetheless, Basaglia acknowledged the affinity of some of his ideas with those generated by the institutional psychotherapy movement, particularly the analysis of power relations within psychiatric institutions.

After receiving a medical degree in 1949, Basaglia's first contacts with psychiatry were typical of those of most young doctors. He did not question the parameters of psychiatry as a science whose objects and instruments were taken as givens, its values as absolutes. This brief scientific period in Basaglia's career is reflected in a series of early publications on psychotropic medication and on psychological testing.[16] Very quickly, however, he began to explore a broader terrain, to search for human rather than merely scientific contexts in which to understand psychiatric disorder.

During the period of his tenure at the Neuropsychiatric Clinic of Padua (1949-1961), existential phenomenonology was the only alternative to the organicist schools that then dominated

Italian psychiatry. Psychoanalysis, which also countered the way in which biological psychiatry objectified the individual,* did not really surface in Italy until the 1970s. Basaglia soon became one of a score of Italian psychiatrists who had embraced phenomenology, particularly influenced by the writings of Eugene Minowski, Ludwig Binswanger, and Erwin Strauss. In reaction to the dehumanization wrought by World War II and, as in the case of Strauss, to the rigid Pavlovian behaviorism of the 1950s, the phenomenologists sought to understand men and women through their diverse possibilities of existence. This precluded objectifying, that is enclosing individuals within any system of fixed psychological or medical categories.

At Gorizia, to which Basaglia went as director in 1961, the phenomenological approach gradually revealed its shortcomings. Faced with the reality of a suffering person rather than with the reified case studies found in the psychiatric textbooks of his medical student days, Basaglia questioned the limitations of phenomenological analysis to cast light on the class nature of the illness and the larger social and political context that determined its modes of expression. "Like psychoanalysis," he wrote in 1967, phenomenology "has yet to modify the nature of the relationship with the object of its inquiry; it keeps [the person who is ill] at a distance, in the same objective and a-dialectical dimension to which classical psychiatry has already relegated it. Both theories have penetrated institutional practices only very marginally."[17]

In fact, like psychoanalysis, phenomenology as a treatment modality was a privileged one, able to affect few people at one time, and on a one-to-one basis only. It lacked the potential to change the lives of large numbers of confined people. As a way of understanding reality, phenomenology had little to contribute to the definition of an institutionalized patient's experience.

Yet, phenomenology exerted a profound influence throughout Basaglia's life, not only in his writings, but also in his

---

*Objectify is a term that Basaglia uses repeatedly. He is referring to the reification of patients and their afflictions through biomedical diagnosis and treatment. For Basaglia diseases (any more than patients) cannot simply be reduced to biological entities. Patients and illness speak to the sensitive and often contradictory aspects of culture and social relations. The objectivity of medicine and psychiatry is always a phantom objectivity, a mask that conceals more than it reveals.—Eds.

practice. Essential to Basaglia's analysis of psychiatric situations, for example, was Husserl's concept of "bracketing": the suspension of judgments in the first encounter with the reality of the immediately given. It was Basaglia's bracketing of mental illness as disease that provided ammnunition to the critics who for many years falsely accused Basaglia of denying the existence of mental illness. Basaglia meant only to imply that we could not know what was the reality of the illness until we could first strip away the many layers created by poverty, stigma, segregation, and confinement which covered and concealed it. He made this point very clearly when he stated:

It is not that we put the illness aside, but rather that we believe that in order to have a relationship with an individual, it is necessary to establish it independent of the label by which the person has been defined. I have a relationship with someone not because of the diagnosis, but because of who she is. In the moment that I say, "this person is a schizophrenic" (with all that this implies for cultural reasons) I will begin to behave toward her in a unique way, that is, knowing full well that schizophrenia implies an illness for which nothing can be done. My relationship will be that of someone who only expects "schizophrenicity" from the individual. We can see how, in this way, the old psychiatry discarded, imprisoned, and excluded the sick person for whom it was believed there existed no recourse, no tools for treatment. This is why it is so very necessary to draw closer to her, bracketing the illness, because the diagnostic label has taken on the weight of a moral judgment that passes for the reality of the illness itself.[18]

In his day-to-day work at Gorizia, bracketing meant paying little attention to the diagnosis but instead listening closely to what the patient had to say. Suspending the most general labels—psychotic, alcoholic, depressive—was difficult, for the trained clinician was then left without any other language. It was often only the lay persons—the *volontari,* who later came to the hospital from the outside— who being innocent of psychiatric jargon and terminology were able to break from the traditional and stagnating way of relating to patients. Basaglia's suspension of psychiatric knowledge also implied leaving behind the batteries of psychological tests, the mental status exams, and the diagnostic and statistical manuals in order that he and those who worked with him could see the patient in a new, evolving manner.

At Gorizia as elsewhere, Basaglia would always search to restore a subjectivity to the way in which patients were viewed. But the emphasis shifted from that of his phenomenological period. Rather than focusing on bracketing the illness, he would take the side of the patient, as a person who suffers and is oppressed. And this inevitably meant praxis, a refusal of the accepted ways of organizing suffering, and an involvement in transforming the patient's life.

It would be incorrect, however, to assume that Basaglia was able to gird himself with this cultural and intellectual armament, and simply swoop down on the institution. The process of moving from a phenomenological (and hence purely analytical or even ideological) stance to collective action was a gradual one. It involved not only a personal trajectory, but the growth of a whole social movement. Two conditions made this possible: the backwardness of Italian psychiatry at the time, and the political and social climate of Italy during those years.

In the first place, Italian psychiatric institutions posed an anachronism in a rapidly expanding capitalist society. There was, as yet, no humanistic or liberal social psychiatry to compete with the prevailing biodeterminist and other positivist models of mental illness that were evolving, in the decades after World War II, in France, England, or the United States and spawning new models: institutional psychotherapy, the *politique de secteur*,[19] therapeutic communities, the community mental health movement, and preventive psychiatry. The traditional asylums, under the aegis of the provinces, were still governed by a 1904 law which linked psychiatry to the criminal justice system, assigning it the function of control and custody (*custodia*) over care and treatment (*curia*). Voluntary commitment procedures were nonexistent, and the current mental health legislation was blatantly concerned with the control of social deviance. At this time, all of Italy's mental institutions were filled with poor, working-class, and immigrant persons—a fact that allowed their reform to become a central issue for the organizations that represented the interests of these disadvantaged groups, especially the unions and the leftist parties. In fact, the entire health care system was anachronistic. There was no comprehensive health insurance, like the programs evolving in other Western countries. In Italy the poor and working class depended on their employers and mutual benefit funds.

Since the late fifties Italy had been experiencing rapid economic growth and had recognized a need to modernize its institutions. Meanwhile, what had been a gradual shift of Italians to the Left was suddenly galvanized into an explosion of activism in 1968 and 1969. A comparison that is often made between the French "May Events" (1968) and Italy's "Hot Autumn" (1969) sheds light on the context in which Basaglia's anti-institutional movement gathered momentum.

In France, the explosion of the student movement was intense: not only did it spread rapidly to the unions and among workers, but the sit-downs, rallies, and strikes cut across class, sex, and generational lines, involving people from many different walks of life. Yet, almost as quickly, the protest was spent. While subtle changes were to be felt for years in the ways people defined themselves in relation to each other, to institutions, and to authority, the effects on the labor movement and on the workplace were mild, with a few rather striking exceptions such as the self-management that workers installed in the Lip watch factory and the resistance of the Larzac peasants to the takeover of their land by the French military.

In Italy, 1968 witnessed a handful of factory strikes, but the real conflict peaked during the more generalized worker and student strikes of the Hot Autumn of 1969. Unique to the Italian movement were two innovations: strikes and workers' councils that largely bypassed union structures, and the sprouting of new, grassroots forms of organization and representation in schools, factories, and neighborhoods, such as the *assemblea*, or spontaneous general meeting. (Its counterpart in the anti-institutional movement will be discussed below.) Finally, the major party outside the right-center Christian Democrats, the Italian Communist Party, embarked on a strategy of social transformation by exercising democratic options within already existing structures, the so-called long march through the institutions. Thus, the Hot Autumn had profound repercussions and Italy changed by great leaps in the following years. Women had not won suffrage until 1946 but the Italian feminist movement became the strongest in Europe. The strong labor movement transformed the workplace. And Italy finally established a national health service and closed its archaic mental asylums.

Basaglia, and many of the psychiatrists who worked to build the democratic psychiatry movement, participated in these dramatic events, and the experience influenced the form the anti-institutional movement later took. Once he began turning away from phenomenology, then, Basaglia turned to the Italian Marxists, who were developing a new language to describe the changes and the social consciousness brought about by '68 and '69. Of particular salience was the Gramscian perspective that emphasized understanding the specific social and historical context within which individual consciousness and action take place.

Destroying the Mental Hospital: The Experience of Gorizia

If we focus on the period from 1961 to 1969, when Franco Basaglia and his colleagues slowly dismantled and transformed the psychiatric hospital at Gorizia, we will have a glimpse of how he worked and how his theoretical writings and his practical experiences interacted. Gorizia is also the emblem of the anti-institutional movement; the methods developed and the issues exposed and worked through, are a microcosm of the multiple experiences that fell under the rubric of the Italian anti-institutional movement.

The microcosm that Basaglia and his colleagues saw in Gorizia was that of the asylum, of the *manicomio,* as a microsocial architectural space that reproduced perversions in human relationships which were not only countertherapeutic, but iatrogenic, creating an illness specific to itself. British and American researchers had already created a name for this phenomenon: institutional psychosis or institutionalism.[20] The *manicomio,* wrote Basaglia in this period, was "an enormous shell filled with bodies that cannot experience themselves and who sit there, waiting for someone to seize them and make them live as they see fit—that is, *as* schizophrenics, manic-depressives, hysterics, finally transformed into *things.*"[21] Elsewhere, he would state about this locus of his practice: "Within its four walls, the pulse of history ceases to beat, the social identity of the individual contained therein is suppressed, and the process of total identification of the individual with its psychic dimensions takes place. The conditions of his life may be offered as proof of his innate inferiority, his culture disregarded as the expression of his irrational deviation. The silence which sets in, in the asylum, becomes both typical of it and guarantees that, from it, no other message will reach the outside world."[22]

Like the American sociologist Erving Goffman, Basaglia saw in this institution clear parallels with the prison. There were doctors, white gowns, orderlies, and nurses just as in a general hospital, but in reality a psychiatric hospital was a custodial institution where medical ideology was an alibi for the legalization of violence. Then at the heart of institutional psychiatry there must be a gross distortion and deception. The institution existed not to answer the real physical and social needs of the patients but rather to serve its own needs and those of the social order whose interests it represented. If the hospital could be compared to a prison, and hospital workers to prison guards, Basaglia reasoned, there must have been a crime. But what crimes had these inmates committed? Unlike ordinary criminals, he concluded, psychiatric inmates were confined not for what they had actually done, but rather for the "phantom of what they *might* do" or for "what is presumed *could* happen."[23] Institutional psychiatry was justified, in the final analysis, by the overprediction of dangerousness of the common mental patient.

In this first period, the sociological writings of Hollingshead and Redlich also played an important role in formulating the Gorizia experience.[24] It was obvious to everyone in contact with asylums that patients were recruited from the marginalized and poorer social classes. But Basaglia and his colleagues—including his wife, Franca Ongaro Basaglia, and many young psychiatrists, psychologists, and sociologists who were attracted to Gorizia as the only alternative in psychiatry—went further in their class analysis of a two-tiered psychiatric system. They recognized that psychiatric diagnoses were rooted in the prevailing economic order, in a moral economy which defined "normality" and "abnormality" in its own rigid and class-based terms. This system of classification explained in part why most of the patients in a public institution like Gorizia were from the working and under-classes of society.

A first step, however, not only had to involve understanding the institutional dynamics, it also had to allow the patient to emerge once again as a person. To facilitate communication, psychotropic medication, just being introduced in Italy at that time, was used. This measure eliminated the more violent forms of physical restraint, enabling psychiatrist and patient to distinguish the damages produced by the illness from those produced by the institution. Chemotherapy, however, produced the first of many contradictions that forced Basaglia to look for alternatives. Psychotropic drugs adversely affected the anxieties of both doctor and patient. They calmed the doctor's anxieties about his or her inability to relate to the patients as human beings, to find a shared language. On the other hand, the drugs increased the patients' level of awareness of their situation, convincing them that they were utterly lost and without appeal.

Medication wears two faces: it can be a chemical straitjacket or it can be therapeutic because it allows a different person to exist. As in the Italian women's movement debate on contraception several years later, the psychotropic drug was seen to have a different meaning when it was controlled and imposed by doctors and pharmaceutical companies than when it was appropriated by the consumer. In Basaglia's work, the very act of taking medication became a moment of critical awareness. For example, a family's request for a patient's sedation became an opportunity to discuss what was behind the request, what the consequences might be, and what alternatives existed. On the other hand, the drug could be a positive "weapon with which to confront the situation." But it was never to gain privilege over other alternatives. It was to be used only when needed during a crisis, and not merely for maintenance.

During these first years, Basaglia and other Gorizia colleagues came into contact with Maxwell Jones and his therapeutic community in Dingleton, England. Back in Gorizia, they began the long, slow process of establishing the "open-door" policy, which involved two main changes in the way the asylum was run.

The first was to open up the wards by creating paid work

in the hospital. To be able to work—at Gorizia this could mean to work in the kitchen, to maintain the grounds and buildings, to cane chairs, or to farm—gave patients a reason to leave the ward; it ended the general stagnation and the emptiness of life where temporality and all contact with the external world had stopped. Eventually, instituting fair standards of wage labor for employed hospital patients also exposed the sham of the earlier "ergo-therapy," (work therapy), through which unpaid labor, upon which the institution had come to depend, had been extracted from hospital inmates. As paid wages replaced token cigarettes (which, generally, only male patients had received), work in the hospital came more to resemble the social reality of labor in the outside world, and patient could feel that they had more in com-mon with ordinary working people. By 1967, over half of Gorizia's patients were working, three times as many as when Basaglia had arrived. But employment of patients also opened up new contradictions, such as the imbalances between equal com-pensation and differing competencies amidst the reality of budget cuts. Many of the discussions between patients and staff on these issues undoubtedly influenced the later development of coopera-tives as a nonexploitative form of work in hospitals in Trieste and elsewhere.

The second transformation at Gorizia was the meetings, and in particular the daily *assemblea,* a gathering of patients and staff with a rotating chairman elected from among the patients. This was a spontaneous event to which anyone—patient, visitor, townsperson—could come and go but which no one was required to attend. No formal distinctions separated nurses, doctors, and pa-tients, and the topics for discussion came from the floor, centering on patients' needs, which they began to express, both collectively and as individuals. The *assemblee* are not to be confused with the general meetings that were part of the British and American thera-peutic community models. The Italian assemblea was a stage for confrontation, for expression by people who had been silent for years, if not confined to bed or back wards. In contrast to the American or British situations, on which a whole literature was making its way to Italy, the assemblea avoided psychodynamic in-terpretations or primary attention to the therapeutic process; the meetings were not run or directed by staff. In fact, these *assemblee* were disorganized, uncontrolled, and open to anger, passion, and unreason. They were anything *other* than safe places for the controlled venting of interpersonal or intrapsychic problems. A coworker of Basaglia described the meetings as follows: "The first *assemblee* were chaotic. They suffocated in a passionate struggle for power, the bitterness and hostility breaking through in both verbal and physical attacks. Certain administrators would scorn this event where everybody had a right to speak their mind, where the first stammering phrases of the most repressed and regressed patients were encouraged, where even delirious speech was accepted without stigmatization."[25]

For some patients the *assemblee* represented the first public occasion at which their angry complaints were recognized for what they were—legitimate demands that human needs be met—rather than essentially meaningless symptoms of psychiatric disease. The recognition was both gradual and collective. For example, the meetings were initially disrupted by a patient who refused to enter the room, but who insisted on shouting through the window. What was first dismissed as the annoying interruptions of a disoriented patient gradually came to be viewed differently by the group. The patient was not shouting through the window because he was crazy. Rather, the man was protesting. He, too, had found a way to use the assemblea to take power through speech, and his protest was henceforth recognized as a legitimate demonstration, an exercise of his rights.[26]

What began to emerge at the *assemblee* was a collectivization of responsibility for the consequences of behavior. Individual problems were analyzed and translated into institutional terms. The dialectical method of negation is perhaps best exemplified in the way problems were solved in the *assemblee*. One woman patient at Gorizia used the assemblea as a vehicle to express her demand for electroshock treatments. Finally, the current president of the meeting, also a patient, asked, "Why do you feel guilty? Why do you want to be punished?" In the heated discussion that followed, participants interpreted the woman's guilt in *institutional* rather than psychoanalytic terms. That is, all the patients had, at one time or another, sought an explanation for their confinement. Since they had been locked up, they must have broken the law, and, perhaps, their punishment was deserved. This perverse institutional logic, now finally brought out and uncovered for the sham that it was, provoked a crisis as the patients' long suppressed anger for their unjust commitment was allowed expression. The hospital as prison had to be negated.

There was a gradual evolution of the assemblea from a place to vent personal problems toward it as a place for translating personal situations into collective and political ones. It was at the assemblea that most of the decisions regarding deinstitutionalization were made, including the timing of individual discharges, community and work placements, and the role of family members. The decisions were not made by a panel of experts using psychiatric criteria. Rather they were made collectively, largely on the basis of common sense and lay criteria.

Without a doubt, the most poignant expression of empowerment, collectivization of responsibility, and anti-institutional practice that emerged at an assemblea took place in 1968, when Basaglia was indicted for manslaughter after a patient who had been released into the community murdered his wife. According to Italian law in effect at the time, the asylum director was responsible for the actions of patients committed to the mental hospital. When officials attempted to close down the asylum and transfer out patients until a new director could be found, students and other community activists arrived and stayed at the hospital to keep it open. For fifteen days there was no mention of "the incident" at the assemblea, until finally one patient exploded, "Why can't we talk about this terrible thing? How can we keep silent when *he* [Basaglia] has to pay dearly for something for which we are all responsible?"[27]

During the anguished discussion that followed, it emerged that everyone felt guilty for what the "bad" patient had done. To both hospital workers and patients the incident represented the frontline, symbolizing everything they had worked for. If there had been an error in judgment, it should be acknowledged, but the responsibility for the error should be shared. The incident provoked a moment of crisis, but also a moment of breakthrough in the anti-institutional struggle. People wanted to stay together, to experience the trauma at one another's side; and so some staff and volunteers began living in the hospital. As a result, for the first time real efforts were made to reach the most regressed, back ward patients, using play, gymnastics where possible, or any simple gesture that might come to mind.

As with the political movements in Italy at the time, the assemblea in the hospital setting was basically about power: decision-making power in and out of the hospital; power in relation to doctors or other staff members; power in the work situation; and power as it excluded and stigmatized persons. The general assemblea was one of about fifty meetings held each week—by nurses, by other staff, by smaller groups of patients. It became an example of critical consciousness that spread to other hospitals. In fact, the assemblea represented one of the most important *collective* moments unifying Italian anti-institutional practice. Critical reflexivity and the creation and exchange of new knowledge went on in these gatherings, as in the cafes and in the spontaneous meetings with families and townspeople, as well as in the more formal political forums. The *assemblee* are essential to understanding how democratic psychiatry could evolve as a practice.

In the assemblea could be seen a second commonality with other Italian social movements—the application of negative thinking that stems from phenomenology and Marxism. Through this dialectical method, Basaglia proposed a series of paradoxes to reveal the contradictions underlying traditional institutional practice and logic: "When you point out contradictions you are opening up a crack. For example, when we demonstrate that psychiatric institutions only exist as an apparatus of social control, the State is forced to create something else to replace it. From the time when the contradiction first explodes into consciousness to the time when it is inevitably covered up, there is a moment, a chance for people to realize that the health system does not correspond to their needs because society itself is not organized to meet those needs."[28] It was in this tiny crevice, this fragile space that Basaglia and his co-workers tried to reconstruct psychiatry as a critical practice of freedom, an alternative psychiatry, as it were, that would help reestablish the excluded, the marginal, the scapegoats of society and help them reclaim their buried history.

Basaglia's method of "negative thinking" was used to continually raise the questions "What is *wrong* here?" "What is the *real* problem?" "Whose needs are being served?" "Whose are being neglected, and why?" as a way of confronting contradictions and piercing through the false consciousness of psychiatric ideologies. The challenge to power was expressed symbolically: patients and staff gave up their traditional uniforms, and with them, their traditional roles, as they relentlessly examined the source and nature of their professional power, the way it was delegated, and in the name of what objectives it was maintained.

Gorizia went far beyond the techniques it had borrowed. Therapeutic communities, as Anglo-Saxon sociological studies of the sixties were revealing, never questioned the underlying structure of power relations.[29] At Gorizia, authority, power, and status were constantly rendered explicit, if not always challenged. In its own therapeutic community the contradictions within the hospital were linked to larger social ones. Basaglia and his co-workers gave priority to an analysis of the global (political and economic) nature of mental problems in place of the traditional micro-analyses of intrapsychic and interpersonal psychodynamics. Knowledge emerged in small fragments that were appropriated by many people in such a way as to bridge the gap between subject and object. Such was the case when, in later years and under the influence of the women's movement, female nurses and patients could finally identify with each other and recognize common problems.

The open door policy construed by this series of changes—the use of psychotropic medication and an end to violent restraints, the elimination of ergotherapy and the emergence of the assemblea as a central body—led to further paradoxes. In fact, in an early piece, Basaglia had written, quite ambitiously that the open door "is the holy terror of our legislators. The destruction of the bars affects patients profoundly and gives them feelings of living someplace where they can gradually regain their relationship with others."[30] But reality moderated such easy optimism. Basaglia discovered that the open door merely reminded the patients of their confinement, and of their rejection by the world outside. Instead of taking the cue to freedom and autonomy offered by the open door, the newly liberated patients at Gorizia remained passive and imprisoned by an internalized image of the asylum. Basaglia wrote: "They sit quietly by and they wait for someone to tell them what to do next, to decide *for* them because they no longer know how to appeal to their own efforts, their own responsibilities, their own freedom. As long as they accept liberty as a gift from the doctor they remain submissively dominated."[31]

And so the open door policy produced another paradox: fewer escapes, less aggressive acting out, and more of the great quagmire of patient gratitude to the benevolent doctor/father. The only immediate solution to prevent this newly emerging therapeutic community from deteriorating into a "cheerful haven for grateful slaves" was for Basaglia to engage his patients in a relationship of reciprocal tension, to challenge their mortified humanity, using as leverage each inmate's potential aggressivity. Basaglia encouraged even his most regressed patients to participate actively and aggressively in what he later referred to as the "destruction" of the hospital: first, to destroy, with their own hands, the noxious barriers that had confined and excluded them: doors, bars, window gratings. An entire hospital wall was dismantled in a collective expression of what Basaglia later referred to as "institutional rage." On another occasion patients and nurses destroyed outmoded furnishings and equipment that were ugly, archaic, or symbolic of punishment.

Once the doors were opened, Gorizia moved to a second stage: the critique of the therapeutic community and the turning toward the outside. As new services sprung up—a mental health center for after-care, a school, a day hospital—more opportunities arose for the collective assumption of responsibility. For example, if an alcoholic, now free to leave the hospital, went off on a drinking binge, his failure was discussed as a shared failure. It became a crisis for the whole ward, not just for the individual, and a collective explanation was sought. The freedom to make choices, including the right to come and go, created a paradox. It left open the possibility of disruption, of crisis (such as suicides) which had previously been suppressed under the hospital-as-total institution regime. For example, patients might address what was to be done about a ruckus caused by an alcoholic who returned from town with a bottle of spirits in his jacket. The patient's action might provoke a collective decision to force another choice. Either the disruptive patient would have to leave or he would have to act more responsibly and with probity.[32]

By 1968 the Gorizia experience had become known

all over Europe. At this time, the team made a conscious decision to multiply the anti-institutional experiences in other regions of Italy—to effect a "molecular revolution." Basaglia left in 1969, along with some other doctors from the Gorizia team. Still more left in 1972 when the experiment was suppressed by the local administration. But it was the difficulties the hospital faced as it became a more open institution, rendering its social control functions dysfunctional, that pushed Basaglia further into working with forces beyond the hospital.

The Diaspora:
Psychiatry as a Cultural Revolution

The antihierarchical and anti-authoritarian nature of the Gorizian experiment corresponded to the new values being expressed in the student and worker movements of 1968. The current of European Marxism, dominated by Sartre on the one hand, and the critical theorists of the Frankfurt School on the other, focused the center of the struggle on groups and institutions that mediate between the individual and the means of production, and ultimately extended to the multiple domains of everyday life. The major unions, also, were turning to issues such as conditions in the schools and health care facilities, and they demanded a whole series of reforms, which would become central in the seventies.

Mario Tommasini, the director of health for Parma, and others, had been aware of the terrible conditions in the institutions in that northern Italian city and elsewhere, where neglected children, juvenile delinquents, the unwanted elderly, and mental patients had collected. In 1967, nurses had demonstrated against the "instruments of torture" used in the provincial asylum by marching through the streets in straitjackets, while the hospital itself, the former stables of Napoleon's second wife, Marie-Louise, was occupied in protest by medical students and Parma student activists. Similar actions occurred in other Italian cities: in Turin students demonstrated against the building of a new psychiatric hospital. The patients themselves went on strike in the sheltered workshops, demanding higher wages and better working and living conditions. Many different organizations to combat mental illness were spawned.

The year 1970 marked a diaspora for the Gorizia group. For several years, Gorizia had provided the only alternative to conventional psychiatric practice. With Basaglia and his co-workers, the anti-institutional practice had become articulated and finally synthesized in their collective product, the book *L'Institutione Negata* ("The Institution Denied"),[33] which was widely circulated in Italy and abroad. Furthermore, political alliances were formed between unions and the more progressive parties. In these linkages, the psychiatric issues merged with a denunciation of segregation of all kinds and a critical examination of the social functions of medicine. Basaglia was actively involved in attempts by workers to gain control of their health care and to change the safety and health conditions of their work place.

In tracing the lines of dispersion outward from Gorizia, like the roots of a tree, we can tentatively reconstruct the early growth of the movement and also highlight the saliency and contrasts between the first experiences beyond Gorizia—Parma, Reggio Emilia, Arezzo, and Perugia. In a sense they represent stages and syntheses in the evolution of democratic psychiatry, the formal organization into which Italy's anti-institutional psychiatrists and mental health workers would converge in 1973. In this dispersion, too, we see fault lines split slowly through the organization as differences in opinion and practice emerge. The internal debates among the protagonists, however, are less important than the particularities of each situation, to which we now turn.

PARMA: "EVERYONE OR NO ONE"

In 1969 Basaglia was called to Parma, in north central Italy, by Tommasini, its commissioner of health. From the outset, two aspects of the situation went beyond those in Gorizia.

It had been evident to Basaglia and his followers that mental patients could not simply be returned to the same, often hostile families and antagonistic communities that had originally rejected them. He recognized that provisions had to be made for them: alternative social and medical services; adequate housing; and employment that was neither exploitative nor demanding. In short, the job of destroying, and, ultimately, closing down the wards of the *manicomio* had to be accompanied by the far more radical and difficult task of opening up communities, making them more receptive, responsive, and responsible, and more than just passively tolerant of the psychologically different, troubled, suffering individuals who would be returned to their midst.

These first steps into the community in and around Parma involved accompanying the patients to the villages or towns of their origin, working side by side with other organizations, such as unions, for broader social changes. Here was a deeply *cultural* as well as political task, for Basaglia, Tommasini, and their coworkers had to confront and do battle with the demons of archaic superstitions and negative stereotypes about the mentally ill. In this respect, Italy did not differ from other Western countries, in which mental illness is a highly stigmatized condition, viewed as incurable, even contagious, sometimes fatal, and strongly hereditary. The stigma, therefore, attaches to the family members of the patient and is particularly destructive to community relations in a society like Italy's, that is still, to a large extent, familial.

But in Parma, the priority was not so much an anti-institutional struggle against psychiatry as one against *all* total institutions—orphanages, reform schools, nursing homes. Tommasini would eventually become identified with this emphasis on all forms of exclusion. A deeply moving documentary film produced in Parma in the mid-1970s by the radical March 11 Film Collective and entitled *Fit to be Un-Tied* captured these two aspects—the outcasts' return to the community and the spurning of all forms of exclusion.[34] In the two-hour film a group of metal workers discuss how they have succeeded in integrating a dozen seriously mentally "retarded" people into the factory in which they work, and how these people are now accepted as workers like any others. A middle-aged man with Down's syndrome, flanked on either side by his new comrades, recounts his first day in the factory, and describes how he now removes the pages of his calendar marked Saturday and Sunday because these are his least favorite days, the days away from his worker-friends. This sequence is followed by a scene in which a militant union organizer apologizes to the camera for not being prepared, but says it seems to him that the way in which he and his fellow workers have approached the problems of those who are called crazy is perhaps more useful than the methods of the psychiatrists. He adds that the new relationships are not just one-sided, but reciprocal, and that the presence of the former patients, their enjoyment of work, and their conviviality has deeply changed something at the factory: "Until their arrival we had lacked a certain dimension of being human."

A second crisis provoked by the reintegration of the mental patient was most certainly to the families of the ex-inmates. Whereas for the older, single patients alternative placements usually lifted the burden of responsibility from their families, younger patients (especially the many decarcerated "troubled adolescents") were generally returned to their over-wrought parents, who often lacked the resources and skills to cope with them. This dilemma was, once again, captured in *Fit to Be Un-Tied,* where the prematurely aged and worn mother of a young delinquent son, Paolo (a boy full of rebellious wit, charm, and boundless energy), tried to explain why her son had problems: "The problems were ours; we were poor, no? I've always had bad luck." The return of her son from one of the institutions closed by Tommasini was interpreted by the harried mother of eight other children as just one more stroke of bad luck. For Tommasini, it highlighted the city's failure to support her through these difficulties.

Tommasini carried on these efforts after Basaglia's departure from Parma in 1971, opening up 250 apartments, farm and light industry cooperatives, and group homes; he began to include, under the umbrella of the excluded, young drug addicts and unemployed persons. Once the focus of struggle had shifted to the community, the asylum itself was left behind. However, after an initial emptying-out period, the process stagnated, pointing to the pitfalls of working either inside or outside, rather than on both fronts.

REGGIO EMILIA
In Reggio Emilia, a city near Parma, Giovanni Jervis, a psychiatrist from the Gorizia team, went to work.[35] Jervis began from the opposite point of departure: the community. The hospital was to remain untouched; it would die a slow death because

the preventive activities outside it would halt the channeling of people in crisis to its doors.

Preventive action here meant intervening whenever a personal crisis appeared. The intervention, however, was political rather than psychological; it spurned the institutional method of social control—hospitalization—for a response that could be arrived at collectively, especially by discussing the problem with working-class and student organizations. Through this "socialization of the therapeutic demand," a sort of psychotherapy emerged, but one based on a notion of class conflict.[36]

At the same time, the Reggio Emilia group refused to create any structure that might become institutionalized, such as a day hospital or an agricultural community. In the long run, however, the need for prevention exceeded the resources available. Even brief hospitalization sometimes had to be turned to. Reggio Emilia eventually left behind two legacies: a very politicized model of family therapy and a hospital still untouched.

AREZZO

Agostino Pirella, who had replaced Basaglia at Gorizia, was named director of a psychiatric hospital in Arezzo, Tuscany, in 1971. This experience was one of the best examples of contemporaneous work inside and outside the institution. Several aspects of Pirella's efforts to coordinate the asylum's destruction with the creation of new services are particularly salient. On the one hand, a favorably disposed leftist political administration gave mental health workers a great deal of autonomy in the creative process of health planning. Secondly, the nurses—a source of resistance at Trieste and other hospitals—were actively supported in their state of constant anxiety and role-flux engendered by the hospital's changes. Then, too, deinstitutionalization went hand-in-hand with depsychiatrization; the process of social exclusion was broken in part by responding to community needs while raising public awareness for the plight of patients.

The creation of a social center illustrates this.[37] A small orphanage had been closed down. At the same time, patients released into the community faced a housing shortage. So the patients moved into the empty orphanage building and began to farm and raise a few animals. But some rooms remained unused. The local neighborhood organization was invited to use them for their meetings. Soon they were showing films there, so the residents opened up a cafe-bar, which brought them some extra income. Then a bowling green was developed, and naturally a bowling club was formed. Soon it was officially recognized as an athletic association and entering competitions, and so forth.

Here was the irony: the institution whose mandate it was to manage what is not normal, provided an answer to the alienation of normal people. In Pirella's words: "In our city, we lack moments of social aggregation and autonomy, which are self-managed rather than technocratic, open at the grass-roots level and not paternalistic. It's hard to believe that it is actually psychiatry, in the moment when it negates itself, that it most succeeds in affirming itself positively and in producing such moments."[38]

With Arezzo, the mental health center and the hospital lost their uniqueness as a locus of mental health intervention. For one thing, crises were managed in multiple settings, wherever they arose. And then, natural support systems were mobilized in place of technically determined or professionalized ones. Finally, a psychiatric intervention gradually gave way to counseling and even common-sense interpretations of problems.

PERUGIA

Perugia, in central Italy, presents a polar opposite to the depsychiatrized ventures of Arezzo, although its beginnings parallel that of Gorizia. In 1965, a group of psychiatrists embarked upon the slow process of humanizing the mental hospital, then deinstitutionalizing it. As elsewhere in the late sixties, the hospital saw a fervent period of *assemblee*. First, the meetings were internal; hospital patients and staff discussed, especially, who should be released, and who should be readmitted.

But one sociologist has remarked on the greater importance of the *assemblea populare,* the large mass meeting held outside the hospital, in transforming psychiatry in and around Perugia.[39] Unlike the regions that have been discussed above, the Umbrian region, of which Perugia is the capital, boasts a long history of populism, activism, and even anticlericalism. The following account of an assemblea held in Umbria in 1969 illustrates its importance as a tool, borrowed from this populist tradition: "A patient who had left the hospital had seriously perturbed the life of the town. He argued with everyone, he would not stop fighting, he went so far as to threaten some people with death. Faced with this situation, the townspeople demanded that he be returned to the hospital, but the psychiatrists refused. With the mayor, they came up with the idea of calling a meeting [*assemblea*], which would be open to everyone, to try to understand, along with the townspeople, what had happened and to search with them for a solution. Given the seriousness of the incidents and their timeliness, a considerable number of people, 1,300, attended . . . their resistances were strong, the discussion rowdy, but eventually the proposition was made that the patient could stay in the village but was to be accompanied by a nurse, at least at first."[40]

Beginning in 1970, Perugia created a network of nine community mental health centers.[41] The patients in the community, and the appearance of new "subjects" undergoing crises—people who had never been hospitalized before but showed up at these centers—pushed the Perugia team somewhat afar from the Basaglian perspective. Basically, team members asserted that psychiatric suffering has its own specificity and hence requires specific responses. For one group of Perugia doctors, this perspective developed into a new psychotherapy, psychoanalytically oriented, though applied in a collective manner.[42]

From this period, new anti-institutional responses sprang up—in Naples, Ferrara, Pordenone, to name a few. But in the four cities described above, one can discern commonalities. The context: a small city or town with a leftist local administration open to change. The issues: a challenge to existing power relations, within and outside the profession of medicine; and a shift to self-managed solutions and empowering organizations; a movement into the community. The method: political alliances, *assemblee,* and cooperatives substituting for sheltered work, and individual entitlements providing a form of financial autonomy. These elements parallel Basaglia's earlier and later work, often growing directly out of it. And they exemplify the practice of democratic psychiatry in Italy.

Two divergences, though, symbolize the major splits within the Italian movement, present to this day. The welfare, or

totally depsychiatrized, model (*assistenzialismo*) is often placed opposite the psychotherapeutic, or "specificity," approach. Similarly, the destruction of the asylum from within is often opposed
to the encirclement theory of prevention.[43] A closer examination
of the issues reveals that these approaches are ideal types that are
much less divergent, to the foreign eye, than first appears. What
critics call *assistenzialismo* often cloaks the fact that Basaglia and
his followers never *codified* what was nevertheless a clear method
of working with people who were suffering: deciphering the messages in psychosis; responding to material needs; engaging the individual's personal network; and using a range of people, professional and nonprofessional, to intervene and create support. On
the other hand, the psychotherapeutic approaches *within* the anti-
institutional movement emphasized a collective approach in
which a team of persons intervened. While not labeled as such,
the methods consisted of a type of networking, often with political overtones. And the practitioners of this approach, with a few
exceptions, continued to integrate advocacy and political activities as part of their everyday work.

    Trieste, where Basaglia succeeded in finally closing
down the asylum, points up some of these divergences. It is to this
experience—the most complete in the anti-institutional movement—that we now turn.

TRIESTE: "FREEDOM IS THERAPEUTIC"
    When he became director of the Psychiatric Hospital of
Trieste in 1971, Basaglia was finally able to eliminate the asylum, and venture into the unexplored territory of the community. Trieste presented a new situation: once part of the Aus-
tria-Hungarian empire, this magnificent city on the northern
Adriatic Sea is home to large numbers of marginal people, including the elderly and refugees from the Istrian peninsula of
Yugoslavia. Despite the presence of a not necessarily sympa-
thetic "white," or Christian-Democrat administration, as well as
organized neo-Fascist groups and parties, the province's administrator, Michele Zanetti, was willing to promote the transformation of the hospital where 1,200 patients were interned.

    Trieste quickly became a crucible of innovations, experi-
ments, and actions. Young people, radicalized by '68 and the po-

litical movements of the seventies, came to work there, often as volunteers or on fellowships. Nonprofessionals were a constant presence. "Freedom Is Therapeutic": this slogan, scrawled on the hospital walls along with other political graffiti, captured the excitement and fervor of this early phase.[44]

But one could not simply destroy the inner space of a hospital, leaving those once confined there at the mercy of the outside world. Alternative solutions had to be found, links had to be reestablished with the community; and patients had to develop new personal and social identities. Ultimately, ex-inmates had to regain a contractual power within the community.

The movement in Trieste, therefore, took place simultaneously on two fronts: in the hospital and in the community. Soon after his arrival, Basaglia restructured the hospital into open communities, organizing them into five zones corresponding to geographic areas of the province. But of primary concern was the reversal of an institutional logic which made the hospital a guardian and the patient its dependent: the establishment of patient rights.

In Gorizia, there had been a problem of a minority of inmates who were either too old or too senile, too physically frail, or too deeply institutionalized to return to the community. Three hundred of these people still remained in the institution by 1968. Of these, approximately one hundred were senile, infirm, and bedridden, and required constant care by the nursing staff. Another hundred were elderly and senile, but ambulatory—patients for whom the hospital was, for better or worse, their only home, and they refused to leave. The final hundred inmates were chronically and actively psychotic persons who were unable to function in the community, or for whom no alternative arrangements could be found outside the hospital. And, some of these patients also preferred to remain living in the institution.

At Trieste, on the contrary, even before most of the patients had left the hospital, a new legal status was created: that of *ospite*, or guest. Some of them were patients who could not yet find housing elsewhere. Others, like the remaining patients of Gorizia, were perhaps elderly or too ill. But as *ospiti* their full civil rights were restored. They were free to come and go as they pleased, with lodging and meals provided on the hospital grounds. Some worked, even in the city. This was a de-medicalized solution; neither medication nor psychotherapy was mandatory.

But more than that, the creation of guest status was part of a whole series of changes "around the organizational and disciplinary pillars of the therapeutic universe. Ergotherapy was replaced by the creation of a cooperative of workers; the ospite's lack of money set in motion a large machine to abolish interdiction and guardianship and to obtain pensions; the criteria for entitlements were modified through successive struggles and vindications; play therapy was ridiculed at [spontaneous] social gatherings; art therapies were turned on their heads by experiments with 'animation,' through which the city began to come into the asylum."[45]

As the wards were unlocked and replaced with smaller units and autonomous housing, such as the apartments where guests lived in buildings that, fortunately, were already scattered throughout the hospital grounds, the flow of traffic through the doors was encouraged both ways: inmates into the city, citizens into the asylum. Staff members went out to talk to families, officials, and administrators. But for citizens to come inside, there had to be strong inducements: film festivals, shows, plays by traveling repertory companies, or performances by musicians, actors, and artists. Once they mingled among the patients, the townspeople could begin to recognize in the distress and suffering of former inmates some of the same problems in living that had plagued their own lives.

Basaglia and his co-workers had a particular affinity for the Italian artists' community, seeing in the works of the surrealists and post-impressionists, in cinema verité, and street theater compatible metaphors of the sick-making contradictions of contemporary society. Through the vehicle of art there existed yet another way of sensitizing the outside world to the violence of segregative control. At Trieste, local and visiting artists were invited to participate in the anti-institutional movement, and some even moved into the vacant wards and buildings. The best-known group was the Rainbow Collective. With the inmates they painted colorful and outrageous murals, psycho-political graffiti ("Psychiatry—the Machine of Peace Crimes"), ironic cartoons with captions such as "Come and get your electroshocks with us; signed Pinochet." Sculptures created by Ugo Guarino were put on display in a former back ward that gave mute but terrifying testimony to the suffering of those patients once imprisoned there. The sculptures were collages created out of the debris left from the stage of destroying the hospital: bits of decaying wood, paint peelings, broken furniture stained with blood, sweat, urine, and feces.[46]

Outside the hospital grounds, a group of actors and ex-inmates formed a company that performed puppet shows and guerrilla theater in the streets and piazzas of the town. They enacted the history of the hospital and its inmates, and they celebrated its demise. In 1975 a group of artists worked with the inmates of Trieste to build Marco Cavallo, a giant, blue, papier-mache horse on wheels. Artists and ex-patients paraded Marco through the streets and squares of the city, as a symbol (reminiscent of the Trojan horse) of the freeing of the captive inmates hiding inside.

Marco Cavallo, "the large theatrical machine," the horse of the patients' desires, became a unifying symbol; it was exhibited in schools, fairs, and marketplaces, and it traveled outside Italy as well.[47] The horse brought with it another side to the transformation of Trieste. On the day of its triumphant entrance into the city, the nurses went on strike, protesting the archaic conditions they had to work in, the long hours, impossible shifts, and the paltry salaries. They complained about the reality the patients lived in, and the poverty that awaited them outside. They were joined in the strike by all employees of the province.

The strike assumed an importance at Trieste that the collective moments—*assemblee,* spontaneous meetings, and such events—already had for the anti-institutional movement.[48] Every extra *lire* for entitlements, every new room for a community mental health center, had to be fought for.

Eventually, Basaglia and his coworkers were able to open six alternative community mental health centers in Trieste by building a power base through sometimes shifting alliances with the provincial administrator, political parties, and labor unions. But when political constellations changed and became less supportive, or when funds dried up, the Trieste mental health workers went directly to the townspeople; they started to collaborate with workers in other institutions, such as in the prison and

the general hospital. By the mid-seventies, the foray of mental patients back into the community had produced a new phenomenon: poverty from the asylum now joined the poverty outside,
that of chronic unemployment and housing shortages, which
were so acute in Trieste. There was also the poverty of human contact, that of loneliness, exclusion, and abandonment. With no existing type of social services, a new response had to be created: a
kind of arsenal of emergency assistance. By obtaining money for
ex-patients—Basaglia and his staff constantly badgered the provincial administration for higher entitlements—they broadened their
choices for community existence.

    By the time Basaglia left Trieste to take over psychiatric
services in Rome in late 1979, the hospital was completely emptied. As in Gorizia, Turin, and other cities, hospital walls and
fences had been literally torn down. In Trieste, the buildings
themselves had been reconverted and incorporated into the definitions and parameters of community life: a beauty shop, high
schools, dormitories for college students, the local alternative radio station, even a cooperatively run day-care center for children
now occupied the emptied wards and corridors. This effect of
blurring the lines between inside and outside was described by a
woman who worked in the day-care center: "The significance of
the presence of children in a mental hospital lies. . .in the hope
that one day we will stop building mental hospitals in and on
the heads of children. The contradiction lies in the fact that 'normal' children are now in a space for 'crazy' people. . .(and the
hope that this space) . . . could be used by the adult to learn to
live with children."[49]

    A structured alternative to the asylum meant both eradi-
cating any possibility for its perpetration and providing a network
of articulated, integrated services to respond to people in crisis. In
Trieste this meant creating a community mental health center
open twenty-four hours a day, crisis-intervention and emergency
services, and beds in the community mental health center.

    Had Basaglia simply stopped with the destruction of the
asylum, had he abandoned the physical space of the institution,
he would have left intact the *idea* of segregative control as a possibility to be rediscovered by other, newer agents of social consensus yet to come. Basaglia was mindful of Michel Foucault's his-

tory of the total institution in Europe and the stages by which each successive generation, each new episteme, recovered the old segregative and penal institutions to incarcerate, in turn, a new category of social outcasts and scapegoats, so that the leper was replaced by the witch and heretic, who were in turn replaced by the debtors and paupers of the eighteenth century, and still later by the sexual deviants and defrocked priests, and finally all of these by the mad men and women. By bridging the gap between inside and outside the asylum, by confronting the contradiction between *custodia* and *cura*, treatment and punishment, and by redefining and resocializing the institution as a positive social space, Basaglia steadily chipped away at the cultural foundations of the old exclusionary logic. But instead of excluding the contradictions, isolating and hiding them away, Basaglia's work returned them to our consciousness so that we might once again recognize that part of ourselves we have for so long denied as madness, as folly, as delirium. Having successfully challenged the special expertise of medicine and psychiatry in the management of human misery, Basaglia also confronted the old and uneasy alliance between psychiatry and the law. Demedicalizing and decriminalizing madness went hand in glove.

Psychiatry and Law: The Law 180

The psychiatric professional [today] . . . so often compared to a ship sinking in a stormy sea, has already gone under. What remains is the tumultuous sea in which we must face, not health and illness, but life itself. It's as if, over the last ten or fifteen years of our work, we had made holes throughout the ship or uncovered already-existing leaks. Once we had established that the ship was not going to sink to the bottom, we began to throw overboard from the hold, the tree, the cables, the pieces of the ship. And we burnt those pieces, although they continue to infest the atmosphere within the logic of an ecological delirium. Our current problem is the same Cortez faced after he burnt his ships: we have no bridges left behind us to help us sail the seas again in safety.[50]

Italy's mental health reform bill, or Law 180, marks a final turning point in Basaglia's itinerary. It was an off-shoot of the anti-institutional movement's concern with breaking the circuit of social control that defined normal and abnormal behavior and which punished and excluded all that could not be understood, domesticated, or neutralized.

Basaglia was the principal architect throughout many phases of drafting the Law 180. In order to understand how he had reached such a level of political influence it is necessary to backtrack and explore the social conditions which aided passage of the legislation. In a fertile climate of changes and experimentation, between the student and worker revolts of 1968 and the end of the left-center coalition in the 1980s, Italians largely redefined the meaning of political. Women, school children, parents, neighbors, workers, youth were the protagonists of the transformation, the "new subjects" united by a common denominator that ran throughout their demands and projects: subjectivity, personal needs, diversity, and autonomy.[51] The women's movement expressed this new current perhaps most clearly in their insistence on control over their reproductive system and the demedicalizing of pregnancy, birth, and the female life-cycle.[52] The labor movement claimed not only a right to occupational safety and health, but also control over health services so as to lessen their dependency on factory and company physicians. Similarly, Basaglia's incessant questioning of the parameters of normality and of reason resonated with women, youth, and intellectuals. In this sense, health was central to the agendas of all these movements.

Health issues, including the questioning of psychiatric power, were taken up by the labor movement very early on. At a landmark congress on "Psychology, Psychiatry, and Power Relationships" in Rome in 1969, health professionals, progressive intellectuals, and representatives from the unions discussed concrete proposals, and the Italian Communist Party presented the first joint health-psychiatric care platform. Then, by the late seventies, democratic psychiatry solidified its political base, gathering a powerful momentum since it first brought together 2,500 people at Gorizia in 1974. Although schisms rocked the organization (especially around the use of specific techniques), members united around the goal of much needed mental health reform. Gradually, local administrations had begun to develop programs out of hospitals, except in the South, where few such

34   INTRODUCTION: THE UTOPIA OF REALITY

initiatives existed beyond Naples. Then in 1976, the heavy gains made by Left parties in the legislative elections boosted democratic psychiatry's influence, especially in shaping national health reform.

Basaglia himself became more politically focused following the en masse resignation of the Gorizia staff in 1972. Although he continued to work within his professional sphere as a clinician and psychiatrist, he also practiced beyond it, as illustrated by his six-year relationship with the Trieste administration, under Michele Zanetti, who translated Basaglia's concepts and ideas into political platforms and programs. In Western countries, the model of a psychiatrist who simultaneously operates on the local level, as director of a transformed psychiatric hospital, while actively negotiating the political system, from a global perspective, is altogether rare. Basaglia, also the archetypal *homme politique* in his ability to maintain the double relationship to popular social movements and to established politics, was to influence directly the sweeping mental health reforms of 1978.

During 1977, most of the political parties drafted and introduced proposals into the Italian Parliament for a national health service. The parties of the parliamentary Left introduced legislation on psychiatric reform that incorporated asylums, and other total institutions (such as orphanages, special schools, etc.); abolition of the 1904 law regulating asylums; establishment of community mental health as the core of psychiatric care; use of the general hospital for acute psychiatric cases; and overhaul of involuntary commitment and guarantee of a maximum of patient rights.

Shortly thereafter, members of the Radical Party, a champion of constitutional and civil rights in Italy, took to the piazzas with petitions calling for a referendum on a constitutional amendment that would totally abolish the commitment procedures and the public mental hospitals that were established by the 1904 law without any provisions for community-based alternatives. Due to general frustration with the pace with which the mental health reforms were taking shape in Parliament, they very nearly amassed the required number of signatures. It was largely out of fear that the Radical Party might succeed, and massive dumping of mental patients result, that Law 180 was quickly drafted and passed through a Christian-Democrat and Communist Party coalition. Basaglia was consulted by the law's sponsors throughout the period of its passage. The Radical Party initiative had separated psychiatric reform from the general health reform by limiting it to a constitutional amendment. To the contrary, the proposal that emerged as Law 180 was later incorporated into the National Health Services Act (Law 833).

Although a compromise measure, the law reflected some basic tenets of Basaglia's work, especially the dismantling of the asylum system and the decriminalization and depsychiatrization of mental illness. The law, however, did maintain a form of involuntary commitment, and forensic hospitals, private hospitals, and university clinics were not placed under its jurisdiction. (For a translation of the law in its entirety, see appendix to chapter 7.)

Law 180 begins from the premise that all psychiatric evaluation and treatment should be voluntary. It put a freeze on all new admissions to psychiatric asylums, and demanded that all current and chronic patients be gradually discharged and reintegrated into community life through a network of new outpatient services. Meanwhile, existing psychiatric hospitals were to be unlocked and patients' civil liberties returned to them. The law prohibited the construction of new psychiatric hospitals or the upgrading of all existing ones. New patients were to be evaluated and treated in the community. If necessary, during an acute phase of illness or distress, a person could be admitted to psychiatric wards of general, district hospitals. These wards could not contain more than fifteen beds, and in no case could compulsory hospitalization last for more than fifteen days, with independent judicial reviews required at the second and seventh days after admission.

The significance of the law is apparent. Its unambiguous goal is the total abolition of the state mental hospital system. More important, the law recasts the relationship between law and psychiatry: dangerousness is no longer the rationale for compulsory treatment and segregation. Nor is the law concerned with the definition and classification of the various types of mental disease (and the degree of threat each is presumed to pose to society). Rather, Law 180 establishes the state's only interest in psychiatry as the supervision of the *forms* and *reasons* for treatment, both vol-

untary and compulsory. The law destigmatizes the psychiatric patient: mental illness is no longer treated as a special case of illness
that allows for special violations of the patient's civil rights. Instead, mental illness becomes, under the law, one of the many
conditions (some infectious diseases are another example) which
might require compulsory treatment or brief hospitalization.
Gone in Law 180 are allusions to the "irrationality," the "mental
incompetence," and the "presumed dangerousness" of the mentally afflicted. Furthermore, the commitment process itself is politicized by assigning responsibility for compulsory commitment to
the mayor, an elected public official, in addition to two new doctors. In other words, the delegation of responsibility to a gate-
keeper who is directly accountable to the public is made explicit.
Commitment is no longer hidden behind a medical mask and con-
founding psychiatric language and expertise.

In 1979, Basaglia moved to Rome to become Director of
Mental Health Services for the Lazio region which included Rome
and four other provinces. Before his untimely death in August
1980, he was able to witness the rather striking immediate impact
of Law 180: the large decrease in public hospital patient censuses
(from 54,000 in 1978 to 42,000 in 1980) and the 60 percent decrease in compulsory admissions. In addition, statistics compiled
by Italy's National Research Center indicated no corresponding increase in admissions to private facilities or evidence of gross dumping.[53] Definitive studies and evaluations of the effects of the law
are yet to come, and few reliable up-to-date statistics have been
published.

After an initial wave of enthusiasm, however, Law 180's
supporters became aware of the problems involved in its implementation, including direct sabotage. The expediency with which the
law was drafted and passed had serious consequences. Opposition
to the so-called Basaglia method which its detractors eventually
identified with the "Basaglia law," came from various sources.
Even in the seventies, Basaglia's work had been contested in lawsuits. Meanwhile, traditional, biodeterministic psychiatrists had
been gaining strength with a resurgence and reformulation of positivist psychiatric models beginning in the late seventies, while at
the same time classical psychotherapies were enjoying their first
broad support. Hospital nursing staffs had gone on strike against

open-door policies, on the grounds that they would have to take the brunt of unleashed patient aggression once inmates were free to move about. And although no jobs were lost when wards or buildings of mental hospitals closed down, many hospital staff members rejected the alternative of working in the community. Like chronic patients, these psychiatric workers were often over-institutionalized, and some of them joined the backlash.

Furthermore, every minister of health since 1978 has consistently avoided providing leadership or support for nation-wide application of the law. The first minister postponed the date for prohibiting readmissions to psychiatric hospitals by three years, while appointing several commissions to examine the question. Then, although no funds were allocated over a five-year period to implement Law 180, a later minister promised ample funds to implement proposals that would move Italy back toward a hospital-based system. There were other obstacles as well.

Five years after its passage, it was possible to venture a typology of regions according to degree of implementation of the law. Those areas where the anti-institutional movement had been most active before 1978, such as Trieste, Arezzo, Ferrara, and Perugia, acted most in accordance with the spirit of the law. There, hospital populations were succussfully reduced, and a network of alternative services, from work cooperatives to free-standing clinics to supervised apartments to group homes, continued to grow. In other areas, especially in northern cities such as Genoa, Turin, and Venice,[54] deinstitutionalization efforts were underway, but success was still limited.

Finally, there were areas (especially in the south of Italy) where implementation of the law was practically absent or, worse, where it was applied in a negative way, guaranteed to provoke a crisis. In some provinces of southern Italy, patient populations in large hospitals had been maintained or even increased, with special regional decrees postponing the date after which readmission would no longer be possible. Elsewhere in the South, deliberate misapplication of the law resulted in a form of dumping that Italians call "wild discharges," that is, patients literally bused off hospital grounds without any discharge plans or material or social resources.[55] As a result homelessness seems to have increased in several cities.

The particular situation in the south of Italy deserves special attention, for the region has always remained locked into a kind of hostile economic vassalage to the more industrialized and politically progressive North. Noncompliance with national laws and programs has been one way in which provincial administrators have maintained their hegemony. So, for example, although the mental health law of 1904 had required each province to establish an asylum, in 1973 only three of the seventeen southern provinces had a mental hospital. Likewise, the 1968 Law ("Legge Mariotti"), which called for the reduction of hospital populations to a maximum of 677 beds and which established community mental health centers, was barely followed. Some hospitals simply subdivided into two hospitals as a way of circumventing the reduced-bed criterion.[56]

In place of provincial hospitals, the southern regions had always favored an alternative: a system of private hospitals under religious auspices to which patients were taken from cities and towns all over the south, and where they were warehoused under minimal public supervision. Hence it should come as no surprise that after 1978 funds for psychiatric hospitals were rarely converted into support for alternative, community-based services.

However, regional differences went beyond the North-South division. The law decentralized the administrative level of psychiatric assistance, holding Italy's twenty regions responsible for planning. As of 1983, however, nine of the regions had not yet designated preventive, rehabilitative, and treatment services outside the hospital (in the *territorio*).[57]

Neglect, sabotage, and incompetency in carrying out the law's intent can explain only part of the problem. It should be recalled that the law was a compromise measure, and at least two structural aspects rendered it vulnerable to misapplication.

First, the only service that is specifically required is the Diagnosis and Treatment Unit (SDC), a ward of no more than fifteen beds attached to a general hospital. Generally, such units are locked and rely heavily upon psychopharmacology as the treatment of choice by the staff. By locating the service in hospitals, the very space determines their medicalized character, which certainly defeats the spirit and purpose behind Basaglia's and his colleagues' work in democratic psychiatry. Because community services, which are not specifically mandated, have either not been funded or else are extremely limited in staff and in hours of operation, the SDC is the only facility in most places that people (or their families) can fall back on when they are in an acute phase of distress. Meanwhile, the fifteen-day limitation (originally intended as a protection to patients' civil liberties) has been subverted by the technique of multiple readmissions. In other words, the SDC has become a new revolving door facility.

Second, the absence of adequate regulations, mechanisms, and funding for community alternatives has tended to produce the distortion pictured above. Perhaps Rome exemplifies this situation the best. Plagued by typical problems of metropolises everywhere—unemployment and a large underground economy, immigration, shortage of public services—it has few community mental health centers for a population of almost four million. Members of democratic psychiatry would challenge the explanation that cost factors prevent the Italian community model from being carried out on a wide scale, contending instead that community care and hospital care cost approximately the same. Nonetheless, the entitlements that allow an ex-patient to obtain housing and the minimum money needed to live outside the hospital are still provided primarily and unsystematically by the provinces. As a result, a major incentive to an adequate standard of living for individuals is limited by the lack of a universal entitlement, such as Supplemental Security Income in the United States.

By the mid-eighties, a new block had arisen in opposition to the law. On radio talk programs and in the newspapers, families of patients pleaded their cause. Some asked for the public mental hospitals to be reopened; others joined with democratic psychiatry to push for an "honest" implementation of Law 180. Family associations were most vocal in Rome. There, with a ratio of SDC beds to general population on the order of two per 100,000 and scarcely any other services available, patients were either abandoned or left as a burden for the family to deal with, most often a wife or mother. Thus in a span of a few years, a visible segment of the general public—families of public mental patients—had become a new force to which psychiatrists and administrators had to respond.

Although conditions in the Italy of the eighties (as elsewhere in much of the West) are not the most conducive to a demedicalized and alternative practice of community psychiatry—as the economic crisis has taken its toll on jobs and housing, and as cutbacks threaten social services and the new health systems—there are still grounds for guarded optimism. Basaglia himself had warned that the anti-institutional movement might be nipped in the bud; yet he also grasped new possibilities emerging. With respect to the passage of Law 180 he said: "Even though it is the fruit of a struggle, a law can only be the result of the rationalization of a revolt. But it can also succeed in diffusing the message of a practice, rendering it a collective heritage. . . . it can diffuse and homogenize a discourse, creating the common bases for subsequent action."[58]

The anti-institutional groups had used conflict and protest as a resource, as had the woman's and youth and other movements. Yet once the government responded to their demands, either through financial resources or facilities or by opening up decision-making bodies, the original conflicts were attentuated. But rather than being co-opted, the movements were destructured and demobilized, as one sociologist has suggested.[59] In place of conflict arose legitimized forms of representation which singled out only certain subgroups as spokespersons for the movement and determined their forms of expression. In the case of psychiatry, alternative practitioners no longer dealt directly with province administrators, but with a bureaucratic tangle of agencies and administrations. For example, in Perugia, at least fourteen organizations and officials, from the local health unit directorship to the committees representing mental health centers (but without patient representatives), are involved in decision-making processes concerning psychiatry.

Nevertheless gains made by Italian social movements in the decade following 1968 were nothing short of astounding: a national health service, anti-pollution laws, the gradual elimination of asylums, free continuing education, and a long list of victories attained mostly by the feminist movement: legitimization of divorce and abortion, publicly funded day care, reform of family law, and the opening of women's health clinics. New forms of protest and politics had won nothing less than an expansion of citizen's rights, an increased participation in government, and a multiplication of social services. Italy had moved from an old system of charity toward a more modern welfare state guaranteeing universal rights, not only to the traditional groups linked to production (workers and their families), but to the various marginal groups, the *emarginati*, that had appeared. It is in this context that the Law 180, too, stands firm.

Legacies and Utopias

No possible alternative to the institution exists unless it is a constant and practical critique of every form of institution: from the mental hospital to the mental health system, from the center to the neighborhood.[60]

In part Franco Basaglia's legacy is with democratic psychiatry and with those community workers in cities where anti-institutional work continues. In part, his legacy is with the alternative psychiatric workers throughout Europe, North America, and Latin America who identify with the spirit of collective human decency, radical tolerance, and de-estrangement that were all hallmarks of Basaglia's vision.

Reflecting on psychiatry in the United States today, we may ask what bearing his legacy has on our situation. Understanding how deinstitutionalization in the United States differs from the anti-institutional movement in Italy should shed light on this.

At first glance, Italian deinstitutionalization does not appear very different from our situation. Indeed the post-World War II trend towards changing psychiatric institutions and, ultimately, decarceration, is common to most Western countries. It has been suggested, for example, that the mental asylum has outlived its usefulness to the state, and that it represented an archaic institution of social control, inappropriate to the goals of twentieth century advanced capitalist nations.[61] Hence we now witness the shift away from large custodial institutions—Scull's "monasteries of the mad"[62]—for absorbing marginals, deviants, the unruly and the unreasonable (the "mad" and the "bad") to a new circuit of social control that includes community-based programs and facilities. Yet the actors in this process, the way in which it was carried out, and the outcome in Italy differ qualitatively from the United States.

At approximately the same time that Basaglia and his co-workers were destroying the institution at Gorizia and deconstructing the logic behind institutional psychiatry, Governor Ronald Reagan was blithely closing down state mental hospitals in California, preparatory to a total "pull-out" of public responsibility for, and commitment to, the care of the so-called chronically mentally ill. Although there were many different rationales behind the policy of deinstitutionalization in the United States (medical, social scientific, and ideological), what motivated Governor Reagan (and other public officials elsewhere) was a concern to save his tax-paying constituency money. He was quite prepared to increase the public coffers by consigning public mental patients to the streets and other forms of abandonment. "Humanizing" and "communitizing" care for the mentally ill really equalled drastically limiting the state's financial commitment to them.

The economic motives for reducing hospital populations had been articulated as early as the 1930s.[63] But in the seventies, actual incentives would become available in the form of income maintenance for indigents, legislated through amendments to the Social Security Act. Supplemental Security Income (SSI), for example, could be used in community health centers, but not in hospitals. Medicaid could be applied to nursing homes. Both allowed a "new trade in lunacy," as Scull refers to the current board-and-care home scandal,[64] to flourish, and encouraged the growth of the nursing home industry.

But financial incentives are only one part of the story. Deinstitutionalization in the United States beginning in the 1950s came about from the convergence of several other tendencies. Public asylums, a legacy of the nineteenth century, were rapidly approaching a state of total physical decreptitude that made their renovation or replacement mandatory. At the same time, investigative journalists, novelists, social scientists, and others legitimized the call for modernization by exposing the cruel and custodial nature of the asylums.

As in other Western countries, the chemical synthesis and marketing of psychotropic medications permitted patients to exist outside the confines of a hospital. This was followed by two decades of legal action and landmark cases brought by civil libertarians and patients' rights activists that pushed their cause against the conditions of psychiatric institutions, if not the very nature of confinement and psychiatric treatment itself. In 1972, *Wyatt v. Stickney* established guidelines for upgrading Alabama's notoriously punitive and repressive mental hospitals—from improving patient-staff ratio to purchasing bed sheets, to new toilet and shower facilities. A few years later, a case won by a long-time hospitalized patient, Kenneth Donaldson, made involuntary commitment and treatment more difficult to enforce. In some states, patients could win the right to refuse treatment. Regardless of the political climate in which these battles were fought, judicial decisions were implemented in such a way as to favor deinstitutionalization, as both a humane *and* a cost-saving policy of reform.

For several years now, observers have recognized that deinstitutionalization in the United States did not fail; it was simply never really attempted.[65] (The American Psychiatric Association's much publicized document on the homeless mentally ill is the most recent legitimization of this view.[66]) Insofar as the closure of state hospitals was never accompanied by the opening up of communities, and in the absence of any redefinition of the meaning of mental illness, or any redefinition of psychiatry as a social practice, deinstitutionalization merely reproduced in the local setting the same exclusionary, institutional logic that was the very foundation of the public asylum system.

The myth, of course, is that psychiatric patients were returned to community life; the reality is that community was defined as any setting outside the grounds of the state mental hospital. What really occurred was the transfer of care from state-run hospitals to federally funded or privately financed community-level institutions. Nursing facilities, the most common alternative placement for ex-mental patients (about half of their residents are reported as having psychiatric disorders) constitute, in many cases, as restrictive and punitive an environment as many state psychiatric hospitals.[67] For other ex-patients, community is the hostile and rejecting inner-city neighborhood where, alone and disoriented, they fall prey to "penny capitalists" speculating in human misery, and to the violence of streets and welfare hotel life.

Finally, the criminal justice system has absorbed still more of a population that would in earlier years have faced involuntary commitment. The 80% increase in the prison population during the past decades is paralleled by increasing reports of psychiatrically disturbed inmates.

We would be remiss if we were to imply that deinstitutionalization in the United States eliminated the asylum while establishing "softer" forms of intervention and control—psychotherapies, mental hygiene programs, or community-based care. For one, the mechanisms allowing softer psychiatric and social interventions have been in place since at least the turn of the century.[68] More important, though, the asylum itself, as a "hard" form of control, persists today as in earlier decades, side-by-side with other forms. And involuntary commitment is now neatly complemented by new, out-patient compulsory treatment and other aggressively controlling social legislation.

Prison, board-and-care and adult home, shelter—these are the components of the new circuit of control that has replaced the custodial institution. To this should be added a last way-station—the streets—and the accompanying unspoken policy of abandonment and neglect.

The problem of homelessness forces the discourse on deinstitutionalization to confront one of Basaglia's major insights: that mental illness is also a problem of poverty, exclusion, and marginality. Of course, not all homeless persons today are psychiatric patients, former or present; in fact the evidence suggests the opposite.[69] Yet once decarcerated, patients face the same problems of unemployment, the obsolescence of traditional industrial and other working class skills, and the disappearance of low-income housing that many other segments of American poor face.

Unfortunately, the organized response to homeless persons who suffer from psychiatric problems is too often either abandonment, makeshift and precarious emergency services, or therapy and medication that turn the social aspects of their problems into mental health needs. This is further complicated when psychiatric labels connote that their bearers, being ill, deserve charity and care, unlike other poor people living in public areas. It is the "difference between being merely disgraced (and disgraceful) and being disgraced but deserving."[70]

Indeed, the very public nature of madness and vagrancy—as the poverty of the asylum joins the poverty of the streets—recreates a modern substitute for Jeremy Betham's Panopticon. Bentham's design for the perfect nineteenth century total institution was one able to induce in the inmate a sense of permanent visibility, an arrangement of space that would render him an object of perfect and continual surveillance. Certainly, the traditional mental asylum exercised control through surveillance from a single, static, vantage point. Today, however, surveillance is no longer contained within a perfectly rationalized architectural space; its gaze is polyvalent, its viewers a multiple public, the colonizers of those homeless street people who transgress the newly privitized terrain of public parks, subways, and shopping malls. And so, the objects of public surveillance and control, no longer confined within a single institution, must circulate from one portal of entry to another. If the so-called mentally ill homeless are described as an eye-sore, this of course implies that they are rendered the objects of our discriminating, incriminating, and hostile gaze.

Italy's deinstitutionalization also creates a circuit of control; yet the fragile spaces and crevices of freedom within it are many. A first explanation for this altogether different transformation of Italian psychiatry are the actors in the Italian movement: a professional leadership committed to radical change, and organized political and community constituencies from the grassroots level on up. In the United States the movers are primarily administrators and psychiatrists who operate from the top down. Unique to the American movement, however, are the ex-patients themselves, whose absence from the Italian movement has met with criticism from other countries. However, the patients' rights groups in North America have rarely formed the alliances with professionals that characterize the successful Italian experience.

The process central to Basaglia's critical discourse and practice—and to that of his followers—is the question of power and empowerment. All changes came about in a political, not simply technological, framework. In the United States, several alter-

native movements led by feminists, gays, minority, and neighborhood groups challenged the absolute power of the medical and
psychiatric professions over their lives in the 1960s and 1970s.
But the major thrust of deinstitutionalization, with the exception
of the community control efforts around mental health centers, occurred in the absense of any challenges to power, professional
and otherwise. Power issues in the United States were a reaction
after the fact, usually limited to one group's self-interest. Meanwhile psychiatrists attempted to regain control over a deprofes-
sionalized system, and communities fought what they saw as an
invasion of ex-patients. In the Italian process, the actors took up
the reins and directed deinstitutionalization. In the United States,
no charismatic leaders stand out as having set the movement in
motion. The process simply eventuated in fragmented and piece-
meal fashion, without a centralized policy.

     In both countries the outcome was the transfer of care.
But beneath surface realities the nature and quality of this care
differs. A corollary to recognizing how central power is to medicine and psychiatry is the valuing of an individual's autonomy.
The contrast between cooperatives and American sheltered
workshops illustrates this point. In Italy a turn-of-the century
law allows economic self-management by patients and other
marginal groups who come together in productive and meaningful work—artisanry in areas where it is traditional, service
work in large cities. While a few such examples exist in the
United States, the sheltered workshop model predominates,
which, as ethnographic research has shown, perpetuates a dependent, infantilized image of differentness.

     Autonomy is allowed to emerge when entitlements,
housing, and other basic needs are seen as human rights. While
patients' rights and other advocacy groups continue to fight for
this in the United States, the overriding tendency is to perpetuate
dependency on care-giving institutions and to divide individuals
into deserving and undeserving categories. The use of contracts,
resocialization programs, creative living programs, and other
therapeutic models that multiplied in community settings all too
often replicate the old moral treatment. The highly regimented
permanent placements in day hospital programs and adult resi-
dences, and the overdetermined life-style of patients who must de-

pend on welfare and mental health programs for survival, have also been analyzed and documented.[71]

This oscillation between autonomy and dependency appears in the so-called young adult chronic, who must often survive by "making it crazy," as Estroff writes of those who bounce off and between day hospital and night shelter, between drop-in clinic and drop-out training programs.[72] With their only form of dependable subsistence, SSI, tied to a damaging and chronic diagnosis, it is little wonder that in the bustling, impersonal marketplace of life on American streets, ex-mental patients now traffic in illicit symptoms, trading their illness for a semblance of economic security through welfare for the totally and permanently disabled. And so we have chronicity born of economic necessity, a new possibility for existence determined by the social welfare bureaucracy. This dilemma was cogently expressed by one ex-patient who said: "I'd like to *do* something with my life, but then I would have to give up being a schizophrenic. And if I gave that up I would have to be something else, and I just don't know what in the world that would be."[73]

Often transient, jailprone, destitute, desperate, and on the street, these people often use drugs and alcohol to self-medicate their psychic pain. Their anger and disorientation can be understood in the historical context, which corresponds to deinstitutionalization, in which they came of age: "Their relationships with institutions have been formed in an era of civil rights and consumerism. Few have experienced long-term hospitalization, and few exhibit the apathy, lack of initiative, or the resignation that numerous studies found to characterize long-term mental hospital residents. These 'new' chronic patients *have not been socialized to docility, to the role of acquiescent mental patient:* they do not use services in the tractable fashion of their predecessors but rather as wary, often angry consumers demanding response to their broad needs for social and economic support."[74] (editors' italics)

An alternative Basaglian view might lead us to explore how deviance and noncompliance can be forms of resistance and acts of autonomy. Difficult to categorize or treat, these young street people are considered the bane of social workers and psychiatrists alike, for they even "resist the contention that they are mentally ill."[75] Rather than recognizing the legitimacy of many of their complaints, and helping them to channel productively their anger and aggressivity, mental health professionals are simply targeting them as prime candidates for reinstitutionalization in the "new asylum."

By contrast, the anti-institutional psychiatry inherited from Basaglia constantly creates situations for socialization—not in the sense of retraining ex-patients in basic skills of relating inoffensively to others and conforming to social institutions, but of bringing people, ex-patient and not, together, allowing them to interact and support one another, and to face their problems together. Unlike the community support philosophy in the United States, this approach does not separate the so-called chronic patients from others. In our increasingly disaggregated society we would do well to facilitate the few such collective instances as have appeared in America in recent years. For example, network therapy and early feminist theory began this task in this country a decade ago.

Inherent in this brief comparison of the United States and Italy are two concepts of deinstitutionalization. In the most obvious American form, a configuration of new institutionalized responses, and not a new alternative psychiatry, is used to *organize* and *regulate* suffering in people who in an earlier era would have been automatically hospitalized. In Basaglia's work we can extract a different meaning for deinstitutionalization: a return to the original relationship between the individual and the social context from which he or she was excluded. Starting at this zero-point, real needs can be deciphered before they are translated into solely psychiatric terms. Autonomy can be valued, and the meaning of crises understood. In this model of deinstitutionalization, participation—by communities, organized groups patients, families, mental health workers, and others—is legitimized as a democratizing element. And, more importantly, the person who suffers is allowed a subjectivity, and there is a willingness to heed Foucault's early call to "give madness back its voice."[76] In Basaglia's terms this means an empowerment through words, an understanding that even delusional or delirious speech may be a febrile voice of protest, the only possible resistance available to those who are usually silenced, disgraced, and excluded.

The Italian experiment, although flawed and riddled

with inconsistencies and contradictions, offers evidence that deinstitutionalization can be done differently and with considerable success. To what extent the Basaglian program and ideology can be exported or imitated in other contexts is debatable, in so far as the Italian experiment—where it succeeded—did so exactly because it was able to articulate with the vernacular culture, with the anti-authoritarian and communitarian ethos of large segments of the Italian working *and* professional classes, at a particular historical moment.

We can, though, appropriate Basaglia's legacy, learning by our own trial-and-error, confrontation, and unmasking. He left us a pedagogy, not for the classroom or medical laboratory, but for the transformation of reality. He taught that power had to be more than an empty attribution; and that in order to challenge conventional wisdoms and reality, one had to be comfortable playing with power, yet avoid being locked into its hold. In this pedagogy, the corpus of knowledge that is created in action as we work in previously unthought of ways can be validated and passed on to others, in a cultural sense.

Basaglia's legacy was utopian, but it was a practical utopia, one that expands possibilities through a daring and dangerously fragile creation: an anti-institutional movement that turned Italian psychiatry inside out. We, too, might unify those practices and places in the American context that tolerate differences, that ensure the rights to basic health care and material needs without medicalizing marginality, and that allow reciprocity and mutuality with those who suffer. An anti-institutional movement transforms cultural norms while it challenges the sick-making and sick-managing structures. We too, can find in the rich potential of American pragmatism and ethnic cultural diversity our own alternative realities and practices.

Susan Sontag writes at the beginning of *Illness as Metaphor* that, "Illness is the night-side of life, a more onerous citizenship. Everyone who is born holds dual citizenship, in the kingdom of the well, and in the kingdom of the sick. Although we prefer to use only the good passport, sooner or later each of us is obliged, at least for a spell, to identify ourselves as citizens of that other place."[77] She is expressing here the intense feelings of marginality and exclusion experienced by the afflicted, especially by the stigmatized afflicted—those from whom it is all too easy to turn away in disgust, revulsion, and pity. It is also, however, a sobering reminder that each of us ambulatory, sane, and whole individuals holds only a temporary truce against illness, madness, suffering, exclusion, and death. We are, as Estroff likes to remind us, the temporarily able, the temporarily sane. It is an essential truth that Basaglia and his co-workers were able to convey to a large populace in Italy. Another was the reminder that a person's differentness, malaise or suffering, are not legitimate grounds for ostracism, exclusion, and confinement. Democratic psychiatry, as developed by Franco Basaglia and his co-workers, implies the creation of a social space in our communities where those who are the veterans of outer conflicts and inner turmoil, of mental prisons and medical wars, can co-exist with, and not apart from, the rest of us.

A member of the film collective that produced and distributed the documentary, *Fit To Be Un-Tied*, touched upon the spirit of the Italian anti-institutional movement when he explained: "What we are trying to say is just this: community life is like a banquet. We want to make sure that everyone has a seat at the banquet table."[78]

Part One DESTROYING THE MENTAL HOSPITAL: WRITINGS FROM GORIZIA

Introduction

Nancy Scheper-Hughes

A. R. Favazza was fond of telling his medical students that "mental hospitals were like cathedrals" and that "once built they are practically impossible to dismantle. Even bombs and conflagrations cannot bring them down for more than a brief moment."[1]

But the public mental hospital has been under a state of siege in North America since the early 1960s, and the old nineteenth century fortresses more resemble silent catacombs than either cathedrals or monasteries for the mad today. Nonetheless, given the current social and political climate in the United States of the 1980s, a celebration of the demise of the asylum may be somewhat premature, and Favazza's pessimistic insight may yet prove to be accurate. The history of psychiatric reform in Europe and the United States has tended to be cyclical so that the mental asylum has been "discovered," buried, and then rediscovered as a utopian premise on other occasions.[2] The search for an institutional solution to the problem of the "homeless mentally ill" offered by the Task Force of the American Psychiatric Association is just one such reincarnation.[3] The possibility for a recovery of the asylum was established from the outset in the United States where deinstitutionalization was mandated by a law, the Community Mental Health Centers Act of 1963, which created neighborhood catchment areas and community out-patient services satellites around the orbit of the state mental hospital. In this way both deinstitutionalization and the hegemony of the traditional mental institution were simultaneously and contradictorily maintained. Mental health advocates such as Leona Bachrach,[4] Richard Mollica in the United States,[5] and Kathleen Jones in Britain,[6] argue persuasively for the integration of the state mental hospital into the new community psychiatry. However, other, more radical mental health/mental patient advocates such as David Rothman,[7] and Lee Coleman,[8] have protested the fallacy that mental hospitals and deinstitutionalization can coexist.

In Italy (and elsewhere in Europe and Latin America where his thinking and practice have been most influential) Franco Basaglia's *abolitionist* position vis-a-vis institutional psychiatry represents the most comprehensive critique of, and attack on, the mental hospital to date.

We have chosen for our opening selections two essays drawn from Basaglia's first major work, *L'istituzione Negata*, The Institution Denied.[9] Through these selections we can begin to grasp the young psychiatrist's growing disillusionment with all liberal proposals to "humanize" the psychiatric hospital. Basaglia struggles with the realization that all reformist proposals (including Maxwell Jones' therapeutic community proposal with which Basaglia was initially quite taken) serve only to bolster a necessarily faltering psychiatry, a psychiatry in crisis.

In the first essay, "Institutions of Violence," Basaglia introduces the mental hospital as one of many violent institutions spawned by a society that increasingly delegates its authority and power to bourgeois social technicians ("agents of social consensus"): teachers, social workers, criminologists, doctors, and therapists of all kinds. Contemporary institutions (including schools, the family, prison, and clinics) are essentially social arrangements that sanction those with power to discipline, punish, and control those without it, so that the very essence of the educative or social work, or therapeutic impulse is pathological. They coerce submerged and powerless individuals into accepting their modified condition as objects of violence.

Within the closed arena of the mental hospital, so structurally impenetrable to interventions that go beyond its custodial functions, the solution is not to be found in humanitarian gestures or impulses which run the risk of glorifying the reformers and increasing the dependencies of the weak, but rather in a long overdue "calling into question" the relations of power and violence that characterize the practice of institutional psychiatry. For Basaglia and his initial *equipe* at Gorizia this "calling into question" translated into an anti-institutional movement designed to "destroy" the mental hospital and to turn the practice of psychiatry inside out and on its head. Basaglia did this by introducing an externalizing discourse on madness, one that interprets mental illness as part of a more general problem of a political nature (namely, the way society responds to disturbing elements in its midst), *and* by envisioning a public psychiatry able to align itself with human suffering outside the hospital walls. Although strongly influenced by Goffman's *Asylums*,[10] Basaglia's analysis of the mental hospital offers a more complex social interpretation of mental illness and a more penetrating analysis of the tragedy of society's institutionalized response to alienated human needs.

The second selection, "The Problem of the Incident," has a curious history. It was written early in 1968 as a hypothetical reflection on the thorny question of responsibility for the violent acts of mental patients both in the hospital and outside. Later that same year Basaglia's philosophy was severely tested: a patient who was released from the asylum at Gorizia returned home where he soon after murdered his wife. The "problem of the incident" was no longer hypothetical. Insofar as the patient was judged incompetent due to insanity, Basaglia was held responsible for the man's crime and he was indicted for manslaughter. The incident, reported more fully in our Introduction, became a kind of watershed in Basaglia's anti-institutional movement, and he and his followers never again waivered in their belief that the real source of patient violence and aggression was not illness but rather sickening and perverse familial, social, and institutional relations. And, as we shall see developed more fully in the latter sections of the book, Basaglia abhorred collusions between psychiatry and the law, and he denied that *anyone*—not even the most skillful forensic psychiatrist or behavioral scientist—could predict human behavior. Hence he maintained that a premonition or a fear of *what could possibly happen* (i.e. "dangerousness") was not sufficient grounds for detaining thousands of hitherto innocent persons against their will in public asylums.

Against this backdrop we might cast a more critical eye on those most vocal opponents of the anti-institutional movement who have argued that freedom for the still psychotic or delusional individual is only the freedom to be crazy, sometimes dangerously so. In the United States, for example, a host of bitter diatribes began to appear in the psychiatric literature during the late 1960s and 1970s in an effort to counteract the growing public consciousness of mental patients' rights and to defend the flagrant and almost casual violations of those rights by mental health professionals. Articles appeared in some of the most prestigious professional journals carrying such malicious titles as: "Drug Refusal and the Wish to be Crazy"; "Dying With Your Rights On"; and "With Liberty and Psychosis for All."[11] They argued against the validity of mental patients' subjective assessments of their own condition, and they labeled as "symptomatic" of their irrationality the patients' refusals of the most modern and scientific psychiatric techniques for their improvement, such as modified ECT and powerful, mind-altering drugs. In the hierarchy of human rights, suggested one well-respected clinician, "the most important civil liberty which can be guaranteed to the seriously ill patient is freedom from psychosis."[12]

If, in the pursuit of this greater (although certainly elusive) liberty, lesser liberties had to be temporarily suspended (through involuntary treatments and forced confinement) then so be it. Other psychiatric writings in this genre stressed the necessity of balancing patients' rights to freedom with "normal" citizens' rights to live in a "safe" environment.[13] Finally, patients had to be protected against themselves, and hospital staff from abusive patients. At a grand rounds presentation during the winter of 1980 presented to the Department of Psychiatry at Tufts/New England Medical Center Hospital, entitled "Psychiatry On Trial," Dr. Michael Gil, former clinical director of Boston State Psychiatric hospital, expounded on the disastrous consequences of a successful civil rights class-action law suit on behalf of patients' rights to refuse treatment.[14] While the hospital was under a court order to suspend the use of involuntary physical and chemical restraints and to curtail the use of seclusion for intractable patients, the frequency of violent acts on the Boston State wards multiplied: patients took swipes at each other, landed blows on unsuspecting staff, and rituals of self-mutilation increased. Gil complained that an injudicious application of civil rights philosophy to the mental hospital context was ill-advised and that it had turned a once orderly and peaceful medical institution into a raving madhouse. Finally, he argued for a special exemption of psychiatrists from normal legal redress; psychiatry, he suggested, should stand outside and "above the law."

It was to just such lines of reasoning that Basaglia addresses much of his writing. He denies that psychiatry can serve two masters, and he exposes the deceit of psychiatric double-agents who claim to represent the interests of both the individual patient and the larger society. He doubts psychiatry's claims of offering involuntary patients "freedom from psychosis," and he understands that protecting the safety of communities entailed the protection of class-based, vested, economic interests. Basaglia's uncompromising position places him squarely on the side of the patient.

In "The Problem of the Incident" Basaglia analyzes patient violence in relation to the structure and logic of the traditional mental institution with its constant and hostile surveillance of the inmate. In a situation of such total objectification and when all responsibility is taken away from the patient, freedom can all too readily become symbolized in the "forbidden act." The logic of the asylum reproduces the very behavior it is supposedly mobilized at every turn to prevent. From the patient's perspective, what else is the implicit message conveyed by locked doors, barred windows, keys, and physical restraints if not the taunting dare to escape? So, too, the constant overprediction of the mental patient's dangerousness to self or to others can elicit suicide or murder as the only possible autonomous act, as the only affirmation of existence available to the damned. Suicide is the final flowering of the institutional logic. A revolving-door mental patient in Boston once told me why she slashed her arms with glass and razor blades with almost predictable periodicity: "It reminds me that I am alive." It is in any case counterproductive to restrain physically a patient bent on self-mutilation or self-destruction. As Peter Breggin observed: "Trying forcibly to prevent suicidal activities leads to a struggle between therapist and patient that encourages suicide . . . involuntary treatment and drug therapy humiliate and harm the patient, often causing greater despair and an even greater likelihood of suicide.."[15]

The dynamic changes in the context of a more open institution, such as the one that Basaglia was trying to create at

Gorizia. There it was hoped that the patient might begin to experience a new subjectivity through which he might see himself or herself as a nonthreatening, nondangerous person. Violent incidents can still occur, but in this context they would represent the failure of the institution to respond to the patient's evolving needs. The open institution, however, leads inevitably to the outside world. Here the situation is more volatile as when the newly released patient responds— sometimes with explosive rage and violence—to a social reality that continues to exclude, reject, and despise him. Such incidents are a potent reminder that the critique of, and struggle against, the psychiatric institution must be carried forth into a relentless critique of *all* social and political institutions that reproduce human suffering, from the family to the schools, from the hospital to the prisons, from the church to, finally, the state itself.

1. Institutions of Violence

In psychiatric hospitals, patients are usually crowded together in large rooms which they are not permitted to leave, even to use the toilet. If they have to relieve themselves, the nurse on duty rings for another nurse, who comes to accompany the patient. This ritual usually takes so long that patients end up soiling themselves right where they are. This natural response to inhuman regulation is interpreted by the hospital staff as the patient "acting out" in spite toward them, or as "incontinence," a symptom of her regression due to the illness.

In a psychiatric hospital, two people lie immobile on the same bed. Under the pressures of overcrowding, the hospital staff takes advantage of the fact that catatonic patients will not bother each other, and assigns two to a bed.

In a school an art teacher rips up a child's drawing of a swan with paws, telling the child that she only likes "swans that can swim."

In a nursery school, the children are forced to sit silently while the teacher works at her knitting. She threatens them—if they move or talk to each other, or do anything that will disturb her work, they will have to spend the rest of the day with their arms raised in the air.

A patient being treated in a public hospital ward, if he has not paid for a private room, is at the mercy of the doctor and his moods, and may be subjected to the venting of anger that has nothing do to with him.

In a psychiatric hospital an "overexcited" patient is given the "stranglehold," a common method of knocking a pa-

Translated by Teresa Shtob.

tient out by suffocation. A damp cloth or towel is thrown over the patient's head so she cannot breathe and then tightened around her neck until she loses consciousness.

Parents often work out their frustration by violence directed against their own children who do not measure up to their competitive aspirations. If a son or daughter is not better than someone else's, this *difference* is experienced as a failure. The child may be punished for poor grades as if physical punishment could resolve the school problems.

In the psychiatric hospital where I work, some years ago an ingenious system was developed by nurses on the night shift to make sure that a patient would wake them every half-hour so they could punch their time card, which was a hospital regulation. The method consisted of having a patient (who had to remain awake) sort out strands of cigarette tobacco which had been mixed together with bread crumbs. The task was designed to take approximately half an hour, after which the patient roused the nurse and won the tobacco as a prize. The nurse punched her time card, indicating she was awake, and then she could resume her nap, giving the same, alienating task to another human time piece.

The following was published in *Il Giorno* some time ago:

An end to gloom! San Vittore prison will finally lose its dark, dismal appearance. Several painters have been working for days and one wing which looks out over Viale Papiniano has been painted a bright uplifting yellow. When the whole job is finished, San Vittore will have a more dignified demeanor, lighter and less distressing than in the past. As for inside the prison? The cells will still be dark, but in the meantime, the bright yellow exterior walls will "lift our hearts."

The examples could go on ad infinitum, touching every institution in our society. The common thread in all these situations is the violence exercised by those who hold the weapons, against those who are hopelessly dominated. Family, school, factory, hospital—all are institutions based on the rigid division of labor: parent or child, teacher or student, employer or worker, doctor or patient. The main characteristic of these institutions is the clear division between those with power and those without it. The division of roles involves a relationship of abuse and violence between the powerful and the powerless, which turns into the exclusion of the powerless from power. Violence and exclusion underlie social relations in our society. The administration of the violence varies depending on the need of those in power to veil and conceal it, and institutions are created ranging from patriarchal family and public schools to prisons and asylums. The violence and exclusion are justified as the necessary consequence of legitimate educational goals (the family and schools), or regulatory functions (prisons and asylums).

This is the recent history of a society organized on the clear division between the haves and the have nots, which leads to deceptive dichotomies between the good and the bad, the healthy and the sick, and the respectable and the disreputable. The situation is quite transparent—paternal authority is oppressive and arbitrary; schools are based on threats and blackmail; the employer exploits the worker; asylums destroy mental patients.

However, the so-called post-industrial affluent society has newly discovered that the open display of violence can actually create internal contradictions that could harm it. The advanced capitalist society has found a new system—the delegation of power to social technicians, who administer that power in its name and who contribute, through covert forms of technical violence, to the creation of new outcasts.

The task of these middlemen is to mystify violence through technologism, without altering its real nature. They ensure that those subjected to violence will adjust to it and fail to develop a consciousness that might allow them to turn that violence against their dominators. Their task is to discover new forms of deviance that have heretofore been considered normal, and thus to expand the grounds for exclusion.

The new social psychiatrist, psychotherapist, social worker, industrial psychologist, and industrial sociologist, to name but a few, are little more than new administrators of violence for the powerful. By easing friction, by decreasing resistance, and by resolving the conflicts caused by the institutions they represent, the new technicians and their supposedly healing, benevolent, and nonviolent activities, permit the overarching relations of violence to continue. Their task, defined as guidance and therapy, is to adapt individuals to an acceptance of their condition as the "objects of violence." The adaptations may vary but violence remains the only reality they are permitted.

With these new technicians, the results are the same as in the past. Technicians promote broad consensus regarding the social inferiority of the excluded, just as, in a less subtle way, they created definitions of biological diversity that sanctioned the moral and social inferiority of those who were different. Both systems try to reduce the conflict between the excluder and the excluded by marshalling scientific evidence of the basic inferiority of the excluded. Psychotherapy, in this sense, is a revised, updated version of previous scientific distinctions which created the "norm," with its sanctions for those who transgressed it.

The only possibility for the psychiatrist is to reject any false solutions and to increase awareness of the situation in which both the excluders and the excluded coexist. The therapist's ambiguous position will continue until we realize the game we are being asked to play. The *therapeutic act* means preventing the patient from becoming conscious of being excluded, and moving from the narrow sphere of persecution by family, friends, and hospital to the global level, where he is conscious of being excluded by a society in which he is superfluous. Therefore we must reject the therapeutic act whenever it acts to soften the reaction of the excluded towards those that exclude them. To do this, we ourselves must become conscious that in the very moment that we are objectified by our role, we too are excluded.

Whenever we compete for power—to become a professor, a chief physician, or to acquire a well-paying private clientele—we are scrutinized by an establishment that wants us to fulfill our task, without deviations from the norm. It wants us to guarantee our support and our skill to defend and protect it. By accepting our social mandate, we guarantee that the therapeutic act is an act of violence against those excluded from power. They are entrusted to us because we can scientifically control their reactions towards the powerful. If we work inside these institutions of violence, we must reject this social mandate, and dialectically translate the rejection into practical activity. We have to disavow the therapeutic act as an act of concealed violence, and combine our own consciousness of being mediators of violence, and therefore ourselves excluded, with the consciousness that we have to arouse in those in our care who are excluded. We must not contribute in any way to their adjustment to their exclusion from society.

A system is *negated* when it is turned upside down, and when its specific field of activity is called into question and thereby thrown into crisis. This is the case with the present crisis of the psychiatric system, which has been turned on its head and called into question by a growing understanding of the specific field, psychiatry, in which it operates. The encounter with the reality of institutions reveals the sharp contrast with technical and scientific theories; that reality itself involves processes having little to do with illness and its treatment. This necessarily brings about a crisis in scientific theories of the concept of mental illness, as well as in the institutions based on those theories, forcing us to try to understand "external processes," rooted in the social, political and economic system.

The incorporation of the mental patient into the body of medical knowledge has been a slow and laborious process for science. In the medical field, the meeting point between the doctor and the patient is the patient's body, considered an object of medical investigation. But when the discourse is shifted to the level of psychiatric encounter, the result is neither simple nor without consequences. The meeting point between the psychiatrist and the mental patient is also the patient's body, but here it is a body that is only *presumed* to be ill and that is objectified a priori, in order to determine what approach to take. In this case, the patient will be assigned an objective role which becomes the basis for the institution that will protect her. This type of objectifying approach ends up influencing the patient's self-concept, so that she can only experience herself as a sick being, exactly as she is experienced by the psychiatrist and by the institution treating her.

On the one hand, science has told us that mental illness is caused by a not very well-defined biological impairment, in the face of which we must passively accept deviations from the norm. Psychiatric institutions became exclusively custodial as the direct expression of the impotence of a discipline which, when confronted with mental illness, could only define, categorize, and shelve it. On the other hand, psychodynamic theories that have attempted to find the meaning of symptoms through investigations into the unconscious have also objectified the patient in a different way, not as a body but as a person. In similar fashion, phenomenological thought, notwithstanding its desperate search for human subjectivity, failed to rescue human beings from their objectification; for human beings and their objectness are still considered as facts which cannot be changed, but only understood.

These, then, are the scientific interpretations of the problem of mental illness. What actually happened to the mentally ill, however, can only be understood from within our asylums, where neither analyses of Oedipal complexes, nor theories about our being-in-the-world have saved patients from the lethal passivity and alienation of their condition. If these "techniques" had really been integrated into the hospital organization, if they had been confronted and challenged by the mental patient's reality, they would have been forced to expand and penetrate every aspect of institutional life. This would have necessarily threatened the coercive authoritarian structure and hierarchy on which the psychiatric institution is based. But these approaches and their subversive potentials are contained within a system of psychopathology, where instead of questioning the fact that patients are objectified, they continue to analyze the various forms of their objectification. They are contained in a system which sees all its own contradictions as inescapable facts. The only possibility [historically] would have been to superimpose individual and group therapy on biomedical and pharmacological treatments, but their combined effect would have been negated by the custodial environment of traditional hospitals or the paternalistic nature of the more humanistically-oriented hospitals. Since psychiatric institutions are impervious to any intervention that goes beyond a custodial approach, a real therapeutic relationship is only possible for the noninstitutionalized mental patient. In their relationship with the psychiatrist, voluntary community patients retain a margin of reciprocity related to their contractual power. Yet even here the integrating and accommodating character of the therapeutic act is obvious insofar as it restores the structure and roles that are are in crisis but which have not been totally destroyed as in the asylum.

The possibility of a therapeutic approach to mental illness is closely related to the larger social system, where each relationship is determined by economic laws. It is not medical ideology which establishes any kind of [therapeutic] approach, but rather the socioeconomic system. If we examine it closely, mental illness means concretely different things, depending on the social standing of the sick person. This does not mean to imply that mental illness does not exist, but it points to an important fact about mental patients in psychiatric institutions: the consequences of mental illness change, according to the established treatment modality. These consequences, the level of institutionalization and destruction of the patient in state asylums, are not the direct result of the disease, but rather of the type of relationship the psychiatrist and society establish with the patient. These include:

1. The Aristocratic relationship—in which the patient has a contractual power to counter the doctor's technical power. Here the relationship is reciprocal only in terms of the roles—the medical role, kept alive by the myth of technical power, and the private patient's social role, which constitutes his only guarantee of control over the therapeutic act of which he is an object. The free "client" patient imagines the doctor as a storehouse of techno-medical power while the doctor imagines the patient as a source of economic power. Since this is an encounter between powers, more than between persons, the patient does not necessarily passively succumb to the doctor's power, as long as he maintains a real economic value. But when that value is diminished and his contractual power vanishes, he then begins the true "career of the mental patient," as a person whose social position has neither influence nor value.
2. Social Security or Health Insurance Relationship—in which there is a reduction in the psychiatrist's technical power but an increased in his arbitrary power. In such encounters the patient is not always aware of his rights or his actual position in the relationship. Here, reciprocity only exists insofar as the patient can demonstrate considerable maturity and social, especially class, consciousness. The doctor, meanwhile, retains the ability to determine the nature of the relationship, reserving

for himself the possibility of calling forth his technical power any time he feels his arbitrary power is challenged.
3. The Institutional Relationship—in which the doctor-patient relationship is so imbalanced and the institutionalized patient is in so vulnerable a position that the power of the psychiatrist is virtually unassailable. The patient is left no choice except to submit to institutional rules and arrangements. He has become a citizen without rights, entrusted to the whims of the doctors and nurses who may toy with him as they wish. In the institutional context there is no reciprocity, nor is its absence in any way concealed. It is in this encounter that we can see unveiled and without hypocrisy what psychiatric "science," as a projection of society, has in mind for the mental patient. The real issue is not mental illness but rather powerlessness. In the complete absence of any form of contractual power, the mental patient has no other way of resisting except through "abnormal" behavior.

This outline for an analysis of different ways of approaching and experiencing mental illness—and we can only know which aspect it presents in a particular context—shows that the problem is not the type, causes, and prognosis of illness itself, but rather the kind of relationship that is established with the patient. The illness as a morbid entity plays a secondary role, even though it is the common denominator of the three situations described above. Uniformly in the last case, and often in the second, the stigma that becomes attached to the illness confirms the individual's loss of social value, already implicit in how the illness has been experienced.

If, contrary to the appearances of our psychiatric hospitals, the illness itself is not the determining element of the mental patient's condition, then we must examine the other factors which play such an important role.

Patients in psychiatric hospitals represent one category of patients whose stigma goes beyond the illness itself. These patients present as people without rights, subject to the institution's power, at the mercy of society's representatives, the doctors, put at a distance and excluded. We have already seen that the patient's exclusion or expulsion from society is closely tied to the lack of contractual power, to their social and economic condition, and not to the illness itself. What is the technical, scientific, clinical diagnosis on which the patient was admitted? Can we speak of an objective clinical diagnosis, tied to concrete scientific facts? Or isn't the diagnosis simply a label which hides, under the semblance of a specialist's judgment, a more profound discriminatory meaning? A wealthy individual with psychotic symptoms treated in a private clinic will be diagnosed differently than a poor person with the same symptoms committed to a psychiatric hospital. The first patient will not automatically be labelled a mental patient "dangerous to himself and to others and a public disgrace," nor will his treatment strip him of a sense of his history or forcibly separate him from his own reality. Private treatment need not interrupt the continuum of the patient's existence, nor does it reduce or irreversibly destroy his social role. Therefore once the crisis is over, he can be reintegrated into society. The destructive, institutionalizing power present at all levels of the asylum organization only affects those who have no choice *but* the asylum.

Can we continue to delude ourselves that the patients in psychiatric institutions include the mentally ill from all strata of society? Can we believe that it is only the illness that reduces them to so miserable an objectified state? Would it not be more fair to argue that these patients are first of all the objects of a prior violence, the violence of our social system that pushes them out of productive life, on to the margins of society, and finally all the way to the hospital door? Are they not the refuse, the disruptive elements, in a society unwilling to recognize its own contradictions? Are they not simply people starting off from an adverse position who have already lost before they have begun? How can we continue to justify our exclusion of these people, and our definition of all their actions and reactions only in terms of illness?

Diagnosis has already become a labelling process that classifies the patient's passivity as irreversible. But perhaps this passivity is not only and always a sign of sickness. In considering the patient's passivity only in terms of his illness, psychiatry confirms the need to separate and exclude him without recognizing that the diagnosis might be discriminatory. So the patient is excluded from the world of sane people, society is freed from the criticism he represents, and society's concept of the norm is confirmed and validated. Given these conditions, the relationship between doctor and patient can only be objectified, since communication between them occurs through the filter of a definition and label which allows no possible appeal.

This approach presents us with a reality turned upside down in which the problem is no longer illness itself, but rather the relationship that is established with the illness. The doctor, the patient, and the society by whom he is defined and judged are all involved in this relationship. The objectification does not lie in the patient's objective condition, but in the relationship between the patient and the therapist, in the relationship between patients and a society which delegates their care and protection to doctors. The doctor needs objective definitions that permit him to assert his own control, just as society needs to discard some and reward others, in order to conceal and banish its own contradictions. The rejection of the inhuman condition of mental patients, the rejection of their objectification, is closely connected to the current crisis of psychiatry and of the society that it represents. Psychiatry, science, and society have defended themselves from the mental patient and from the problem of their presence among us. When we psychiatrists exercised power over those who have already been violated by their families and at their work place, our defense inevitably turned into an infinite crime, as we concealed the violence we used with the hypocritical mask of necessity and therapy.

What kind of relationship can we have with patients, now that we have identified what Goffman defined as the "series of career contingencies"[1] which lie outside the illness? Does not the therapeutic relationship act as a new violence, as a political relationship directed at integration, since the psychiatrist as a representative of society has a mandate to cure patients by therapeutic acts which only help them to adjust to being "objects of violence?" Does psychiatry convey to the patient that this is the *only* choice she has?

If we passively accept our mandate, aren't we psychiatrists ourselves the objects of violence by a technical power which determines how we will act? This is why our present work must be a *negation*, an institutional and scientific reversal that leads to the rejection of the therapeutic act as the resolution of social conflicts. The first steps towards this reversal have been achieved by proposing a set of institutional reforms that have been defined as a therapeutic community, according to the British model.

The first experiences with the therapeutic community model date back to 1942 in England. British pragmatism, free of the very ideological thought of German-influenced countries, moved away from the hardened view of the mental patient as incurable, and pointed to institutionalization itself as the primary cause for the failure of psychiatric asylums to restore patients to health. Main's experiences, and later those of Maxwell Jones, were the beginning of what was to become the new institutional community psychiatry, based largely on sociological assumptions.

At the same time, in France, a large psychiatric movement, led by Tosquelles, was beginning. An anti-Franco exile since the Spanish Civil War, Tosquelles began his career as a nurse at the Psychiatric Hospital in St. Albans, a small town in France's Massif Centrale. There he received his second medical degree and eventually became the head of the Institute. Here, as well, it was in a small hospital and not in a psychiatric research institute, that a new language and a new kind of psychiatric institution could arise, based on psychoanalytic premises.

These two efforts, which had different theoretical origins, showed in practical terms how effectively they could overturn an ideology, which talked of mental illness as an abstract entity, clearly separate from the patients and their experiences in psychiatric institutions.

German-speaking countries, however, tied to a rigid Teutonic ideology, are still trying to resolve the problem of psychiatric asylums by erecting ever more perfect structures in which the custodial mentality still dominates. We need only cite the example of Gütersloh, Herman Simon's hospital, now headed by Winkler, devoted solely to technically perfecting Simon's ideology of ergotherapy. Social psychiatry has come into fashion in Germany as well, but there it does not encompass an understanding that psychiatric asylums have failed or that they violate and objectify patients. The German interest in social psychiatry is superficial and ephemeral, based on the perceived necessity to keep German psychiatry abreast intellectually. One unfortunate consequence is the construction of new institutions of social psychiatry, such as the one that will be built at Magonza, the new Brasilia of German psychiatry, under Haefner's leadership.

In Italy as well, where mainstream psychiatry has been influenced by German thought, institutions have changed very slowly, lagging years behind England and France. Although there were precedents to refer to both with the French experience of community mental health[2] and the British therapeutic communities under discussion, we also felt the urgent need for contributions that would be relevant to our own social and cultural reality, and not just adaptations of other models. Because of this, we chose the community therapy model only as a general reference point to help us begin *negating* the reality of the asylum. Inevitably, this was proceeded by the negation of any formal classification of mental illness, since the categories were considered ideological in terms of the patient's real condition. The English model provided a good starting reference point until the asylum changed and our work was necessarily transformed.

Later on, the definition of our institution [at Gorizia] as a therapeutic community was confusing, since it might be misunderstood as a model for the resolution of the negation. If the therapeutic community model is absorbed and incorporated into the system, it loses its oppositional function. When we trace the steps in our transformation of the institution, what emerges is the need to continually question and to change the course of action, as each effort becomes part of the system and is negated or destroyed.

Our therapeutic community arose as the denial of a situation that was proposed as a fact rather than a product. Our first contact with the asylum immediately showed us what forces were really at play. The patient, rather than perceived as a sick person, was the object of an institutional violence that acted on all levels, because any opposition was defined as a symptom of the illness. The degradation, objectification, and annihilation of the patient does not derive from the illness, but is produced by the institution's destructiveness in its attempts to protect the sane from madness. But even if we strip the patient of the superstructural and institutional overlay, he is still the object of society's violence. In addition to being a mental patient, he is a man without economic, social, or contractual power—a simple negative presence, reduced to being

nonproblematic, noncontradictory, in order to mask the contradictions of our society.

In this situation, how can we treat illness as a fact? How
can we recognize and locate illness, except as an unknown, that
we can not yet define? Can we ignore the distance that separates
us from the patient, and blame it on the sickness itself? Mustn't
we first remove all the layers of objectification, and find what lies
beneath?

If the first step in this subversive activity is an emotional
one—the refusal to see the patient as a nonperson, the second
must be a realization of the political nature of this activity. Every
approach to the patient continues to fluctuate between a passive
acceptance or a rejection of the violence on which our social and
political system is based. The therapeutic act is a political one, oriented to integration. It tries to resolve an ongoing crisis by turning
the negation that provoked the crisis into an acceptance.

This is how our process of liberation began, emerging
from a violent and highly repressive reality, and attempting to
overthrow the institution. Going back over the gradual stages in
this process, we will present excerpts[3], in chronological order,
from our conceptualizations of the work we were engaged in. Perhaps it will then be easier to understand our work, and our refusal
to set up a model for resolving conflicts, that might only have res-
cued the institution.

August 1964:

In 1925, a manifesto signed by a group of French artists calling themselves "the surrealist revolution" was sent to the directors of mental
asylums. It ended by saying: "Tomorrow, when the time comes to
visit your patients and you try to communicate with them without a
lexicon, remember that you have only one advantage over them:
force."

Forty years later, the situation has barely changed; most European countries are still ruled by the old laws that hover uncertainly
between welfare and safety, pity, and fear. Coercive limits, bureaucracy and authoritarianism still rule mental patients' lives—those
same patients for whom Pinel had vociferously demanded the right of
freedom. . . . Apparently psychiatrists have just rediscovered that the
first step in curing the patient is for them to restore the freedom they
had stripped away. In the closed asylum, where the mental patient

had been isolated for centuries, the need for a system of administration for the complex hospital organization meant that doctors were only required to guard, protect, and curb the excesses that mental illness could produce. The value of the system overrode the value of those it was supposed to cure. But today, psychiatrists realize that attempts to "open" the asylum produce a gradual change in the patient's presentation of self, his relationship to his illness and to the world, and a change in his perspective, which had been restricted and diminished by both the illness and the long hospitalization.

From the moment the patient enters the asylum, he enters a new emotional vacuum. . . . He enters a place orginally intended to cure him and render him harmless, but which now seems created to completely destroy his individuality and to objectify him. . . . When the first steps are taken, however, to transform the asylum, the patient . . . no longer appears resigned and submissive to our will, intimidated by the force and authority of his keepers. . . . He now appears as a sick person who, although once objectified by his illness, now refuses to be further reduced and objectified by the doctor's gaze, that tries to keep him at a distance. The random aggressivity which would occasionally break through patient apathy and indifference in the past was an expression of the illness and even more of the institutionalization. In many patients this was now replaced by a new aggressivity born of the dawning recognition that they had been unjustly stripped of their humanity and their freedom. It is at this point that the patient, with an anger that transcends his own illness, discovers his right to live a truly human life. . . . Once the asylum's alienating aspects are gradually destroyed, it is then necessary to prevent the institution from deteriorating into a cheerful haven for grateful slaves by using the only possible leverage that we psychiatrists have at our disposal in order to have an authentic relationship with our patients: the individual's aggressivity. This can be the basis for a relationship of reciprocal tension which alone is capable of breaking the bonds of paternalism and authority which up until now have maintained their institutionalization.

March 1965:

Our hospital is extremely institutionalized in all its aspects: patients, doctors, and nurses. . . . Therefore we have tried to provoke a situation in which all three groups can break out of their rigid roles, creating tensions and countertensions involving us all. This has meant taking a risk—which was the only way to put patients and doctors, and patients and staff on the same level, united in a common cause. The new structure we would create had to be based on this tension, and if it slackened, everything would have reverted to the old levels of institutionalization. The new organization of the asylum had to emerge from the bottom up, instead of from the top down. Rather than presenting a plan as a fait accompli that the community was asked to support, the patient community itself would create a structure born of its needs and necessities. Likewise the organization of this structure would not be based on rules imposed from above, but would itself become a therapeutic act. . . . But illness is almost always tied to social and environmental factors, and tied to the degree of opposition to a society that ignores human beings and their needs. The solution to illness must therefore also be social and economic, so that those who for whatever reasons have not succeeded, who could not stand up to the pressure, can be re-integrated into society. Any attempt to address the problem of mental illness which does not include basic structural changes will prove meaningless. Any real solutions must deal with what happens to mental patients when they are released, their difficulty in finding work, the social environment which rejects them, and all the circumstances that force them back into the psychiatric hospital. Reforming current psychiatric laws means not just new systems and rules that establish a new institution, but confronting the basic social problem linked to that reform.

June 1965:

If we examine what social forces were able to annihilate so totally the mental patient, we realize that only one is capable of such damage: authority. An institution based exclusively on authority, whose primary goal is efficiency and order, has to choose between the patient's freedom, with its potential for resistance, and the smooth running of the asylum. Efficiency has invariably been chosen and the patient has always been sacrificed in its name. . . . Now that drugs and their effects have made it obvious to psychiatrists that they are not dealing with a sickness but with vulnerable people, they should no longer consider the mental patient as a threat to society. Nonetheless, *this* society will always defend itself against whatever frightens it and will always impose its restrictions and limits through the institutions designed to treat mental patients. Psychiatrists should not participate any longer in the destruction of their patients, who have been transformed into objects, reduced to *things* by an institution which communicates with itself instead of reaching out to the patients. . . .

For their rehabilitation, the patients vegetating in our asylums need a new nurturing and welcoming environment. But more importantly, they need a reawakened feeling of resistance to the power that has defined and institutionalized them. Once this feeling reawakens, the emotional vacuum in which they have lived for years will become filled with personal strengths—reactions, conflicts, and the aggressivity which constitutes the only leverage for their rehabilitation. . . .

We are faced with both the need for an institution and the impossibility of making it materialize; the need to sketch out a system we can refer to, only in order to immediately transcend it; faced with the impatient desire to initiate change from above, and the necessity to wait until it develops from below; faced with the search for a new kind of relationship between patients, doctors, staff and society in which the protective role of the hospital will be equally shared. . .; faced with the necessity to maintain a level of conflict so that every individual patient's anger is stimulated and not repressed.

October 1966:

The creation of a hospital run by the community and based on nonauthoritarian principles puts us in a position that diverges from the rest of society. This tension can only be maintained if psychiatrists take a radical position aimed at demolishing the values underlying traditional psychiatry. We must free ourselves from our roles and try to outline something which may contain the germ of future errors, but which will help us to break out of the fossilized present situation. We cannot wait for laws alone to sanction our actions. . . .

The truly therapeutic community stands in opposition to the social reality in which we live. It is aimed at destroying the principle of authority, and it is antithetical to all the principles of a society that is completely identified with rules that relentlessly carry it towards anonymity, impersonality and conformity. . . .

In Italy, however, we are still unjustifiably lazy and skeptical. The only socioeconomic explanation that can be given is that our social system, far from offering full employment, is not really interested in rehabilitating mental patients; how can they be assimilated into a society that has not yet resolved the problem of work for its healthy members? The demands that psychiatrists make will lose their most important social meaning if their work inside a disintegrating hospital system is not linked to broader structural changes, that take into account all the social problems connected to psychiatric services. The therapeutic community is a necessary first step in the progress of the psychiatric hospital, necessary above all for its function of revealing how the mental patient was traditionally perceived, and for identifying new roles that did not exist in the authoritarian hospital.

Yet the therapeutic community is not a final goal, but only a transitional stage, while we wait for the situation to develop further and provide us with new understandings. . . .

All the members of a therapeutic community—doctors, staff and patients—are united in their total commitment, and the contradictions of reality supply the fertile ground from which a reciprocal, therapeutic activity will arise. It is in the play of contradictions—between doctors and patients, between nurses and patients, and between doctors and nurses—that new possibilities and new roles will emerge. The therapeutic aspect of our work is this dialectical experience of contradictions. When these contradictions are dialectically confronted instead of ignored or covered up, and when the technique of finding scapegoats is dialectically discussed instead of accepted as inevitable, the community may be called therapeutic. But a dialectic exists only when there is more than one possibility, when there exists an alternative. If the patient has no alternative, if his life is predetermined, and his only participation consists of obedience, then he will find himself imprisoned by psychiatry, just as he found himself imprisoned by the outside world, unable to confront dialectically its contradictions. Just as he could not challenge that reality, he cannot challenge the institution, which leaves him only one escape—refuge in psychosis and delirium, where there are neither contradictions *nor* a dialectic. . . .

Changing the interpersonal relationships inside the institution is the first step, and it is both a cause and an effect of moving from the custodial ideology to a more therapeutic one. This change tends toward the creation of new roles which are totally different from the old ones. In this uncharted land, which is the starting point for a new therapeutic institutional life, each individual will create his or her role.

In the therapeutic community, the doctor is constantly challenged by a patient whom he can neither ignore nor remove. The patient is always there, expressing his needs, and the doctor can not withdraw to some detached position where he can ignore the problem of the illness. Nor can he resolve it by simply giving generously of himself. In fact, his transformation into an apostle with a mission would create another kind of distance and difference, no less serious and destructive than the previous kind. The psychiatrist's only possibility is a new role, created and then destroyed by the patient's need to fantasize about him. The patient first sees him as protective, and then negates that, so he can experience himself as strong. While the medical aspect of their relationship would remain the same, this new role would allow the psychiatrist to better understand the patterns that emerged, and he would be able to represent, in this relationship, the dialectical pole which both controls and challenges, and is controlled and challenged in turn.

The ambiguity of the psychiatrist's role will continue, as long as society does not clarify his mission. He has a precise role bestowed on him by society: to control the hospital organization in which mental patients are protected and treated. We have seen how the concept of protection, and the security measures needed to contain the dangerous patients, is in sharp contrast to the concept of treatment aimed at the patient's personal growth. How can the doctor reconcile these two contradictory needs, as long as society does not clarify whether it wants psychiatric assistance to be directed towards custody or cure?

December 1966:

Every society based on cultural and class distinctions and on competition, creates areas where it compensates for its own contradictions, and where it fulfills its need to objectify a part of its own subjectivity. . . .

Racism in all its forms is an expression of this need for compensation, just as the asylum, as a symbol of what we might call "psychiatric ghettoes," expresses the desire to exclude whatever is frightening and incomprehensible. This desire is justified and scientifically rationalized by psychiatry, which considers those that it studies incomprehensible, to be relegated to the ranks of the excluded. . . .

The mental patient is an outcast, but in our present society, he can never oppose those who exclude him, since all his actions are circumscribed, defined and finally, dismissed, by his illness. Yet psychiatry, in its dual medical and social role, can help the patient understand his illness and how society has excluded him in response to that illness. The mental patient can rehabilitate himself out of his institutionalization only if he becomes aware of being rejected and excluded. . . .

In the asylums, traditional psychiatry has demonstrated its failure. Faced with the problem of the mental patient, it has resolved it negatively, excluding him from his social context and therefore from his humanity. . . . Any human being, regardless of his mental state, placed in a coercive environment where humiliation and despotism is the rule, will begin to gradually identify with the laws of his captors and will begin to objectify himself. He constructs a facade of apathy, disinterest, and insensitivity which is only an extreme defense against a social world which first excludes, then humiliates him. It is the last personal resource that the mental patient, like the inmate, uses to protect himself from the unbearable experience of consciously living as an outcast.

If he becomes aware of his exclusion, and society's responsibility for it, only then will the emotional vacuum the patient has lived in for years be gradually replaced by a surge of self-righteous anger. This will turn into an open opposition to his reality, which he now rejects not because he is sick, but because that reality really cannot be endured by any human being. He will win his own freedom; it will not be a gift from someone else.

March 1967:

Originally, the patient suffered a loss of identity, but the institution and psychiatry gave him a new one, through objectifying him and surrounding him with cultural stereotypes of mental illness. The patient in an institution that insists on relating to him as a sick body, adopts the institution itself as his own body and assimilates the self image that the institution imposes. . . . The patient, who already suffers a loss of liberty by being sick, has to obey a new body which is the institution, negating any autonomous desires, actions, and aspirations that would make him feel alive and still himself. He becomes a body lived through the institution and for the institution, so much so that he can be considered a part of its physical structure.

"Before going out, all locks and patients were checked." These are the words found in a note left by one shift of nurses for the next shift, to show that the ward was in perfect order. Keys, locks, bars, patients—they are all part of the hospital furnishings, without even a minimal differentiation among them. . . the patient is merely an institutionalized body. Sometimes, until she is completely tamed, she "acts out" and tries to reacquire the characteristics of an actual, lived body, and she refuses to identify with the institution.

An anthropological approach to institutional life gives us different interpretations of the behaviors traditionally associated with mental patients. The patient is "indecent" and "disorderly;" she behaves in an unseemly manner. These can be interpreted as aggressive symptoms that show that the patient is still trying to escape the objectifications which she feels confine her, to show she is still alive. Within the institution, there is a pathological reason for each action and a scientific explanation for all behavior. Therefore the patient who is not successfully objectified when she enters the asylum, is finally tamed and labelled with all the blessings of official science. . . . The patient finds herself in an institution that systematically invades her personal space, already invaded by the illness itself. The passivity that the institution forces on her does not let her experience events according to her own internal dialectic. It does not allow her to live and to be with others, so that they can all protect and defend themselves. The patient becomes an undefended body, moved around, like an object, from ward to ward, concretely prevented from creating a body of her own, and prevented from making her reality dialectical. . . . It is a community that can only be described as antitherapeutic, an enormous shell filled with bodies that cannot experience themselves and who sit there, waiting for someone to seize them and make them live as they see fit—that is, as "schizophrenics," "manic-depressives," "hysterics"—finally turned into *things*.

April 1967:

We have seen how pathogenic the asylum is. A transformation which is not accompanied by an inner struggle, a calling into question of the entire structure, will only be superficial and illusory. It is not a particular tool or a technique that is destructive and antitherapeutic, but rather the entire hospital organization which focuses on efficiency, and which inevitably objectifies the patient, who should have been its raison d'etre. The introduction of a new therapeutic technique into the old institutional context would be both destructive and self-defeating. The institution, understood as a problem to be solved, could be quickly covered up again so the problem appears less dramatic. Even the so-called psychosocial therapies used by psychiatrists as the "path to social integration," run the risk of obscuring problems. Like the Emperor's new clothes in Anderson's fairy tale, they provide no cover-up at all, since the underlying structure will only negate or destroy them.

January 1967:

The problem of the mental patient can no longer be denied . . . so now they try to maintain him within a society that still fears and scorns him, through a series of institutions that protect society from the human diversity that he continues to represent. . . .

The choice is clear. There are two paths to follow. We can decide to confront the mental patient without projecting on to him the evil[4] we fear will contaminate us, and we can start to see his problems as an unavoidable part of our present social reality. In this case the problem of "mental illness" can no longer be contained within the restricted definitions of a "science" like psychiatry. Rather it becomes a more general problem of a political nature, involving the kind of relationship our society wants or does not want to establish with some of its members. Or we can continue to pursue the current path: we can *sedate* our anxieties by creating newer and better barriers to increase the distance between *us* and *them*. We can run right out today and construct a beautiful new "model" psychiatric hospital.

June 1967:
Traditional psychiatry, which treated its categories as universals, has shown itself inadequate to its task. But once we call it into question, we run the risk of falling into a similar impasse, unless we maintain a critical stance in our practice. . . . If we want to begin from the "mental patient" as the primary reality, there is a danger of approaching the problem in an exclusively emotional way. A simple reversal of the negative image of the coercive, authoritarian system into a positive image through humanitarian gestures would relieve our sense of guilt towards the patient, but would only confuse the issue. . . . We need a psychiatry which constantly checks itself against reality and finds in that reality elements by which it can challenge itself. . . .

Asylum psychiatry knows that it has failed in its encounter with reality. Once it lost contact with reality, it did nothing more than write "literature" and develop its ideological theories, while mental patients suffered the consequences of this split—segregation. . . . To fight the effects of an ideological science, we also have to fight to change the social system that sustains it.

Psychiatry has played its role in excluding mental patients, by confirming that their symptoms are organic, random, or incomprehensible. But it also is the expression of a system which believes it can negate or erase its own contradictions by pushing them away, rejecting the dialectic, and trying to portray itself as a science without contradictions. . . . The patient is our only reference point, and we must consider both aspects of his reality. He is a patient with a dialectical series of psychopathological problems, and he is a socially stigmatized outcast. For a community to be therapeutic, it must take this dual reality into account—illness and stigmatization—in order to gradually reconstruct the patient as he was before society acted against him with all its negative force.

In actual practice, the so-called therapeutic relationship unleashes a dynamic that has nothing to do with the illness, but which nonetheless serves an important function. In the power relationship that is established between doctors and patients, the diagnosis of illness is fortuitous, an opportunity to create a power strategy which will be crucial to the development and life history of the illness itself. Whether it is the almost absolute "institutional power" granted to the psychiatrist in an asylum, or "therapeutic," "technical," "fantasized" or "charismatic" power, the psychiatrist has advantages over the patient that inhibit the reciprocity of their interaction and the possibility of a real relationship. The patient, precisely because he is a mental patient, adapts all the more easily to this object-like relationship, as he tries to escape from a problematic reality he does not know how to confront. In the relationship with the psychiatrist, he will be objectified and relieved of responsibility for himself, through an approach which fosters his regression. . . .

The psychiatrist has a power which has not served to increase his understanding of mental patients and their illness. Instead, he has used it to defend himself from them, with one of his chief weapons: the classification of syndromes and pathologies. . . . Because of this, the psychiatric diagnosis has inevitably become a value judgment and a label. Faced with the incomprehensible contradictions of our reality, there is nothing to do but unleash the accumulated aggression on the incomprehensible objects that it produces. The patient has been isolated and ignored by psychiatrists so that they can devote themselves to abstract definitions of illness and to the classification of symptoms, unafraid of being contradicted by those who were ignored. . . . Through diagnosis, psychiatry avails itself of a power, a technical terminology that sanctions society's exclusion of those who are not integrated into the system. This sanction has no therapeutic value however. It is limited to sorting out who is normal and who is not, and the norm, once scientifically established, is not a flexible and debatable concept, but something rigid and tightly connected to the values of both doctor and society. . . .

The present problem in psychiatry is therefore what choice to make. Psychiatrists could once again use their tools to defend themselves from patients and from the problems they raise. There is a continual temptation to calm the anxiety provoked by their relationship with the patient, yet even this is a sign of the reciprocity of the relationship. . . .

Psychiatry is thrown into a real crisis. Looking beyond the divisions that this crisis has produced, it should be possible to begin to see the mental patient, stripped of the labels that have until now covered him over and classified him into a fixed role. But psychiatric reformers are already prepared to attack us with new solutions, which usually mean new labels for old psychological structures. Learning the language is easy but the words do not necessarily correspond to the work that has been done or that remains to be done.

Psychiatric crisis, or institutional crisis? The two are so tightly interconnected that we cannot separate cause and effect. Both have a common denominator—the type of objectifying relationship established with the patient. Science, by seeing the patient as an object of study, to be dismembered according to an infinite number of classifications; the institution, by seeing him, in the name of efficiency, or in the name of scientific labelling, as an object of the hospital structure. . . . At this point shouldn't we just dismantle what has been done? Otherwise, we will remain entangled in the pathology of this science, which has invented patients, in the image of its own definitions. Reality cannot be defined a priori. The moment we define it, it vanishes and becomes an abstract concept. The current danger is that psychiatrists want to resolve the problem of the mental patient through technical improvements. . . . This would mean that the psychiatrist, through modern, well-equipped institutions, or through perfectly logical but destructive conceptualizations, would perpetuate a relationship between objects, where reciprocity would still be systematically withheld.

Psychiatry has no understanding of the nature of mental illness, which requires a relationship diametrically opposed to the present one. At all levels—the psychiatrist, the family, the institution, the society—the present relationship is characterized by violence, as the mentally ill are first attacked and then pushed away. . . . Nothing but exclusion and violence makes the so-called healthy members of a family take out their accumulated frustrations on the weakest member. Nothing but violence motivates a society to exclude those who refuse to play the game according to its rules. Nothing but violence and exclusion underlie institutions that, for efficiency and self-protection, establish rules to destroy the individual's remaining personal dimension. . . .

Let us confront the world of terror, the world of violence, the world of exclusion. We do not want to recognize that we constitute that world, because we are the institutions, the rules, the principles, the standards, the codes, and the organizations. If we do not realize that we partake of the world of threats and lies which overwhelm the patient, then we will never be able to understand that the patient's crisis is also our crisis. . . .Above all, it is the patient who suffers. His only choice is to live unproblematically and undialectically because the contradictions and the violence of our society surpass endurance. Psychiatry has reinforced this choice by showing the mental patient that she is allowed only one place—the one-dimensional institution created for her.

October 1967:

It is not the therapeutic community, as a new fixed, unchanging institution, which guarantees the therapeutic nature of our activity. It is the type of relationship that is initiated in this community that will

82 DESTROYING THE MENTAL HOSPITAL

make it therapeutic, to the extent that it succeeds in focusing on the institutional dynamics of violence and exclusion, and creates the basis for a gradual awareness of this violence. This will then allow the patients, doctors, and nurses to confront and combat those dynamics and to see them as closely tied to a specific social structure, and not as unchangeable facts. Scientific research on mental illness will only be possible after we have eliminated all the superstructures that range from the violence in the asylum, and in the family, to the violence in society and all its institutions.

These excerpts on the radical changes going on in our institution [Gorizia], were not intended as a description of a particular technique, or of a system that is more efficient or more positive than any other. The reality of today will differ from the reality of tomorrow, and in trying to freeze it, it either becomes distorted or irrelevant. The excerpts are only conceptualizations of our practice, that gradually developed as the original concentration camp environment gave way to more human relationships. The problems and the approaches have changed gradually, as our work has become clearer and broader.

However, since we are working in a therapeutic institution, we are usually asked whether community control is the answer for psychiatric institutions, what the statistics tell us about our results, and whether more patients are cured. This is difficult to answer in quantitative terms, and I am not sure that this is the right way to frame the questions.

If we look at psychiatric hospitals, we find, for example, that chemotherapy has produced both surprising and disconcerting results. Drugs have an undeniable effect, and we have seen their results in our asylums with the reduction in the number of patients "associated" with a hospital. But with hindsight, we can begin to see their negative effect, both in terms of the doctor and the patient, since drugs affect the anxieties of both, producing a paradoxical situation. The doctor, through the drugs that he administers, soothes his own anxiety about a patient with whom he cannot communicate or find a shared language. He compensates for his inability to handle the "incomprehensible" situation with a new form of violence, while still continuing to objectify the patient. The "sedative" effect of the drug ensures that the patient will remain in his passive patient role. The only positive aspect of the situation is that it creates the possibility of a relationship, even if that possibility is dependent on the doctor's subjective judgment. On the other hand, drugs affect the patient by making him perceive others as less distant, so he assumes the possibility of a relationship otherwise denied him.

Ultimately, what is changed by the drugs is not the illness, but the doctor's apparent attitude toward it. This confirms what we said before, that mental illness is not an objective condition, but one whose nature is created by the doctor that classifies it and the society that negates it. This is supported by the fact that in 1839, before the age of psychopharmacology, Conolly succeeded in creating a free and open psychiatric community.[5] The effect of drugs has made clear what doctors were not able to understand, so concerned as they were with the abstract concept of illness than with real patients. Looking at the issue closely, chemotherapy presents a challenge to doctors and their skepticism. Once that challenge is met, perhaps we can initiate an approach which may or may not include the use of drugs.

At a time when our work is being examined and judged by the public, we are faced with a fundamental choice. We could emphasize our method of work, which after a first destructive phase, was able to create a new institutional reality, and we could propose our model as a way to resolve the problem of psychiatric institutions. Or we could propose negation as the only possible approach to a political and economic system that co-opts every victory and uses it to strengthen itself. With the first choice, we would only end up with another aspect of the same reality we have destroyed. The therapeutic community as a new institutional model would be a technical improvement, but would remain within the traditional psychiatric system, and a part of the general sociopolitical system.[6] In our work, we have tried to show that mental patients are excluded, and are scapegoats for a society riddled with internal contradictions. Now society itself has begun to show an understanding of this blatant exclusion. The therapeutic community, when it resolves conflicts and adjusts its members to society's violence, can carry out society's task of integration and can play into the hands of those it originally fought. In its first and clandestine stage, which was supposed to be the first step in a long process of radical change, the therapeutic community managed to avoid being controlled, classified, and fossilized. But now the therapeutic community has been "discovered"—it cures patients better just as Ivory washes clothes cleaner. Doctors, nurses, and patients—all those who have contributed to creating this new, improved, *good* institution—may find themselves locked in a prison of their own making; excluded from the reality they had thought to influence; waiting to be reintegrated into a system that plugs up its most obvious leaks and ends up causing even bigger ones. The only possibility we have is to maintain the patient's link to his own history, which is always a history of abuse and violence, and to remain clear on the sources of that abuse and violence.

We refuse to propose the therapeutic community as an institutional model, a new technique for resolving conflicts. The meaning of our work must continue as a negation that entails both a destruction and an overcoming of the coercive prison system of psychiatric institutions and psychiatric ideology, so that we can move on to the violence and exclusion of the whole socio-political system, and not let ourselves be exploited by that which we want to negate.

We are perfectly aware of the risk we run, of being overwhelmed by a social structure based on rigid norms and social sanctions. We can allow ourselves to be co-opted and integrated, so that the therapeutic community would be limited to a struggle inside the political and psychiatric system, without attacking its fundamental values and assumptions. Or, we can continue to undermine, today through the therapeutic community, tomorrow through new forms of struggle, the dynamic power as a source of regression, illness, exclusion, and institutionalization.

Our position as psychiatrists means we must make a direct choice. Either we accept our mandate of power and violence, in which case any act of renewal which stays within the limits of the norm will be enthusiastically accepted as the new solution to the problem. Or we can refuse this ambiguous position, trying as much as possible to confront the problem in a radical way, positing it as part of a global approach that rejects partial and deceptive solutions.

By calling into question the present reality, we have made our choice to stay connected to the mental patient. We must force ourselves to constantly check our work and push it forward, even though this is often interpreted as a sign of skepticism or inconsistency on our part. But only by checking our work against the contradictions of our reality, can we avoid falling into the ideology of the therapeutic community, and avoid schematic, categorical work.

In the meantime the psychiatric establishment defines our work as lacking seriousness and scientific respectability. Their judgment only flatters us. Finally we come to share in the lack of seriousness and respectability that has always been the mark of the mental patient and of all those excluded from society.

An Asian parable tells of a serpent that crawled into the mouth of a sleeping man. It slid down into his stomach and settled there, imposing its will on him and depriving him of his freedom. The man now lived at the mercy of the serpent and he no longer belonged to himself. One day the serpent finally left; but the man no longer knew what to do with his own freedom. During the long period of domination the man had become so used to submitting his will to the serpent, all his wishes and impulses to the creature, that he had lost the capacity to wish, to strive, or to act autonomously. Instead of freedom he found only the emptiness of the void, for the serpent had taken with it the man's new essence which was acquired during the period of his captivity. The man was left with the awesome task of reclaiming, little by little, the former human content of his life.[7]

The analogy of this fable with the mental patient's compromised condition is obvious. It presents itself as a parable about the patient's assimilation of an enemy that destroys him with the same lies and violence that the serpent presumably used to dominate and destroy the man in the story. But our encounter with the mental patient has shown us that we are all slaves of the serpent and that unless we attempt to destroy him, or expel him, we will never be able to reclaim the humanity of our lives.

2. The Problem of the Incident

Any violent incident that occurs in a psychiatric institution is immediately attributed to the patient's illness,* the presumed single cause of unpredictable behaviors there. Insofar as psychiatry has defined the mental patient as incomprehensible, the psychiatrist, who is legally bound to supervise and protect the patient, is permitted to abdicate all responsibility for violent or seemingly chaotic behaviors. The psychiatrist is responsible to society, which has delegated to him the control of abnormal and deviant behavior along with the means for transferring to the illness all responsibility for those behaviors, without taking into account therapeutic risks and failures as in all other branches of biomedicine. The psychiatrist's task consists of reducing the patient's subjective experience to a minimum by totally objectifying her within an institutional system oriented to providing against the unanticipated, the unforseeable. The psychiatrist secures his control of the situation by firmly establishing institutional roles through legal maneuvers (the jurisdiction of the Attorney General), administrative regulations (that concern relations with the Provincial Administration), and scientific nosologies that define the patient's chronic malaise.

In this institutional space where abnormality is normative, the unruly, unbalanced, or disturbed patient is tolerated and excused according to the gross stereotypes of mental illness, just as, in the same way, murder, suicide or sexual assaults in more open institutions are justified and explained as expressions of the unknown, unpredictable mechanisms of psychiatric syndromes. Hence, neither psychiatrist nor the environment can be held ac-

Translated by Teresa Shtob.

*The word *incidente* may be translated as "incident" or "accident." We vary it according to the context in which at appears.—ED.

countable for what are defined as *incomprehensible* acts. The abnormal and uncontrollable impulses of the disease are considered sufficiently explanatory.

However, once we become closer to the patient, no longer viewing him as an isolated entity enclosed within an incomprehensible world, but rather as an individual forcibly removed from the social reality to which he once belonged, and uprooted by an institution that assigns him only a passive role, then the institution itself becomes implicated in his behavior. Every event becomes reconnected to the environment in which he lives.

The problem of the violent incident can therefore be considered from two contrasting perspectives, each corresponding to the different ways the institution views the patient.

The primary goal of the classic, closed, custodial institution is *efficiency* and the patient is, therefore, treated primarily as an object. If the patient wants to survive the abuse and destructive power the institution inflicts on her, she must identify with its norms and rules. Whether she conforms to it with servile and submissive behavior or whether she resists it with deviant and insolent behavior, the patient is nonetheless *determined* by the institution. The rigidity of its rules and the one-dimensionality of its reality continue to lock her into a passive and dependent role that allows no alternatives beyond objectification and adaptation.

Thus it is that by establishing a reality with no alternatives other than regimentation and fragmentation that the institution dictates to the patient how she must presumably act. These signals are implicit in the absence of any goals or a future for the patient, which in turn reflects the absence of any alternatives, goals, or future for the psychiatrist, who is appointed by society to control abnormal behavior with a minimum of risk.

Everything in this coercive environment is provided for and controlled in order to avoid *that which must not happen.* In a reality that exists solely to prevent it, freedom can only be experienced as a *forbidden act,* impossible to achieve. The shaft of light from an open door, the unguarded room, the half-open window, the knife left lying about, all present an open invitation to destruction. The patient's identification with the institution means that he can only interpret freedom as an act of violence against himself or others. This is the message and the logic of the institution.

Where there are no alternatives and no possibility of autonomous behavior, the only future is death. Death presents itself as a rejection of an unbearable life; as a protest against objectification; as an illusion of freedom; as, in short, the only possible plan. It is far too easy to see this death wish as part of the nature of the illness, as traditional psychiatry would have us believe.

In this context, every action that in some way breaks the iron grip of the institutional regime gives an illusion of freedom, but is nonetheless equivalent to death. The escape from an institution is an attempt to avoid that other future which is death and to experience the sensation of controlling one's destiny. But inevitably the escape ends in capture and continued enslavement or in a death.

Paradoxically, the only responsibility that the institution attributes to the patient is responsibility for the incident which it hastens to blame on the patient and his illness, rejecting any connection to, or participation in, the tragedy. The patient, who has been stripped of all responsibility throughout the long hospital stay suddenly finds himself *totally* responsible for his one "free" act, which almost always coincides with his death. The closed asylum, a dead world that objectifies patients with dehumanizing rules, offers only one clear alternative: death, as the illusion of freedom. In this sense, any accident is merely the expression of a patient's experiencing institutional regulation to the bitter end, taking its message to its most logical final conclusion.

We could shift this discussion from hospitalized mental patients to *any* people without alternatives, without a future, who cannot find a place for themselves in the world. Their exclusion indicates to them the only possible step to take—an act of rejection and destruction.

In the case of the open institution the goal is to try to maintain the patient's subjectivity, even if this is to the detriment of general organizational efficiency. This goal is reflected in every institutional act. When there is a need for patients to identify with the institution, they identify because they see their personal goals and their future reflected in it. It is an open world which offers alternatives and a real sense of possibility to the patients.

In this environment, freedom becomes the norm and the patient becomes accustomed to exercising it, which means taking responsibility, self-control, managing one's life, and understanding one's illness, without the biases of medical science. For this to occur, the institution must be totally involved in the material and psychological support of the patient. This entails breaking the rigidity of roles; ending the objectifying relationships where one person's values are taken for granted, while the other's are not even recognized as values; the creation of alternatives that allow the patient to fight against the closed world of institutional rules, and that give him a sense of existing in a space that fosters his continued existence. This means that the only way the institution will now protect itself is through the participation of all its members in developing a community, in which institutional limits are set by the presence of the community and the possibility of reciprocal struggle.

This is, of course, a utopian description of an open institution. There are contradictions within such a reality just as there are outside it. What is essential is that the institution does not try to mask or hide the contradictions, but rather tries to face them with the patients and point them out when they are not immediately obvious.

In this context, the incident is no longer the tragic result of a lack of *supervision*, but rather an indication of the institution's lack of *support*. The actions of the patients, nurses, and doctors can sometimes fail or there can be discontinuities where accidents can still occur. Omissions, comissions, failures, and betrayals of trust have logical consequences, but in all these instances the illness plays a relatively minor role.

The open door becomes a clue to understanding what the door—and the isolation and exclusion of patients—mean in our society. The open door acquires a symbolic value as the patient comes to realize that perhaps he is not after all dangerous to himself and to others. This discovery then leads him to ask why he has been forced into such disgraced and excluded conditions in the first place.

In this way the open institution fosters the patient's recognition that he really *is* excluded. Its sole symbolic function is to demonstrate what has been *done to* the patient and the social significance of the institution that has locked him up.

On the other hand, the open door represents a contradiction in a society that bases its safety and equilibrium on rigid and tight social categories that maintain a division of classes and roles. Psychiatrists and nurses inevitably become aware of this contradiction as they find themselves in situations where they are part accomplice, part victim, forced to uphold a social order they now want to destroy. The open door makes the psychiatrist aware of his own enslavement to a system for which he serves as the silent, unknowing double agent.

What possible meaning do escapes and accidents have in *this* context? They are directly related to the institution's degree of openness to the outside world and to the social nature of that world. The alternatives that the open institution offer can still come up against society's refusal to carry them out. The open door leads, inevitably, to the outside world where society and its violent rules, its discriminations, and abuses continue to reject, deny, exploit, and exclude the mentally ill, who represent one of many disturbing elements for whom public institutions exist.

In such a situation, who is responsible for unfortunate incidents? A mental patient can be released and then find that he is rejected by his family, friends, and co-workers—by a reality that violently dismisses him as superfluous. What can he do except either kill himself or whoever symbolizes that violence against him? When this happens can we *really* speak only in terms of mental illness or of "accidents?"

Part Two DEVIANCE, "TOLERANCE," AND MARGINALITY: WRITINGS FROM ITALY AND AMERICA

Introduction

Naomar Almeida-Filho
and Nancy Scheper-Hughes

Basaglia was concerned that his radical proposals in and for Italy, a nation still very much on the periphery of the world economy, not be confused with liberal proposals originating in "core" capitalist countries, especially in England and the United States. So, in his writings on the destruction of the psychiatric hospital, Basaglia's foil was Maxwell Jones and the British therapeutic community. Here, in his writings on deviance and marginality *outside* the hospital, Basaglia's foil is American community psychiatry and its theoretical foundations in bourgeois sociology of deviance literature. The selections chosen represent Basaglia's interpretation of developments in the United States during the late 1950s and 1960s when a variety of new social "institutions of tolerance," fostered by social psychiatry, were mobilized to defuse violence in the ghetto and to suppress expressions of legitimate outrage. "The Artificial Patient" (Letter From America) was addressed to Basaglia's workers in Italian Democratic Psychiatry as a warning. Even the most radical breaks with old techniques of power and control could all too readily be co-opted and put in the service of an old reality, as the American experience of deinstitutionalization and community psychiatry demonstrates.

Community psychiatry represents one of the most powerful movements in the history of psychiatry, just taking into account the financial and human resources that were involved in its implementation. The movement emerged in central capitalist countries, most strongly in the United States, Canada, Great Britain, and France following World War II in response to a series of social, political, and economic events. A number of important epidemiological surveys indicated a high prevalence of mental disorder in the general population, especially in metropolitan areas. Meanwhile, there was a recognized need to maintain the health (and work capacity) of a labor force that was rapidly becoming scarce and expensive. The cost of psychiatric hospitalization was rising dramatically, while the efficacy of psychiatric treatments in hospital was being questioned. It was apparent that new ways of dealing with the seemingly pervasive mental health problem were needed. At the same time, public denunciations of the terrible conditions of public asylums provided strong moral justification for the proposition to "communitize" mental health care. Hence, community psychiatry represented a practical answer to a humanitarian critique of traditional psychiatric treatment, an answer that promised to go to the *social* roots of the mental health problem.

Community psychiatry coincided, not incidentally, with the increasing intervention of the government of these advanced countries in all aspects of civil society as a result of the historical development of the welfare state. Given the diffuse regulatory social control apparatus of the welfare state, it had become possible to transfer authority for the control of social deviance from the psychiatric institution to the community. In France, with the advent of *"psychiatrie de secteur"* and in Great Britain with the organization of the National Health Service, the events summarized above represent the most important determinants of the so-called deinstitutionalization process. In the United States, however, other, more crucial political factors must be added as relevant to the emergence of the community psychiatry movement. During the early 1960s American society was experiencing one of the most critical periods of civil unrest in the century. Discrimination against ethnic minorities, student unrest, drug addiction, delinquency and violence, urban decay and crime, suicide and homicide, and illegal immigration were identified as serious social problems. The urban ghetto was seen as a crucible of seething unrest and, therefore, as a permanent source of danger to the rest of society. Poverty was identified as a target for public action: as the object of a "war." In such a context of social malaise, the state gradually organized a complex of policies, techniques, and agencies within which community psychiatry emerged as the official project for the prevention of social pathologies. For the first time on a grand, public scale the language and concepts of psychiatry were extended and applied to a broad range of social problems and community issues.

The contributions of sociological labeling theorists and the sociology of deviance literature,[1] were used as scientific rationales for legitimizing community interventions in order to detect early "symptoms" of social and mental pathologies so as to provide prompt and preventative treatment. In its American version, community psychiatry discourse stressed the need to utilize all available resources such as churches, schools, voluntary associations, and political, ethnic, and recreational organizations in the target community which could be identified as potentially therapeutic. In addition, community psychiatry programs solicited the help of identified community leaders in solving mental health and related community problems (crime, prostitution, drugs, etc.) through the vehicle of so-called community participation.

The primary targets of community psychiatry were always clearly acknowledged: marginal social groups. Its alleged objective was to deal in direct and practical ways with such troubling phenomena as norms and their deviation, prevention and cure, and sickness and health. In reality, the complex of techniques and practices acted to foster an extremely broad definition of psychopathology and to justify more forms of surveillance and regulation of "problem" populations in the ghetto. Community psychiatry, then, offers a good example of what Gramsci meant when he spoke of the way in which the state can manipulate scientific discourses as a means of furthering its hegemony. As an organic ideology, neither closed nor static, community psychiatry experienced a historical development riddled with contradictions which eventually gave rise to the development of more progressive ideas among some of its own organic intellectuals.

In the following selections, Basaglia treats community psychiatry as if it were a reverse mirror-image of the movement of democratic psychiatry that he was then developing in Italy. The main thrust of Basaglia's critique can be found in his comments on Jurgen Ruesch's apology of community psychiatry.[2] Basaglia points out the dangers inherent in an expanding definition of deviance which only serves to legitimize norms that are directly linked to productivity in advanced capitalist societies. His critique strikes deeply at the heart of the contradiction of community psychiatry with its extreme flexibility in the objects of intervention, so that in the name of mental health, ethnic minorities, women, drop-outs, old people, the poor, children and other marginal sectors of postindustrial society come increasingly to be identified with the deviant. The key to their disvalued social status is their low or nonproductivity. Under industrial capitalism normality becomes equated with productivity. This explains why, to Basaglia's satisfaction, community psychiatry was born in affluent societies characterized by a high degree of economic surplus accompanied by a decrease in human participation in the productive process. The gradual formation of a nonproductive majority becomes synonymous with the ideological formulation (under community psychiatry), of a deviant majority, a *maggioranza deviante*, which must be controlled and neutralized through ideological and political means. Basaglia introduces the concepts of "primary and secondary deviance/maladaptation" in order to explain the political mechanisms through which the control of the deviant majority is achieved. Basaglia's notion of *primary* deviance roughly corresponds to what some American social scientists refer to as "marginalization" (exclusion from mainstream social, political, economic institutions). *Secondary* deviance refers to the ideological reformulations of marginalization as a mental health problem, and the consequent proliferation of "illusory solutions" that act only to stabilize the primary maladaptation. It is essential to grasp that Basaglia's concepts, despite their superficial similarity to concepts in use in American social deviance theory (i.e. the terms "primary" and "secondary" deviance, for example),[3] are always grounded in his understanding of the class struggle. Primary and secondary deviance appear in Basaglia's analysis as mediating elements in the process of social and economic exclusion specific to the class formation process of advanced capitalist societies.

Basaglia suggests that the social functions of community psychiatry are an answer, at the ideological level, to the contradictions occurring at the economic base. In order to reproduce the economic and social formation, individuals suffering from primary maladaptation need to be controlled, but not destroyed. It is a central contradiction that must be resolved. A concrete problem, such as the increase of a surplus population which is a necessary condition for the expansion of capitalism, must be transformed into an ideological question and eventually achieve the status of a scientific problem calling for an effective technology to solve it. In addition, the fact that the economic system has to select and exclude people according to the logic of capital accumulation has to be concealed. In short, deep structural problems must be transformed into delimited problems that can be managed by instruments and techniques of manipulation such as community psychiatry.

In connection with Basaglia's critique it should be noted that the concept of community in community psychiatry discourse is a highly idealistic one, implying a conception of society built on relationships of harmony, consensus, and comprehension, and free of conflict. Community, in this sense, would be understood as a self-regulated system, homeostatic, ahistoric, and therefore, abstract. There are obvious advantages for the dominant ideology in entertaining an idealized conception such as this as the basis for such an important strategy of social regulation as community psychiatry. The demand for full economic and political participation, a basic manifestation of the class struggle, is safely channeled into safer forms of expression, such as community participation, which do not threaten the status quo. This is also achieved when collective social problems are redefined as smaller, localized problems, giving people a false perspective about where the problems originate and how they might be resolved. When superficial changes are made at the community level, the larger social and political issues that are at the root of the oppression and the deviance of marginal groups are depoliticized and atomized in order to insure the hegemony of dominant groups. In the final analysis, then, according to Basaglia, the deviant majority tend to be forced into a participation that is *false* in order to prevent them from a participation that is *real*.

3. The Disease and Its Double and the Deviant Majority: Critical Propositions on the Problem of Deviance

This article does not pretend to be a methodological study nor does it offer a classification of deviants; for that, the reader is referred to the categories created by official psychiatry whose function it is to define and classify different pathological conditions. We are neither analyzing the therapeutic relationship with deviants nor suggesting other possible psychiatric solutions to the problem.

We want to focus on how traditional psychiatry classifies deviance within a category that barely manages to contain the phenomenon. Thus deviants are doubly misfits, maladjusted both in terms of a reality where they cannot fit in, and in terms of an ideology that defines them. Psychiatry still labels them within psychopathology, but the labels are no longer capable of encompassing the problem, which breaks out of the overly narrow limits of medical ideology. Sociology, which similarly tries to apply new categories to behavior at the outer limit of norms, imposes its own ideology on deviants like a new, tight-fitting jacket.

Translated by Teresa Shtob. The corpus of Basaglia's writings is characterized by frequent repetitions and redundancies. Such is the case with two very important, but considerably overlapping essays on deviance, "The Disease and Its Double" and "The Deviant Majority," which originally appeared in *La Maggioranza Deviante* (Torino: Einaudi, 1971). We have chosen to graft sections of "The Deviant Majority" on to the body of "The Disease and Its Double," and we note the two places where this integration occurs with asterisks and ellipses.—EDS.

The crucial thing is to understand how this problem is rationalized through an ideology that circumscribes it, keeps it under control, and reduces its threat. In the social and behavioral sciences, theoretical and scientific topics under study often do not originate from practical problems, but are imported from other cultures. These topics, which are typical of countries at a different socioeconomic level, are introduced into a context where there is difficulty in understanding their assumptions and relevance. This process of identifying at an ideological level is typical of subordinate cultures that play only a marginal role in terms of the economic and political forces that control them. These cultures conform on the ideological level before they conform on the material level. Different stages of cultural development correspond to different stages of socioeconomic development, so that problems arising in technologically developed countries are first adopted as artificial issues in less developed countries.

An example of this phenomenon can be found in the language of our intellectuals. It rarely corresponds to a practical reality, but comes from having borrowed cultural traditions from different realities, which are then applied to a context where their relevance is minimal. The new language which develops, because it doesn't come from a visible, recognizable practical reality, becomes the property of a narrow elite—a kind of code for the few privileged individuals who can decipher its message. In this fashion, purely ideological experiences appear to be real and the nature of problems becomes more confusing, since they are in part real, in part artificially produced by the ideology that precedes them. Anything that is introduced as a problem is turned into something other than what it really is by the rationalizing process it undergoes.

A current example of this is the problem of social deviance. This has already become a crucial problem in technologically developed countries, but hasn't yet burst on the Italian scene as a well-known concrete reality. It has been imported into our culture more as an ideological issue than a real problem. This is corroborated by the fact that sociology, and not psychiatry, has taken it up as a problem under the direct influence of British interpretations of deviance.

In Italy, the deviant individual, who lives on the outer

margins of the norm, is still labeled a psychopath and is enclosed within the parameters of a specific medical typology. Given the relatively small number of "abnormal" behaviors, as defined by the British, this typology is still able to contain the phenomenon. The custodial ideology is marked by a violent and repressive science that corresponds to a primitive stage of capitalist development.

In the United States, however, the problem has already been rationalized into a multidisciplinary approach, where medical typology is flanked by sociological ideology, so that total control is ensured. The phenomenon of deviance in the United States is clearly shaped by both exclusion and self-exclusion from production, supported by welfare institutions, as part of the tolerant climate of advanced capitalism. . . .

[*The following three paragraphs are taken from "The Deviant Majority" as revised by Franca Ongaro Basaglia in 1984, for this volume—*EDS.]

The pressure from these contradictions caused a major policy position, embodied in Kennedy's 1963 law which recognized that mental health was an important social problem. There was an understanding that, in terms of production, the incidence of disease, just like the incidence of health, can become a decisive aspect of a country's economy. New therapeutic welfare institutions were created, drawing groups previously excluded into the productive cycle, and thereby ensuring social control over them through technical control.

Scientific theories of deviance developed in English and American cultures in response to an already existing situation. They are imported into Italy without being tested against our reality, and without having their premises, limits, and consequences defined. They thus become a new sociological "replacement ideology," added on to the older psychiatric ideologies, ready to act as a potential reserve of ideological formulations. The general stigma of deviance replaces the more specific, violent one of psychopathy and criminality. The rigid parameters of science are softened by the entry of the so-called human sciences into this field. These sciences do not change the nature of the phenomenon, but they enlarge it into a false, undifferentiated totality that seems to unite opposites, without really confronting the differences and their relationships.

In Italy, the development of capital hasn't yet taken on a total dimension, and a totalizing kind of control isn't yet required. The definition of innate abnormality and the structure of the deviant psychopathic personality is based on the "ideology of diversity," and in Italy that still suffices to ensure the integrity of its values.

This would seem to make the comparisons with the United States impossible. The two countries are at different levels of economic development and are characterized by different problems and ideologies. Nonetheless, the very ambiguity of the situation in Italy, the fact that what are concrete issues elsewhere arise artificially here, should enable us to discern how scientific ideology functions when it has little to do with the specific reality it hides behind. The situation in Italy may make things clearer, since we find ourselves, at a different stage of economic development, with a different range of corresponding problems, and with an ideological cover-up that exceeds our present needs and requirements [with respect to resolving contradictions—Ed.]. This cover-up tries to conceal the gap between ideology and practice, a gap which shows how the totalizing process of capitalism either uses specific ideologies to hide its contradictions, or creates artificial contradictions. These then, in turn, produce a reality that adheres to the ideologies that have already been created. The comparison between the United States and Italy should help us understand the function and meaning that ideologies assume, as they both veil and create problems.

Our intention here is to analyze the problem of deviance by trying to see the phenomenon as it first arises, and then as it develops, so we can understand the process that creates and then resolves the problem. Usually the whole set of rules that define the values of a given society, in terms of its beliefs, social organization, economy, and technological and industrial development, constitute the line of defense that marks the limits of what is normative. It is a body of relative values that takes on an absolute importance if someone acts against it.

In this sense, it is difficult to define the specific terrain of deviance, since its definition is dependent on a value judgment. With the "psychopath," the problem is already defined, since there are specific medical parameters that classify the behavior. But the "deviant" does not fit into any precise description or at least has not yet been scientifically classified. Deviance is to some degree unclear and can provoke misunderstandings and abuses, but its true nature is still partly visible, since it has not become completely identified with the ideology created around it.

Our comments on the definition of the norm in our industrial society come more from our analysis of everyday life than from theoretical definitions. The definition of the norm clearly coincides with production and this means that whoever remains at the margins of society appears as a deviant. Deviant behavior implies a breach of values, so those same values must be upheld and strengthened by scientifically classifying as abnormal all those who infringe against them. Since the values are not absolute ones, they need a scientific justification for their discriminatory attitudes. Thus begins the search for negative and inferior personality characteristics for both the deviant and the psychopath, and the process of stigmatizing a behavior that often starts out less deviant than what it becomes. Through the appropriate scientific ideology, those who do not play a role in production or who refuse to be consumers, by choice or necessity, must be forced to uphold the norm and its boundaries.

The analysis of the role of deviants in the United States allows us to understand how much their existence seems to threaten and call into question the typical values of an advanced capitalist country, whenever they are not reassimilated into society. When the person who calls the norms into question is able to maintain an active social presence in the community, the danger is continuous, and increases when the community lacks the strength to keep under control an antagonistic presence in its midst.[1] When the number of deviants increases, so they can no longer be controlled, it is necessary to assimilate them differently. They are forced as deviants into an ideological category that defines them, continues to create them, and controls them. The deviant as a real problem, which points to the losing side of capitalism, a rejection of its values and an expression of its partial failure, must become the "problem" of the deviant, with all the ideological characteristics of any "scientific" problem that requires technical and ideological solutions. The deviant, as the expression of the losing side of capitalism, is turned into one of the many sides of a victorious capitalism which has appropriate technical solutions for all its problems.[2]

The ideology of deviance under advanced capitalism functions to confirm that what arises as opposition (conscious or not) is reintegrated into society. Capitalism is strengthened, as it manages to eliminate the forces opposed to it and to rationalize them as an ideological problem.

This phenomenon is also visible in other aspects of American life, for example the problem of the poor and of blacks, both different forms of the single problem of social deviance. These are both real problems rendered ideological by a rationalizing process that changes their nature.

The vast amount of American writing on this subject is astonishing. There seems to be a sudden awareness of what lies beneath the "affluent society," and a ruthless analysis of its evils. But in reality, just when these aspects of American society are being revealed and made known so they can be confronted, they lose their threatening character and become abstractions for which only abstract solutions are sought. The ability to take a problem to an ideological level which will create a new ideological reality is a sign of the strength of capitalism, which tries to completely control production and society itself.

American poverty lost its threatening character when the President of the United States declared a "War on Poverty" as a national program, and organizations were formed (FAO, UNESCO, Peace Corps, etc.), each to resolve one dimension of the problem. The visible hand gives out what the invisible hand then comes to take away. The fact that scholars, sociologists, anthropologists, psychiatrists, and social planners then devote themselves to dissecting the issue, is merely a matter of subsequent rationalizations that increasingly obscure the real nature of the problem.

This new role of the social sciences in everyday life is recent, and is a sign of the discovery of a deeper, more effective form of social control, rather than a desire to help the poor or to resolve the problems of a social system that is still accepted as a natural fact. The increase in social services therefore has another side to it—it helps to manipulate an ever increasing number of persons who escape from the traditional kinds of institutional control.

The problem of blacks is similar. They are less threatening when their rights are recognized and the fact of their segregation is acknowledged. This does not mean that a real change occurs. The black, the mental patient, the deviant, and the poor person all represent different forms of the same problem. Through the ideologies created, they are now recognized even by the new sociology as an "integral part" of the social system, but this does not mean they achieve active participation in the social system. Instead, they become useful tools to the entire society because they appear to become part of a single "middle class," in which differences and differentiations are increasingly hard to identify, and all are reduced to a homogeneity completely controlled by an ever narrower center of power.[3]

In advanced capitalism, the earlier ideology of diversity that confirmed one's own superiority and the inferiority of others, is no longer necessary. The principle goal is now the levelling of everyone into a single middle class which will be easier to control. The ideology of the sick society, with which capitalism tried to hide its contradictions, has been abandoned. In fact, in this later stage of capitalism, the distance between the sick and the healthy has diminished. In the first place, a form of productivity has been discovered in illness itself—for example, the institutions that treat illness are part of the productive cycle.[4] Secondly, production itself has gradually assumed the form of social control.

This process of ideological rationalization is visible in the growing field of deviance. In the United States, the ideology of *deviance* is made to coincide with the problem of the *deviant;* primary deviance, which corresponds to exclusion from production, is confounded with secondary deviance, which is ideological in nature.

The most current interpretations of deviance[*] can be summarized as follows:

*Here Basaglia is most probably referring to the writings of Thomas Scheff, *Being Mentally Ill* (Chicago: Aldine, 1966) and Edwin Lemert, *Human Deviance, Social Problems, and Social Control.* (Englewood Cliffs, N.J.: Prentice-Hall, 1967). American labeling theorists were primarily concerned with society's responses to, and treatment of, deviants and misfits. Scheff and Lemert, like Goffman, traced the social processes through which "primary deviations" (rule-breaking) were stabilized into a deviant career. According to Lemert, secondary deviation occurs when a person learns the deviant role and accepts the identity of a deviant as a "life style." Basaglia's criticism of labeling theory is that it draws attention away from the real social conditions and the productive cycles that promote deviant acts in the first instance.—EDS

1. *deviance* as a limitation of functions and the ability to participate in social life due to the handicaps of an individual with psychological or physical defects leading to their exclusion, or to *secondary* deviance resulting from the primary difficulty.
2. *deviance* due to the lack of necessary social skills for acceptance, or the lack of education and culture that would acquaint them with the necessary social resources: secondary deviance due to the absence of social status, a necessary prerequisite.
3. *deviance* found in individuals who because of either choice or age are excluded, or exclude themselves from social relations (hippies, vagrants, the old, the young): secondary deviance due to a freely chosen or forced rejection of society.

The problem of deviance is managed by collapsing primary deviance into secondary deviance, so that the main concern can be the latter, and the former can be ignored. This means that only the ideological dimension of the problem is confronted, and it is both created and resolved at the same time.

A constant element present in all three cases, which is never emphasized, is that all the forms of deviance occur in individuals who do not participate in production. They have either lost, or never had, contractual power with those in charge of production. Indeed, if the norm is defined in terms of productivity, deviance should be defined in a similar fashion. If it were, we would see the *ideology* of deviance as a social and psychiatric problem which only contributes to the production of an ideological problem and the creation of illusory solutions, without ever confronting the *real* and material problem.

In the United States, the measures adopted by social psychiatry to deal with the problem of deviants only confirm this analysis. The new community mental health centers function to control any form of deviance both by giving it a social psychiatric definition, and by the expansion of preventative and after-care services. In terms of our hypothesis, even though there is recognition here of the social definition of deviance, this only leads to an interdisciplinary rationalization for something which has direct socioeconomic causes. The social misfits who are supervised by these community mental health centers are poor blacks, Puerto Ricans,

Italians, or Jews who are marginal to production, maintained by welfare and deprived of a future beyond the survival ensured them by welfare institutions. It is obvious that these mental health centers act to control people who are marginalized, and who cannot be integrated into productive institutions. The social psychiatric problem of the deviant is created as an ideological issue that is identified with the real one, and this then becomes part of medical ideology. The patterns and the limits of deviant behavior are set so that any inherent meaning in deviant acts will be reduced or eliminated. A way must be found to use the deviant's existence, with its implicit critique of the values of our society, as a further confirmation of those same values.

In American culture, the deviant is absorbed by an interdisciplinary ideology that is supposed to both ensure greater objectivity in his treatment, and identify the social nature of human problems. But the social dimension is limited to the totality of psychological and psychodynamic interactions. What first appeared as a further expansion of the field has actually meant going around in circles without ever expanding its closed parameters.

The function of the ideology of the deviant corresponds perfectly to the ideology used for those psychopathic personalities that are controllable through medical techniques and institutions. What is different is the kind of institution, but this changes when the number of psychopaths increases and control through medical techniques alone would mean locking away an enormous number of people. At this point, new forms of social organization are needed to ensure domination, through the new interdisciplinary approach. The problem then moves into the area of sociological ideology which can suggest more effective and suitable methods for manipulating groups than those proposed by traditional psychiatry.

Returning to Italy's economic development, we find that official psychiatry has stayed at a level consistent with the most backward economic level. The definition of mental illness and the institutions assigned to treat it are still based on violence and repression, since tolerance marks the strength and consolidation typical of a later stage of capitalist development.

The problem of deviance, which was introduced into Italian culture as an ideological subject within sociology, is completely absent from Italian psychiatry, where the deviant is still labeled as the psychopathic personality, a condition to be medically treated. In Italy, the general issue of abnormality is still part of a precise clinical symptomatology that observes traditional, positivistic diagnostic boundaries. The traditional academic classifications, borrowed from German culture, only confused the issue by their obvious value judgments, and eventually they were discarded when psychodynamic and other theories came on the scene. But the tendency to classify psychological abnormalities has been maintained by medical ideology, resulting in the creation of new and different labels to stigmatize any behavior that deviates from the norm and from the descriptions of traditional psychiatric syndromes.

The issue of the psychopathic personality remains, in Italian medicine, one of the most obscure, vague, and controversial chapters in the history of psychiatric diagnosis. It has always been difficult to classify it with an exact list of symptoms. The term "psychopathic personality" usually refers to individuals who are grouped together according to several specific characteristics: a) an unstable social adjustment, accompanied by largely anti-social behavioral disturbances; or b) a clinical history which may not always be defined as pathological, but which does not allow these individuals to be considered normal.

Psychopathic personalities are defined as personalities at the outer margins of the norm, characterized by disturbances in behavior and emotions, with a tendency toward antisocial behavior—all of which are generally traced to character flaws and to particular personality typologies. Italian psychiatry still goes back to Schneiderian categories of pathology, with his ten groups that are then separated into subgroups, and where the preoccupation with classification overrides all other concerns.[*]

Nonetheless, even in the case of later definitions of the sociopathic personality, where the social aspect was also consid-

---

*In the third edition of the Diagnostic and Statistical Manual (the "DSM-III"), published by the American Psychiatric Association, the diagnosis of "Borderline" and of the "Unsocialized Aggressive" personality type correspond to aspects of the earlier psychopathic personality type.—EDS.

ered as a cause, abnormality still referred to violations of a set of medical, psychological, or social values that was always considered natural and unchanging, rather than as relative to the individual's social system. Even when the social aspect begins to penetrate the medical field, it is still clear that it is used mainly to refer to the social *effects* of the psychopathic personality, rather than the effect of social factors on a vulnerable personality. This is in keeping with the custodial ideology that still underlies psychiatric institutions, which exist to protect and defend society from the abnormal, rather than to treat the patient and his illness.

Elsewhere, particularly in Anglo-Saxon countries with a pragmatist tradition, psychiatry, flanked by sociology, had to find technical solutions to new social and economic needs.[5] In Italy, where the medical profession remained backward and subordinate, the first steps were taken to go beyond the rigid Kraepelian categories. But this effort remained largely an ideological one; like any imported cultural phenomenon, it took up themes from psychoanalysis and phenomenology that were distant and unrelated to Italian reality.

Only in the last few years have there been attempts to bring this totally ideological discipline down to a practical level. While not yet acknowledged by official psychiatry, these efforts have called into question the assumptions of psychiatry and have revealed the theoretical and institutional connections between socioeconomic factors and the human sciences, especially psychiatry. Except for these very recent experiences, which are still rejected or ignored by official psychiatry, Italian psychiatry is still bound to an old positivist cultural tradition, even though there is a new ferment in many institutions.[6]

The deviant in our culture is still labelled a psychopath, with all the echoes of Lombroso's classifications,* clearly aimed at protecting the sane from "crazy moral revolutionaries," "zealous radicals and political criminals," and from "anarchists," to cite just a few of his definitions of those who wish to subvert the established order, just as he firmly wished to defend it.

*Cesare Lombroso, the late nineteenth-century Italian criminologist, who convinced a generation of social analysts that there existed a "criminal type" that could be identified by inherited physical characteristics.—EDS.

These definitions are unambiguous—medical ideology acts to protect a political and moral judgment that has little to do with medicine. This imbues scientific definitions with a genuine class character, free of ideological masks or screens. Dominant ideas are always the ideas of the dominant class, which tolerates no one in its midst who does not respect its rules. If the transgression were not punished, why would anyone else have to obey rules in which they have no interest and see no value in their enforcement?

These definitions and judgments can be excused because of the era in which they were made—Lombroso's *L'uomo delinquente* (*The Delinquent Man*) was written in 1897. However, when a recent treatise on psychiatry makes similar statements in 1969, it is a little harder to justify. The continuing classification of psychopaths makes clear that the essential goal is to stigmatize those who deviate from the norm with value judgments that focus on their amorality and licentiousness.[7] Whatever the psychopath does is always wrong because the label and the judgment *precede* his behavior. For him, an act is wrong but its opposite is also wrong—the error lies in not having accepted the rules of the game.[8] So that whoever is exuberant is labelled overly emotional. Whoever shows excessive altruism causes serious concern. Whoever stands up for himself suffers from a combativeness that could turn into protest and contentiousness, but because of his own instability he often gives in. (Here both the presence and absence of contentiousness have an identical negative connotation). The depressed person has characteristics that are the opposite of the overly emotional individual, and his behavior, too, is stigmatized. Then there is the fanatic who wants to impose his own ideas on others, promoting them with all his energy; his antithesis is the fanatic who professes his own ideas with the greatest certainty and scorns everyone else. Perhaps the paranoid psychopath should be included in this group. He has the following basic characteristics: excessive ego, mistrust of others, egotism and hypersensitivity.

These classifications are only slightly different than Lombroso's. There are the unstable psychopaths; the anetic psychopath lacks any sense of ethics or higher sentiment; in fact, the concept of the anetic psychopath is similar to the old idea of moral madness. The histrionic is defined as someone obsessed with grandiosity. In short, "the psychopath has no will power, adjusts poorly to his sociocultural surroundings . . . has inadequate empathy or sharing with others . . . he is distant and has no morals (even if he hides behind deceptive theoretical pronouncements that seem inspired by an intense moral life); he never shows a sense of guilt, is incapable of loyalty and stability . . . everything he does seems unexpected, fragmentary, inconsistent . . . his whole existence and how he acts in the world lack any sense of coherence or 'style.' "

These are the definitions of psychopathy from the most recent Italian treatise on psychiatry. A recent contribution to an international conference of social psychiatry on the subject of deviance draws conclusions that are not radically different.[9] In fact the kind of ingenuous classifying of the former coincides perfectly with the multidisciplinary shrewdness of the latter, as if to indicate that every stage of capitalist development corresponds to a turning point in psychiatry.

As long as muscular energy and individual skills were the foundations upon which any civilization was built, illness or inability to work excluded a person from the spoils that society had to give. But in the middle of the twentieth century *atomic energy* and *automation* have changed the work-oriented ethics of Western civilization. Nowadays people are encouraged to retire early; earnings from labor are taxed higher than capital gains; and modern welfare and unemployment compensation make it attractive for people to stay off the labor market. From an action culture we have moved to an image culture; and from judging people's contributions and productions, we have shifted to an assessment of their consumption. . . . As the human being became obsolete as a form of muscular energy, standards for human behavior were lowered and tolerance for psychopathology increased. . . . In the modern world responsibility for one's own actions and informal control by the ingroup have been replaced by impersonal collective responsibility and control by the outgroup. . . . Thus the chronically ill, the socially marginal, and the disabled who have no families and who formerly fell into the domain of the charitable and religious organizations now have become wards of the state-supported health and welfare institutions. . . . This shift in responsibility means a change in status for unproductive persons. With the old vertical stratification in society, every caste and class had a large central group and a smaller marginal group. If someone tried to become a member of the next higher class, he had to first accept a marginal status and then at a later stage could hope to become a member of the central group. Social mobility consisted of combined horizontal and vertical movements. But in the classless postindustrial society, social mobility consists of horizontal moves toward and away from the central structure of power. The modern population is formed of a central group, including government, industry, banks, science, engineering, the military and the educational system. A circle of consumers of goods and services, organized by those in the center, revolves around it. At the periphery, there are those that are marginal and who have no important function in our society.

Once this total unification around the center of power has been achieved, facilitated by an interclass ideology that preserves a technocratic elite, the author* notes that a subdivision in the stratum of marginal people emerges—hippies and protestors. The hippies "rebel against the consumer society, scorning its material goods and pursuing the attainment of personal fulfillment and inner experience. Their interest in perception and imagination was sustained by mind-expanding drugs. . . . In many cases hippies lived off welfare and constituted a danger to public health because of their anti-hygienic behavior, their venereal diseases and their drug peddling."

Protestors, on the other hand, "pounded at the door of the Establishment, and demanded a vote in the running of the universities. They opposed the technologizing of the human being, and they demanded frank confrontation. When their demands weren't met, they indulged in destructive acts and tried to tear down the structure of the institutions."

In Ruesch's eyes, those who are marginal are neither constitutionally depraved nor organically impaired. His analysis goes beyond those obsolete categories and involves the social organization that determines individuals. His is a clear and ruthless vision of the "point we have reached in contemporary society" where ideological screens have been temporarily removed, so reality can be examined and more adequate measures taken to meet its needs. The obvious limit of this analysis, which is otherwise extremely useful in its clarity, is that contemporary society is considered a "fact," and not the product of a certain kind of economic

*Jurgen Ruesch—Eds.

and social organization. Otherwise, the analysis is ideal, without any illusions or deceptions and, we can sense its importance.

The core of the post-industrial society, is made up of people who possess symbolic skills, both verbal and mathematical, and who can use those skills in the fields of advertising, computer programming, financial control and social organization. The characteristics distinguishing the modern symbolic monopoly from the cultured classes of the past is that its new task requires intelligence . . . Now that the machine has replaced physical labor, and we have unlimited energy sources, physical skills have no value, whereas rational thought and information gathering have become paramount. Unfortunately, not everyone is endowed with an intelligence suited to dealing with complex symbolic systems, nor do they grow up in environments favoring this kind of development . . . Unfortunately, many enter high school or college believing that the institution will teach them symbolic skills. But an institution oriented toward mass education can't provide teachers able to pass on rules of correct behavior, or interpersonal and symbolic skills. These human skills must be learned in the first ten years of life, within the family. What can be learned in the second or third decade are variations of what was learned earlier. College courses are usually difficult, and if students don't already have symbolic skills, they can't take advantage of what is offered them. Their response is one of disappointment, which they express as the demand for teaching that is of greater relevance to their everyday experiences. They don't want to learn what is within their reach, and what they demand to be taught will not prepare them to be part of the center of post-industrial society. That is the dilemma.

This analysis has arrived at an apparent paradox in terms of the deviant, yet it goes on to consider the statistical questions. "How many are social misfits, how many are marginal, and how many belong to the center of our post-industrial society?" The statistics that Ruesch cites are chilling.

According to a Statistical Abstract of the population of the United States in 1965, in a total population of 193,818,000 inhabitants, 6.6 percent, or 12,759,884, were identified as social misfits (the mentally ill, those with physical disabilities, prisoners, suicides, drug addicts, alcoholics); while 13.2 percent, or 25,622,743, were defined as potential misfits (old, unemployed, immigrants, slightly mentally retarded or in rehabilitation).

According to Ruesch's statistics, taken from the United States Census and the National Committee Against Mental Illness, the overall total number of people excluded from production, or in danger of being excluded, amounts to 19.8 percent of the population, or 38,382,627 persons.

"Let us now take a look at the core of our society," Ruesch continues.

The qualifications for admission to higher education are very stringent. Selection procedures decide who is enrolled in college, professional schools, preparatory courses and civil service jobs. Those with high grades go on to prestigious schools and end up in the military-industrial-scientific complex. Those with poor grades end up in government, the educational system and small business. Both these groups constitute the modern core of society. . . . Presently, those at the center, who have IQs above 111, administer and service our technological civilization. Forty-nine percent of the population, those with at least a year of high school education, revolve around this core, perform various services and consume capital goods and services.

Now let us proceed to those at the periphery, who are marginal. About 33 percent of the adult population has only an elementary school education and in the modern economy only a few jobs are within their reach. Together with the misfits, the ill and the disabled, the unemployable live off of public and private largess. Their role is essentially the consumption of welfare and health services.

The figures speak for themselves.

If we translate the percentages of the adult population into percentages of the entire population, the core represents only 10 percent, while the middle group comprises 25 percent. . . . The sick, the old, the misfits, and the young comprise about 65 percent, or about two-thirds of the total population. This group can be defined as the "world of leisure."[10]

His practical conclusions:

1. We must increase our tolerance for deviant behavior in human situations while decreasing institutional tolerance for deviant behavior in technical situations. No one should suffer because of incompetence, negligence or ill will.
2. We will have to replace the old routines, which were for peo-

ple with limited intelligence and interpersonal skills, with new
routines that give them a place in our new society.

3. Since the highly skilled core of the technological society will re-
    main geared toward work, while the masses will be oriented
    toward leisure, we should change our educational curricula to
    prepare society for this reversal of roles. In the past the upper
    classes played while the lower classes worked.

4. In the transitional stage between the old ethic, which valued
    private enterprise, skilled services, knowledge and individual
    superiority, and the new ethic which values collectivism, the
    machine sensation and images, there will be many who can
    adapt neither to the old world nor the new one. It is this mar-
    ginal group that has become a new challenge to the mental
    health disciplines.

The reality described by Ruesch is the reality produced
by capitalism, which is usually hidden by screens that mask its
true nature. The deviant as a real problem is turned into the ideology of deviance, which in turn becomes the systematic establishment of institutions for deviants, increasingly answering the need
for manipulation by presenting the false choice between the
anomic society and the therapeutic community. The material and
ideological world that Ruesch describes is *the immense anomic society as a therapeutic community*. Its apparent interclass nature conceals the strength of a narrower and narrower center of power,
which establishes a kind of technocratic feudalism.

In comparison with the older feudalism, the enormous
middle class that is dominated by the central power no longer has
any awareness of being enslaved. Their enslavement is the new
concept of control, and the new master is merely the totality of all
the slaves. The number of deviants suggested by Ruesch, ranging
from 6 percent to 65 percent of the population, corresponds to the
25 percent that aim to systematically destroy them through the appropriate ideologies and institutions.

We must therefore examine and understand how capitalism manages to transform this contradiction which it inevitably
produces as part of its dynamic, into something which heals and
strengthens it. We must understand in practical terms how reality

is transformed into an ideology that then produces a dual reality, with all the conditions to ensure this perpetual transformation of reality into ideology. Human beings are forced to become what they are not, since what they are forced to become is not part of their human nature. We experience what we become as the real reality and science merely supplies the justification and proof of that real unreality. In this context, our task is to expose the stages of this process, refusing to recognize ourselves in that double which we are forced to become.

[*The remainder of this essay is taken from "The Deviant Majority."*—Eds.]

In a developing society, the goal is to fit those who are abnormal into the boundaries of the norm. In affluent society, the close connection between medical ideology and the law is broken, to create a new kind of multidisciplinary approach. This change does not occur in order to improve life and the human condition, but to discover a new type of productivity and efficiency that manages to utilize those who are unproductive and inefficient, and give them a new social role. Social function is always adapted to social structure and technical assistance is effective only when that connection is maintained. For every level of economic development, there is an appropriate scientific language and institutional reality. Vanguard scientific theories can create a structural crisis in society when it is impossible to advance their practical and theoretical ideas. Otherwise they can be incorporated into a purely ideological language which serves to justify the current stagnation, while awaiting the ideological reality appropriate to the next stage of economic development.

Our psychiatric bureaucracy continues to defend its own conservative positions, which are strictly in keeping with the socioeconomic situation in which we live and work, a reality which still requires control based on the ideology of diversity. At the same time, they cannot ignore the importance of certain current experiences. It would be easier for them to adjust to a new language which arises from abstract theoretical expectations than to accept a language stemming from a concrete situation. Technical function must correspond to social structure to be effective. This implies that psychiatrists, in carrying out their function, are clearly appointed to protect order and defend the norm, and that they accept this mandate. When technical assistance tries to respond to real needs, then this correspondence is destroyed and the implicit meaning of that connection and that mandate is revealed. If not, the intervention inevitably results in increasing the problem that the assistance was trying to prevent.

This process is obvious as diseases spread just when new services are created to treat them. This statistical increase in illness is attributed to socialization to the new service now available to all patients. Yet in terms of health policy, any new service should reduce illness, since it was created to meet an unfilled functional need. Instead, like every institution within the productive cycle, the new service can only look to its own survival. Its goal is production and the patient becomes an object in its grip, and not the subject for whom the service was created.

In a different social structure, when the goal is not production but human beings and their lives, and when production becomes a tool for survival, the new service can provide quite opposite results. In Cuba, for example, except in Havana's large hospital which is being torn down, psychiatric health services function through the organization of small out-patient centers in the different regions of the island. Initially, these new services saw an increase of mental patients being treated, followed later by a decline in their numbers. Does this mean that in Cuba mental illness does not exist or that it is rapidly declining? Certainly not. It's just a different way of organizing a service within a social structure that responds to people's needs and not to the needs of capital. Once again, this underlines the importance of the social aspect of illness in determining the illness itself.

Mental illness is a human contradiction that can occur in any society. Each society shapes illness according to its needs and the social aspect that is constructed will then determine the future development of the disease. In that sense, we can speak of a close relationship between psychiatry and politics, because psychiatry protects the boundaries of the norm that are defined by the political and social organization of society. It is not politics that cures mental patients but paradoxically, it is sickness that is labeled with a specific political definition which helps to preserve those values that are being questioned. Those who are strictly punished whenever they step out of bounds are always those who lack a private space in which to safely express their deviance. This is just the logical consequence of the implicit premises of our social organization.

Those who urge us to be cautious about disclosing the meaning and function of the institutions protecting the norm in our society, are asking us to maintain the clear division between the normal and the abnormal, and to endorse the close connection between psychiatric assistance and public order. The issue of psychiatric assistance is not just a technical issue, since technical skills are used to defend the boundaries of the norm, which have no objective value.

The psychiatrist always acts in his double mandate as a scientist and a policeman. But these two roles are in obvious contradiction, since the scientist should try to protect and treat the sick person, while the policeman should protect and defend the healthy person. Which of these two competing loyalties prevails in the psychiatrist's role? How can you expect to treat those who deviate from the norm, if our chief preoccupation is to adjust to the norm and to maintain its boundaries?

We are not arguing that mental illness does not exist, but scientific concepts that define it are abstract, since they do not confront it as a real phenomenon. Schizophrenia, psychopathy, and deviance are only the absolute form of our lack of comprehension of the contradiction within us, which is the illness itself. Definitions are only the attempt to resolve these contradictions into abstract concepts, which are then reduced to commodities, labels, names, and value judgments that serve to confirm differences.

The language of our technicians is still dominated by the ideology of diversity. The exaggeration of differences serves to protect and defend the expansion of economic development. The ideology of diversity finds itself in agreement with the ideology of equivalence when in fact they correspond to two different theoretical and practical stages linked to different periods of social and economic growth. The development of science is based on these two different ideological rationalizations, and its effectiveness depends directly on the correspondence between socioeconomic structure and specific institutional functions. Any scientific or technical intervention constitutes a new theory which calls current reality into question. Its proof will lie in its being functional to the next stage of socioeconomic development, yet along with that proof it will encounter its own death as the original theory turns into an absolute.

The entry of the new social sciences into the field of deviance has caused an expansion of the issue, the area of study and the treatment of deviance. Older theories and practices that corresponded to previous forms of control have been replaced, having become obsolete and unnecessary. The old custodial and punitive ideology no longer suffices for the total control that is required by the development of capital. It is now possible to expose, through sociological and sociopsychiatric analyses, that which no longer has to be hidden.

Within the dynamic of advanced capitalism, the ideology of deviance serves to reaffirm that contradictions are functional when they undergo a rationalizing process. When Parsons, in *The Social System,* maintains that the function of ideology lies in the relationship between culture and counterculture, he focuses on a crucial aspect of social organization, without, however, giving it a correct interpretation.

If, however, the culture of the deviant group . . . remains a counterculture, it is difficult to find bridges by which it can acquire influence over wider circles. This bridge is above all furnished by the third element, the development of an ideology—or set of religious beliefs—which can successfully put forward a claim to legitimacy in terms of at least some symbols of the main culture.[11] But the problem is how the ideology arises, who promotes it, and how it is used. In reality, the ideology of deviance does not seem to act as a bridge between culture and counterculture, in the sense of the counterculture having influence over culture. . . .

Never before, when it is life itself that is in question, has there been so much talk of culture and civilization. And there is a curious parallel between the generalized collapse of life that is at the root of our present demoralization and our concern for a culture which has never been compatible with life, which in fact has been devised to tyrannize over life. Before speaking further about culture, I must remark that the world is hungry and not concerned with culture, and that the attempt to orient toward culture thoughts turned only toward hunger is a purely artificial expedient.[12]

This understanding is difficult. The conflicts that are produced and stimulated by experience are met with ever more advanced techniques, which then become new forms of social manipulation. These real/ideological limits destroy experience, making behavior uniform, under the guise of the collective organization of well-being. But what is created is only the double, the ideological reality that is most appropriate to maintain and develop the existing social system. We experience this reality as real, and science merely supplies the justifications and proofs for the unreality of what is created.

The role of the human sciences in this process is clear. They have gone so far as to establish a "science of war" (polemology), which attempts a psychodynamic analysis of unconscious conflicts that might create war, along with the appropriate therapy. Or they create the "science of death" (thanatology) in which they reduce death to a mere organizational problem.[13] This is obviously the ideological manipulation of real contradictions—conflict and death—through the definition, creation, and identification of their doubles. Illness, deviance, hunger, and death must become something other than what they are, so that the contradictions they represent can be turned into endorsements of the [social] system. For death the answer is the science of death; for hunger, the organization of hunger. In the meantime, death is still death and hunger is still hunger. Needs are not met and all they try to do is organize and rationalize them. The Food and Agricultural Organization, as an ideological response to the reality of hunger, does not change the reality of starving people, because it does not change the process that simultaneously produces hunger and abundance. The organization of illness does not respond to those who are ill. Whoever tries to directly respond to primary needs—to illness itself rather than its definition and organization—is accused of negating the existence of both the need itself and the illness, since he does not acknowledge the double that has been constructed from it.

Through this rationalization and organization of needs, the individual is deprived of the possibility of self-mastery—of possessing his own reality, his own body, his own illness. In this sense, self-mastery is automatically transformed into possession by others. A contradiction isn't transcended, but instead becomes rationalized in terms of production. In this dynamic, the individual cannot achieve mastery over his illness, but experiences himself in the world as a sick person; he lives a passive role that is imposed on him and which confirms the split between himself and his own experience.

The sickness is turned into a sick behavior—a false relationship which replaces a nonexistent one and which offers the opportunity for the confirmation of domination. The ideological reality thus created is no longer illness or deviance as a primary experience or contradiction. It becomes the subject matter of polemology, thanatology, or social medicine—those sciences of illness, conflicts, deviance, and death.

The patient and the deviant exist just as illness and deviance exist. But when the goal of every act of assistance is control and domination, and the ideology of diversity is no longer sufficient to define and delimit the contradictions, there are other ways to incorporate abnormality into the system of production. The equation of more and less, health and sickness, the norm and deviance is merely the productive organization of diversity.

Into this new terrain, the excluded, the different, the "poor poor" can only become the "social deviants" for whose contradictions Oscar Lewis openly suggests psychiatric treatment as a form of control. This totalizing process, although it defines the equivalence of opposites, maintains their separation and creates an illusory universal middle class that includes everyone. Yet the existence of those differences that underlie the apparent unity creates the conditions for the new poor poor that our social system needs. In this reality, where the deviant majority are excluded from the symbolic language used by those in power, can we expect them to recover some hope of having their own symbolic language?

In July 1967, at a congress in London attended by over 2,000 intellectuals, David Cooper concluded his keynote address as follows: "At this Congress, we are concerned with new ways in which intellectuals might act to change the world, ways in which we might move beyond the 'intellectual masturbation' of which Stokely Carmichael accuses us. We recognize that radical groups in the first world have been conventionally split, not only on ideo-

logical but on personal lines. There is always some kind of spuri-
ous messiah who arouses hope and then disappoints hope. This is
not the 'fault' of the messiah—it is the fault of 'hope'. Hope has to
have another appointment."[14]

But in our Western world, the intellectual is—to use Cooper's words—the false Messiah, who raises hopes and then destroys them. The Messiah remains within the limits of the ideological reality that is constantly produced and transformed, without
ever influencing practical truth.[*]

The fault does not lie with hope, as Cooper somewhat
contradictorily maintains when he wishes us another appointment, but with the false Messiah who every so often creates a new
false hope for new groups of manipulators. In the name of a revolutionary ideology, these groups have the illusion of being a vanguard movement fighting this process and this logic from within,
but they end up participating in a narrow center of power. In this
ideological reality, what arises as a rupture can only end up being
reestablished as a new weapon of domination. The logic of this reality uses the contradictions and differences it produces and ratio-
nalizes them to the next successive level. What creates the false
Messiah is not only "mental masturbation," as Cooper says, but a
reality that tries to maintain the same nondialectical character of
the ideological reality it seeks to affect. If the intellectuals' actions
do not change practical truth, then they remain rooted in ideological reality, where contradictions are once more rationalized in the
name of a metaphysical faith that postpones the "solution" to an
ever-desired, never-achieved tomorrow.[15]

In August 1970, Fidel Castro, faced with a great setback
in the sugar harvest, spoke to the Cuban people about their concrete problems:

We haven't been able to simultaneously fight on several
fronts . . . The heroic struggles to increase production, to increase our
buying power has meant a series of imbalances in the economy. . . . Our
enemies say that we're having difficulties and they are right. They say
we have problems and they're right. They say there's dissatisfaction, and

[*]See Basaglia's use of this term in "Crimes of Peace": "Practical truth which verifies
whether hypotheses are real responses of need," p. 22 of translated text. —EDS.

they're right. . . . Even if our enemies exploit some things that we say and this causes us deep embarrassment, we should welcome this embarrassment, these troubles, so long as we know how to transform the shame into strength, dignity, a working spirit and moral energy! . . . We have obligations towards poverty, towards underdevelopment and towards the suffering of our people. When we're faced with a mother and twelve children, all living in one room and who all have asthma and who knows what else; when we see people suffering and asking; when we see these things with our own eyes and know that our reality is determined by the fact that we need a million houses, so that people could live decently. A million! With all that's needed to get a million houses! . . . How can we resolve the contradictions between the urgent needs we have just described in terms of our population growth and the labor force, and our need for workers? How will we work things out from now until 1975, and then from 1975 to 1980? It's simple: our only choice is to resolve these problems and we must resolve them! Our only choice is to resolve them!

These words are too simple for our minds, corrupted by concepts, words that are too demagogic for all our different, divisive individuality. Our theories are not useful for life, and life serves only to confirm our theories. Projects seem too ingenuous for our knowing judgments, accustomed as we are to ideological games and the illusions of self-criticism. Yet in Cuba they are trying to respond to the practical truth, to a reality "that is more bitter, but also more honorable and dignified," where contradictions are considered constitutive of that reality—to be confronted and not merely defined and organized. Is this also a false hope proposed by a false Messiah?

For us, imprisoned by a life that must be made to appear without conflicts and contradictions, this message is our hope for a reality which does not resolve contradictions ideologically and where they preserve their essential, dramatic quality of necessity. Victory and defeat, success and failure are terms that disappear when there is a shared struggle for a human existence. What we want for human beings is not divisions, and definitions of talent, privilege, rewards and punishment, but a life that creates the same totality for human beings that capital creates for itself: the more and the less unified with value and respect for the existence of everyone.

The deviant majority is now the latest ideological discovery in our world of production. Production must be saved. If this means that three-quarters of the world end up abnormal in terms of this absolute value, then three-quarters of the world are deviants. The totalizing process of capital also involves another totalization—of its own contradictions. The limits of capital are capital itself, and its totalization should coincide with its own death, with the possibility of total deviance from its logic and an escape from its rationalization. We are capable of continuing to discover this process. We must continue to break apart the ideological double that is used to transform reality and to make it conform to its own ideological nature.

4. Letter from America: The Artificial Patient

I was given the opportunity to visit the United States by a psychiatric institution included in the Kennedy program for the mentally ill and mentally retarded. The Kennedy Community Mental Health Bill, which calls for the construction of small psychiatric units within the communities which they have been delegated to serve, has been in operation since October 1963. Numerous centers are already functioning throughout a vast area of the United States. As for the rest of the psychiatric situation in the United States, it is generally that of traditional asylums and mental hospitals despite the emphasis on social psychiatry, which is limited to a few privileged study centers designated to confirm experimentally the Establishment's most functional hypotheses.

My interest in this kind of experiment comes from the fact that it is a result of new legislation in the psychiatric field in a country with a high level of technology, thus representing in concrete our [Italy's] political and institutional future. A direct analysis of such a situation would allow us to verify in reality what a technical action (a specific action in a specific sector) can be and to understand the political significance (or institutional functionality within the limits of this overall system) of a *new* institution, within the *old* social context in which it has been inserted. That is, in order to verify the limits of a new technical action that is maintained within a given political structure, the analysis could show us in concrete terms the extent of the tie between an institutional technique that is defined as "innovative" and the socioeconomic system that supports it.

Translated by Anne M. Lovell and Kayla Conrad.

We must remember that these psychiatric units have not arisen from the necessity on the part of those who work in the traditional mental hospitals to turn the institution upside down (that is, they are not born as an immediate answer to an immediate need), but are the direct expression of a new legislation which tends to resolve technically the contradictions of the reality in which it operates. Here *institutions of violence,* with their explicit significance of destructive and discriminatory exclusion, and *institutions of tolerance,* with their technical resolution of social conflicts, through a new interdisciplinary concept of social and community psychiatry, work side by side and in a complementary fashion under the federal legislation which guides them both. The former are still explicitly delegated to exclude socially disturbing elements; the latter are delegated to readapt the ever increasing fringe of "marginal persons" this socioeconomic system continues to produce. Mental institutions, expressions of the prejudiced concept of incurable illness, allow then, by their very existence, for the rise of psychiatric units intended to confront mental illness even in its social and economic aspects. The new psychiatric units are in fact open—and open to everyone. This enters into the framework of the War Against Poverty which seems to characterize the present American reality as ready to absorb poverty itself as an object of a new productive cycle.

Institutions in our system are one of the many instruments of social integration. In the case of psychiatric institutions, the asylum used to perform its duty (and still does) by excluding disturbing elements in order to keep the healthy society and its values intact. Now the new psychiatric institutions, the therapeutic community in particular (the latter created as a rejection of the traditional mental hospital reality), proposes itself as an organization that maintains its therapeutic nature to the degree to which all of its components participate directly in the process of change, this having become a movement of negation of the traditional institution. But once the reality of an asylum has been destroyed within the institution, and if it has been proposed as an nondialectical reversal of the preceding reality, the process of change stops. In other words, the therapeutic community is proposed as a new institution, having its own rules and dogmas and prepared to carry out with a different technique an institutional function within a social system.

In the case of new psychiatric institutions (the concrete expression of new health legislation), the negation of the preceding mental hospital's reality is already given as institutionalized; within the hospital organization this negation reveals itself only as the process of adaptation and integration of a new model which is typical of any institution. The community technique, born as an institutional answer to the reality which is the mental hospital is assumed as a new psychiatric technique in a specific sense. Identified in this way, it lacks the margin of freedom necessary to perpetuate a process of change, and this margin is the only guarantee of therapy in the institutional situation. In this case the institution, from the beginning, performs its function as an instrument of social integration and hence of regression in view of the patient. The new psychiatric institutions thus present a one-dimensional terrain where the absence of an internal dialectic impedes any possible therapy.[1] This is the general premise.

As for the institution in which I worked, we can begin by saying that there the negation of the mental hospital reality is only superficially apparent. The mystification of roles, the elimination of violence, the affirmation of democratic values in human relationships (these being the therapeutic community's new dogmas) are only one side of the reality which must be dialectical. The different hierarchical levels are hidden by unified action in the name of "commonality;" democratic values are affirmed in a struggle for goals which are common to all levels. Even the violence is destroyed as a means of maintaining the new psychiatric reality. To negate the asylum dimension, one must destroy above all the very existence of the mental hospital which is hidden behind the open psychiatric ward and the therapeutic community. But as long as the asylum continues to exist as a place for unloading disturbed patients, then everything else is mystification. Either the in-patient and out-patient community organization succeeds in creating sufficient help for patients from the district to which it has been delegated to serve, or this community game serves only the staff—for its survival and for its own psychological conflicts. In the latter case, it is the mental institution itself which, by its very presence and actions, enables new and apparently more open and undiscriminating psychiatric units to rise. But if the harsh existence of traditional asylums remains present behind the new units, then the latter can be allowed to dedicate themselves to mental illness even in its social aspects, thus widening its sphere of action, without being absolved from its primary duties. What we must analyze here is the new category of patients to which these units dedicate their psychiatric services. What social and economic factors are evident in this new social trend in psychiatry? How does social psychiatry deal with these factors once they are spotted? We must understand how all of this enters into the framework of a productive regime which has discovered that it can absorb poverty as object of a new productive cycle without changing its very role or condition.

Although I haven't at my disposal all the elements necessary for a complete analysis of the situation, I think I can formulate a first critical hypothesis, of both a particular and a general character, which necessitates further verification.

1. The institution in which I worked serves an area of 120,000 inhabitants (Italian, Jewish, Scandinavian, black, and Puerto-Rican), many of whom are on welfare.
2. The psychiatric unit consists of a hospital center of forty beds with a staff of two hundred (for external and internal service).
3. Behind the new unit the old state hospital continues to exist and operate as a place where patients considered "chronic" and "acute" can be sent. There are 6,000 patients. The unit's action has a preventative character that does not affect the culture of mental illness, but continues to maintain the prejudice of its incurability, which it presumes to fight.
4. The artificiality of the institution is revealed concretely in that it does not perform its primary function (curing the mentally ill in its designated area), but through preventative treatment, created a new category ("emotional patients") from among the marginal persons and misfits—so defined as a result of their socioeconomic position—and thus increases the number of psychiatric patients.
5. This institution creates a new kind of unproductive, marginal

individual who can be rehabilitated only by incorporating him into the new institution, within the productive cycle. The institution justifies its existence through these marginal persons. The economic system thus produces a new kind of misfit who can recuperate by creating an institution in his name, within the productive cycle. Prevention, in this case, serves to broaden the conceptual field of "illness" rather than to reduce it.

6. Given that a new hospital organization is dedicated to pseudo-realities which it creates in its own images, the significance and function of the institution in the general context are unchanged with respect to the asylum reality. A psychiatric institution based on such premises can only exist to organize and perpetuate its own survival, exactly as happens to mental hospitals in which there is no therapeutic goal and in which the patient must identify himself with the institutional reality.

7. By creating a new category of patients, the so-called pilot unit thus takes on a highly regressive character, narrowing the concept of norm and including "deviants," "marginal persons," and "misfits" within the realm of mental pathology. In this way a dialectical movement and meaningful opposition are denied to maladjustments; instead they are incorporated into the institution assigned to control it.

8. Lacking a final goal towards which to direct the actions of all the elements which compose it, and further facilitated by the confusion created by new anti-authoritarian and nonrepressive psychological orientations, the institution is reduced to an anomic ground. Here where violence has been reversed into a situation of sterile tolerance that does not serve as a reality confrontation for the patients, individual psychological motivations have the upper hand and determine the power games of various internal factions, thus increasing the basic antitherapeutic functions of the field.

9. A staff of two hundred persons (with an in-patient hospital service of forty beds) in a situation of total anomie, occurring in institutions without a final goal, is reduced to experiencing problems that come from the uncooperative team work of the medical staff. If the community's in-patients and out-

patients are not the institution's goal, the staff then becomes its only justification and every action is but an attempt to maintain the staff. The institution moves (as always) as a function of the general staff and of the distorted group dynamics of the medical staff that survives only through continual and sterile self-analysis, necessary to justify themselves and their presence in the institution.

10. In this sense it is understandable how a new institution that cannot answer real needs is forced to create, for its own existence within the productive cycle, a giant artificial reality which justifies itself by its giant size.

11. The presence of a staff with new roles such as "community social workers" and "community organizers" (expressions of a social policy carried out by psychiatric institutions) reveals explicitly the social function of the institution. If traditional institutions acted (and continue to act) as instruments of control and exclusion of socially disturbing elements, the new organizations, with the multidisciplinary capillarity with which technologically advanced nations are endowed, succeed in creating much more subtle and penetrating networks of technical-social controls, the line between norm and deviance becoming ever more fragile and indistinguishable.

12. In this light we can understand the artificial omnipotence that these institutions breathe: psychiatrists, social workers, and community organizers are a sign that the new direction in psychiatry can be a source of tremendous power; because through such a network of control they will soon hold in their hands the reins of society's game. This new movement therefore does not have the minimum innovative and revolutionary significance that we like to define it as having. The technicians simply accept playing the game of the general political system, agreeing to act as instruments of social control, hidden under the mystification of technical control.

13. If the mental patient suffers from the impossibility of living his own reality dialectically,[2] such therapeutic institutions will never help him recover the capacities he has lost (or never had). New ideologies are ready to mask the contradictions which become evident as they emphasize now one, now the other, pole. *The technicians are responsible for this.*

Conclusions

We discuss the problems of power. We talk about the concept of authority; we appeal to the democratic principles on which the new psychiatry is founded. We call the institution a therapeutic community and define the new psychiatric orientation as social only because it serves as an instrument of control in favor of the system. All this simply means that a new frame has been put around an old game whose moves and aims we already know.

The tolerant institution, the other nondialectical side of the institution of violence, reveals its giant artificial efficiency as a cover for a fundamental and intentional inefficiency. *To confront real problems we must put into question the whole of reality.* But in our social system technicians in every sector continue to accept their role as promoters of new ideologies that produce artificial problems to be undertaken; this because reality continues to seem unmodifiable to those who submit to it.

Poverty has become an industry. It is a question of domestic colonization, with different tactics for the same strategy: the preservation of the general economic status quo. With its old social service system, welfare attempts to soothe the sore of unemployment, while at the same time weakening the forces of revolt. If revolt is defined as an "illness" and if there are institutions for its cure, then the cycle is complete and the system is protected from any surprises, at least for a while. The luxury hospital for the poor is only the tolerant face of the system which has devised a new means of survival and a new object (at the same point of distance and of objectification) to absorb into the productive cycle.

If we are aware of the part the new institution of tolerance plays in the system as a whole, then obviously it is a mystification to speak of revolutionary, communal, democratic, and innovative techniques when in fact referring to a situation of social control. Language (born in a moment of real negation) is always rapidly co-opted, learned, and consumed, so that it may be used to express exactly the opposite of what it means. Either the situation in which we live preserves a dialectical margin so as to make possible an awakening of consciousness and a process of change, or the new terminology is used only to cover up an old reality. An ever more subtle and penetrating manipulative force, almost dictatorial in its commands, is hidden under the illusion of democratic relationships. The technique of reaching a consensus, used to resolve social conflicts, is merely the expression of an underground manipulation that seeks to obtain the spontaneous subordination of the groups it manages.

The condition of anomie characterizing the institution I have analyzed is the proof of what I have just maintained: that if an institution tends towards a finality that unites the elements that make it up, there are no problems of authority, democracy, or sense of community as absolute categories. The psychological group dynamics are unleashed at every level when no common action exists. Those in authority fear a confrontation and the revelation of their real face. The tolerant fear the revealing of their harshness. The subordinate fears being instrumentalized. The boss fears being disobeyed. In this game everyone is under the illusion of democracy, of sharing power. Everyone can only cut a slice off for himself without thinking of the common use to be made of all the pieces, and so confirm once again the triumph of the division of labor.

In this case what is the use of talking about therapeutic institutions? How can a technical intervention obviate its technical and political contradiction, if we are aware of the finality of the institution as such and of its function in the social context in which it operates?

This is a brief glimpse of our [Italy's] political/institutional future. The United States is our forerunner, with its technological advancement, suggesting technical/institutional solutions to every social problem, so as to gradually reduce the whole society to an enormous subtly controlled institution of tolerance. In Italy we are still in the violent repressive phase and only in some areas have the explosive contradictions forced new proposals. But the example of the United States as a distorted mirror of our reality can put us on our guard against any partial and nondialectical solution, which is but the reversed side of the same system; thus confirming in reality the refusal to recognize any anti-institutional action by the proposal of a new technological model that will help cover up with a new ideology the barely evident social conditions.

Part Three PRACTICING KNOWLEDGE: REFLECTIONS ON THE ROLE OF INTELLECTUALS

Introduction

Anne M. Lovell

Three years after becoming director of the psychiatric hospital at Trieste, Franco Basaglia collaborated with his wife, Franca Ongaro Basaglia, to publish a volume of essays by several prominent intellectuals on the relation of the social sciences to contemporary society. Entitled *Peace-Time Crimes*, the book had contributors ranging from Michel Foucault and the French "voices" of 1968 to Noam Chomsky to such diverse antipsychiatrists as R. D. Laing and Thomas Szasz.

Nowhere is the influence of Antonio Gramsci (1891–1937), founder of the Italian Communist Party and major theoretician of Italian Marxism, so strongly felt in Basaglia's writings as in Basaglia's contributions to *Peace-Time Crimes*, from which part 3 is taken. Particularly important here is Gramsci's theory of technicians and intellectuals.[1] According to his schema, intellectuals could be divided into two types. Traditional intellectuals (such as the literati and scientists) appear to derive their status from a knowledge and profession not linked to any class; in reality, they function to maintain the interests of the dominant class. Organic intellectuals are identified with the class whose thinking they direct rather than with their professional function. To Gramsci all men and women are potentially intellectuals because every human activity involves some form of intellectual endeavor. This implies both that a working class can produce its own class-conscious organic intellectuals and that technical and other types of knowledge can be shared in a democratic way.

Following on this, *Peace-Time Crimes* unfolds the theme that technicians (traditional intellectuals) legitimate and justify a social order that can maintain domestic peace because its violence is institutionalized, often in subtle ways. One example of this, of course, was the Basaglias' earlier analysis of the asylum (see section I). In the following selections, however, the Basaglias broaden questions about how institutions function in fields other than the psychiatric. Technicians and intellectuals, whether they worked in prisons, industry, or hospitals, should understand the mechanisms they used to manipulate people into accepting an oppressive situation. Even more importantly, they should make this knowledge readily available to everyone.

The selections published here are unified by a concept that emerges from the particular political climate in Italy in the seventies: the technician and intellectual's conscious assumption of a radical role. French Marxists had already defined a "new" European working class to include white collar workers and technicians, and placed them, alongside the so-called manual workers, at the head of the movement to transform society.[2] Italians agreed with other Marxists that technical labor, like all labor, is alienated, or cut off from its product.[3] However, they defined technicians in a slightly different manner. They emphasized, as the criterion of this new status, the specialized body of technical and scientific knowledge which, in advanced industrial countries was used to manage social relations, both in the workplace (e.g., scientific management) and in nonwork spheres (e.g., principles of conflict resolution in the political arena).

Exclusion and the conditions patients endure could therefore be changed only by organizing those health care workers the Basaglias call "technicians of practical knowledge," especially doctors, nurses, and students preparing for the health and social science fields. To understand the following such a project could have at the time, we can point to the newly-formed alliances, beginning in the late sixties, of Italian white collar workers with blue collar workers, students, and intellectuals, as well as the emergence of forces on the New Left (*nuova sinistra*). Included in the New Left was an extraparliamentary party, the Manifesto, founded by a group of intellectuals, strongly influenced by Gramsci, and highly critical of the prosoviet line and traditional alignments of the Italian Communist Party (PCI). Eventually expelled from the PCI, the Manifesto developed its own political agenda, specifically incorporating technicians into the larger working class movement. In 1969 they published a widely distributed major position paper on technicians which explained their relationship to the working class movement.[4]

They called on technicians to contest their roles in the workplace, and to refuse to see what they do as an isolated technical function rather than as part of the larger social progress. Much of the history of *Psichiatria Democratica's* activism parallels some of the Manifesto's suggestions: the defiance of one's role; the creation of new norms and objectives that served the majority of people, and not the alienating goals of production or consensus; and the sharing of technical knowledge. The Manifesto was also concerned with a Gramscian transformation of consciousness and social organization.[5] After the "Hot Autumn" of 1969 these new areas became the stage for a fervent, diversified political opposition, especially among young people. It was in this context of political activism, with its new strategies and crises, that the Basaglias were writing, which explains the note of urgency in their language and tone and their more schematic than usual analysis— one that could be generalizable beyond the hospital.

In the first selection, "Technicians of Practical Knowledge," the Basaglias apply the Gramscian concept of technician and intellectual to their critical analysis of the role that doctors, nurses, and students play in the anti-institutional psychiatric movement and, ultimately, in the broader attempts to transform society. These theoretical reflections on the day-to-day work in hospitals like Trieste help the non-Italian reader understand how the anti-institutional movement in Italy was able to attract the active participation of hospital nurses and of the major union federation (C.G.I.L.), as it amassed local and, eventually, national political support. The position taken by Italian mental health workers contrasts with that of mental health workers in the United States, Great Britain, and France during the early seventies.

Unions in those countries focused on the need to ensure jobs in the face of a changing psychiatric system and the cutbacks of hospital personnel during the early phase of deinstitutionalization. Unfortunately, this culminated all too often in a reinforcement of custodialism and its accompanying stereotypes of mental patients. In Great Britain, health worker trade unions went out on strike to prevent psychiatric hospitals from closing. In one case, nurses publicly opposed accepting court-referred patients, labelling them as necessarily "dangerous." They also refused less repressive ways of working with patients.[6] In the United States, state employee unions consistently opposed hospital closures throughout the seventies, through lobbying efforts. In California the State Employees Association also used scare tactics through public statements and reports warning against the violence ex-patients would bring with them into the community.[7] A different approach was taken by the American Federation of State, County, and Municipal Employees who published a widely-read, scathing critique of deinstitutionalization.[8] While French hospital workers joined doctors, students and patients in actions against the discipline and practices inside psychiatric hospitals, this post-'68 fervor was replaced in the seventies mainly by concern with salary issues.[9]

Organized opposition to liberalizing the asylum was not unknown in Italy. In 1972, Trieste witnessed a series of strikes by nurses against the opening of the wards. While most nurses belonged to the conservative trade unions (affiliated with the Christian Democrat Party) and, at times, were supported by neo-Fascist groups, the nurses' actual participation in changing hospital conditions later on did not appear related to union membership.[10] As the hospital changed, many nurses began to unlock the wards voluntarily, taking on the consequences. Some decided to renounce their uniforms, a symbolic refusal of their "pseudo-power"; others began to help patients integrate into normal life such as by accompanying them into the city, without formal passes.[11]

The C.G.I.L. federation became very involved in the reform of health services in the early seventies as nurses continued to question both their roles and the professional dominance of doctors.[12] First, they refused to maintain and create specialized or hierarchical roles within nursing. At Trieste, for example, nurses managed to abolish the position of head nurse (capo-reparto), and took on the coordinating of shifts among themselves, through self-management. Second, they demanded a reform of nursing education. A review of nursing manuals written by psychiatrists at the time revealed that they were based on outdated organicist concepts, which focused on methods of controlling the patient, or on modern psychosocial theories that had little relevance to helping patients in institutions that were still traditionally custodial and violent.[13] In other words, the knowledge base available mainly enabled nurses to exercise power over their patients. Finally, the nurses began to emerge as an autonomous group, separate from the psychiatrists. Their needs and demands included, but were not limited to, better wages and recognition of their status in the place of old voluntaristic and service notions. In Trieste, for example, nurses eventually refused the responsibility for deciding how psychotropic medication was to be administered, handing back to the doctors a form of control that was fraught with feelings of ambivalence about using treatments with such pernicious effects. At the same time, they demanded courses on the uses and properties of these pharmaceuticals.[14]

All of these actions were linked by an underlying shift from demands solely concerning their interests to changes that benefited patients as well and linked nurses to the labor movement in general. By 1979, mental health nurses had caught up with the other unions, which had been fighting for a decade to change work conditions.

The Basaglias' discussion of students in the anti-institutional movement is influenced directly by the Marxist tenet of unifying theory and practice. Whereas nurses took on hospital jobs out of economic necessity, the students' involvement stemmed from a political formation gained from the student movement. The Basaglias also contrasted their suggestion that students use their specialized skills to change their future fields of work with the French, post-'68 position in their conversation with Jean-Paul Sartre, included here. French intellectuals in the fifties and sixties had limited their political activity to (usually Communist) party membership and activism. But many young intellectuals, influenced by the anti-authoritarian themes of the May '68 Events, decided to give up their privileged status (usually a middle-class background and university education) and "join the masses," usually by working in factories. The Basaglias, unlike Sartre, do not separate the intellectual from the technician. Furthermore, they advocate using one's own power against the system, rather than abdicating and remaining outside.

Frequently, the anti-institutional praxis of the Basaglias is mistakenly interpreted as an Italian current of antipsychiatry. Differences between the Italian anti-institutional movement and one branch of antipsychiatry represented by the British psychiatrist, R.D. Laing, are explored in the "Dialogue with R.D. Laing." While both Laing and Basaglia were heavily influenced by phenomenology and by Sartre's Marxism,[15] their practical work soon diverged radically. Laing's exit from the national health system and his organization's dependence on self-supporting and privately-financed alternatives is juxtaposed to the Italian insistence on the need to work within the old institutions and to change the public psychiatry system, rather than to create elitist alternatives that will only be available to a few people. By the time this dialogue took place, Laing's interest was focused on the subjective experience of the individual—where Basaglia's had begun. Laing was also on his way to more mystical concern with prenatal influences. Although Basaglia himself did not describe the way he and his co-workers related to patients, their ability to be with (or to stand by) someone during a crisis, and the accompanying malaise and anguish of not denying the patient's experience by forcing it into preconceived definitions, is to be found in the literature on the movement.[16] However, the anti-institutional psychiatric workers never used the concept of psychosis as "voyage" or other drug-free techniques that were developed by Laing and the offshoots of his Kingsley Hall Community. Such methods implied to the Basaglias a denial of the reality of mental anguish and were meaningless in the context of large institutions.

Basaglia's rejection of the antipsychiatry label is also his "conscious assumption" of responsibility for his (and all mental health workers') professional role. As organic intellectuals, they felt they must undo institutionalized violence that suffocates the economically disadvantaged classes of society.

5. Peacetime Crimes: Technicians of Practical Knowledge

The intellectuals are the dominant group's "deputies" exercising the subaltern functions of social hegemony and political government. These comprise:

1. The "spontaneous consent" given by the great masses of the population to the general direction imposed on social life by the dominant fundamental group; this consent is "historically" caused by the prestige (and consequent confidence) which the dominant group enjoys because of its position and function in the world of production.
2. The apparatus of state coercive power which "legally" enforces discipline on those groups who do not "consent" either actively or passively. This apparatus is, however, constituted for the whole of society in anticipation of moments of crisis in command and direction when spontaneous consent has failed (Gramsci 1930).[1]

When we first read the definitions which Gramsci gave of intellectuals, of their function in production, and their relationship to the dominant group, it was easy to interpret them as an historical analysis of the status of intellectuals in a bourgeois state, one that did not involve us directly, either as we are or were preparing to become. With the [Second World] war over, we believed it was possible to build a world different from the one we had fought against, with each of us making contributions in our own field. We readied ourselves for carrying out a positive role in the building of a new society.

Our hopes only lasted briefly. Almost immediately we found ourselves once again imprisoned in our usual roles; every-

With Franca Ongaro Basaglia. Translated by Teresa Shtob.

one was reestablished in his or her own place and class. Workers and the underclass once again fell into the role of an oppressed class that can realize its gains only through struggle. The bourgeoisie was reestablished, its values, economic laws, and property reaffirmed. Technicians and intellectuals returned to their professional careers and to their middle-class origins. As we set to work to create something which would take into account the needs and the rights of all citizens, we came up against the reality of class struggle and the division of labor, which maintained the unchanged roles and rules of the game. The Resistance, as a people's movement, was neutralized by the new ruling class that gradually divested it of its original meaning of participation and popular consent.[2] They cheapened it, turning it into an abstraction, and, in its name, reestablished their own domination.

In this ambiguous situation, where the gap between what we were and what we wanted to be was determined by the impossibility of acting to transform reality, intellectuals could side with the oppressed class, without having to question any of the values they automatically supported by virtue of their jobs or professions. Their intellectual or professional life could remain faithful to the values and ideology that the dominant class transmitted with the official seal of scientific objectivity; and they continued, whether consciously or not, to be "deputies," "functionaries."[3]

The ambiguity is clear to us now, but then it was not so evident. The intellectual or technician who was a militant in a leftist party carried on a professional life which was contrary to his political activity. An engineer in a factory, a doctor in a hospital, a psychiatrist in an asylum, a judge, a teacher—each upheld in their professional life what they disavowed elsewhere, without an awareness of what it meant to be functionaries of the dominant ideology in their work. The intellectuals were once more the theoreticians, and the technicians were the practitioners of the dominant ideology; neither their political consciousness nor their political activity made a dent in the ideological character of their theory and practice.

After years of theoretical arguments about the function of committed intellectuals and the nature of their political commitment, intellectuals began to become conscious of being deputies and functionaries for the dominant group in a direct clash between their ideology and practice, which arose from their practical work. They were what Sartre called "technicians of practical knowledge," whose duty is to concretely implement both ideologies and the crimes of peace that those ideologies legalize and justify. It was the lower level intellectuals, those who confront practical and theoretical problems and translate theoretical abstractions into an institutional practice, who first began to question the role they played in their professions, and its relationship to the scientific ideology represented in their work.

This awareness began to arise in areas in which professional technicians (or intellectuals, in keeping with Gramsci's quote) usually have the task of legally enforcing discipline on those groups who do not consent either actively or passively, thus dealing with problems of public order and the urgent social needs to "discipline groups who don't consent," even though this mandate is often masked by scientific theories that justify the measures taken. One of these areas is the asylum, a therapeutic institution for control, rehabilitation, and segregation, where the consent of those to be disciplined is obtained beforehand through the mystification of therapy and rehabilitation.

In this field where we work, the gap between the ideology (the hospital as a care-giving institution) and practice (the hospital as a place of segregation and violence) is clear. Moreover, the class origin of the patients contrasts explicitly with the supposed universal function of hospitalization. The hospital is not a place for those suffering from mental problems—it is the place for controlling certain deviant behaviors in those belonging to the working class.

How is the deviance of these patients different from that which we encountered elsewhere, in our years of training in university clinics, consultation rooms, and private clinics? What is the common denominator between the first type of patient and the second, and what is the essential difference? What therapeutic function does an asylum have if it manages to destroy anyone who enters it? Who are the psychiatrists if they lend themselves to this destruction? In whose name do they perpetuate crimes by applying scientific theories that function only to eliminate individuals who are unfortunate enough to be their objects? What is the social function of the asylum which even the psychiatrist usually fails to understand? What is the purpose of this hospital organization when it fails to respond to a single need of those crossing its threshhold? And to what needs should it be responding? Is the psychiatrist, who represents the values and verities of the bourgeoisie, capable of individualizing and recognizing those needs? Does not the service that he provides to patients really consist of exercising the power delegated to him to control an undefined violence about which he knows little? Are not this power and violence inherent in the tools that psychiatric science offers him to ensure the control and the consent of those who are coerced? What then are psychiatry and the illness we find in the asylum? How can we not see that expanding and contracting the definitions of the norm depend on the class of the disturbed person as well as on economic expansion or recession, or that the country's ability to integrate rehabilitated people means that scientific judgments, which from time to time change their irreversible definitions, are relative in nature?[4]

   These questions, arising from our practical encounters with the reality of the asylum where we worked, led to the slow erosion of "scientific truths" and raised the issue of their direct relationship to the social structure and dominant values. The technicians, who normally represented those values, began to reject their role as functionaries of consent, refusing to endorse and legitimize class discrimination and the transformation of their work and assistance into violence. In creating the conditions for a patient's needs to resurface and be met, a crisis was produced for those who had entrusted the technician with an opposite mission. Control and segregation are the answer not to mental illness but rather to society's need to eliminate the problem by delineating boundaries around the space in which it must be contained. By refusing to be the keepers of these suppressed individuals, by trying to stimulate those vital subjective capacities that had been destroyed or forgotten, the technicians had already chosen to side with those they were delegated to oppress, even with the uncertainty that this choice involved. The service providers remained technicians belonging to the bourgeois class, with all the power and status inherent in their role; the patient who used that service was still the proletarian, or member of the underclass, dominated and objectified by that status and power.

Nonetheless, the technician's refusal undermined the basic harmony between the mission of the sciences and the mission of society. Mental illness is incomprehensible and incurable, hence the only choice is to contain it in a suitable place. "Free" society needs to isolate and separate those who are a social disturbance, and appoints scientists to supervise their containment. Destroying this harmony meant exposing how science is subordinated to the interests of society that do not represent the interests of all its citizens. It became clear that science in this area legalizes the goals that a so-called free society cannot openly declare. The bourgeois state protects bourgeois interests, and others are always a social disturbance if they do not accept the rules created for their subordination. They can assert their rights only through struggle. When they reveal that the factory is harmful to health, that hospitals produce illness, that schools create illiterates and marginal persons, that prisons produce crime, that asylums create madness, and that this inferior form of production is reserved for the lower class, then they destroy the technician's unity with the bourgeois state. They destroy his assigned task of scientifically proving that criminals, the mentally retarded, and the mentally ill are what they are by nature, and science and society cannot change processes deeply rooted in human nature. When it is made clear that scientific ideologies act as a falsely neutral prop for the dominant ideology, then the real needs of health consumers can be freed from the artificial needs that are created to ensure control over the subordinate class.

The movement that arose, under the impetus of consumers' needs, to attempt to analyze these issues, found neither support nor understanding. Technicians who rejected their role as functionaries of consent had to be eliminated, all the more so when the means for bringing about this consent became clear to the consumers as well. The ways of dismissing them ranged from flattery, used by the more enlightened, to accusations and lawsuits, on the part of the more backward. The logic of control required that the protectors of the established order defend themselves from defectors. Moreover, consumers who together with rebellious technicians were seeking the path toward liberation understood these processes, but those who represented their class politically had only a partial and confused understanding. This was the limitation of a symbolic act which demonstrated how scientific ideology functioned in terms of class discrimination, but which created a common goal between the technicians and the oppressed class only inside and not outside the space they wanted to liberate.

During those years when political groups representing health consumers were fighting to demand rights for the oppressed, they discussed the supposed neutrality of science in general terms, and maintained that the issue should be subordinated to the primary contradiction between the working class and capital. For them a critique of science arising from the crisis of scientific ideology that would affect the primary contradiction was not valid or politically incisive. Until the primary contradiction had been resolved, they thought, the objectivity of science in certain fields, its technical instruments, and its interpretive theories had to be accepted, as if they were not ways of manipulating and controlling the lower class.

Elements for understanding these processes could, at that time, only come from the technicians as they discovered them in their practice. Technicians were learning to reject what still had an objective, scientific value for the political representatives of the subordinate class. The language of this understanding could not be communicated, and required an analysis and interpretation of the practice being carried out. The technicians needed autonomy for this analysis, or else they would have been caught again in institutional politics, unable to examine critically what they were doing in their own work. Once again they would have been intellectuals who sided with the oppressed class but in their own fields continued to protect the dominant values. The technicians' demand for autonomy, however, was easily interpreted as a bourgeois demand, and their actions remained isolated amidst mistakes and misunderstandings. In fact, these actions constituted an expansion of the territory for struggle. By refusing to be a deputy for the dominant class, technicians proposed analyzing the meaning and function of a particular scientific ideology in a practical area, which could spread the struggle to other areas and enrich it with new content and new activists.

In 1968, while reflections on these experiences began to be publicized, with all the accompanying misunderstandings ("mental illness doesn't exist; it is a bourgeois invention," etc.) a rebellion exploded as students began rejecting their future as "functionaries of consent." Between 1960 and 1970 the worker's movement had resisted Tambroni's neo-Fascist attempts, leading to the struggles in autumn, 1969 [the "Hot Autumn"].[5] Technicians began to reject the authority and power inherent in their knowledge while students refused to acquire that power. Despite the ambiguities typical of bourgeois movements, the technicians did not act merely as intellectuals who possess "knowledge" and guide the masses; they recognized that their role in the social system was to manipulate consent through the ideologies that they create and enforce. What was at stake was the relationship between the technician, science, and the application of science which objectifies the masses.

It is clear that the intellectuals and technicians of a bourgeois society exist to protect the interests and the survival of the dominant group and its values. It is not so clear how intellectuals and technicians continue, in their work, to produce new ideologies that maintain the same function of manipulation and control. Members of the subordinate class, even the most politicized one, cannot automatically perceive science and ideology as controlling and manipulating their lives; they see them as absolute values that they accept as beyond their comprehension or because they are too manipulated to understand. The technician's task, then, is to facilitate an understanding of how ideology manages to make the subordinate class accept measures that seem to meet its needs, but which in reality is destructive. Perhaps that is politically more effective for us than pretending to be workers, which we are not, or borrowing their motivations for struggle, when our profession often involves us as invisible accomplices. Rejecting one's role and authority means using one's role and authority dialectically, through a critique of the science and ideologies that as technicians we will no longer protect. This practical and theoretical critique of science as an ideology, or tool for manipulating consent, involves knowledge of the direct relationship between the dominant group, the functionary (both the intellectual or the theoretician who produce the ideology and the technician who translates it into practice), and the dominant group's use for the ideology.

The processes by which the dominant group delegates authority and uses scientific ideology are not clear and obvious.

For example, people manipulated and controlled by a branch of science like medicine have difficulty identifying either diagnosis or treatment as forms of manipulation or control, if not destruction. At most, they might consider them insufficient responses to their needs, but even those needs themselves are manipulated and dependent on the possible responses they might be given. The patient in a psychiatric hospital is traditionally thought to be mad if he does not see his confinement as a response to his ailment. In reality, given the current condition of almost all our mental asylums, only he is in his right mind. In order to identify and analyze how this manipulation takes place, the critique of science must be accompanied by political activity which enables the subordinate class to take possession of this knowledge and ultimately reject their manipulation.

On this battlefield, the bourgeois technicians can no longer delegate or mediate; they are on the same level as the consumers of the service they offer, with whom they must meet those needs not usually recognized by psychiatry and medicine. Because of their training and class, technicians only know those needs that are constituted by and dependent on ideology.

Unless technicians and consumers work together and express their needs jointly, the responses of the former will not diverge very much from the culture they have assimilated. Locked into an ideology, the technicians translate their actions into repressive measures towards those they should be serving. But the health services that are provided objectify patients and consumers, robbing them of their history. The technicians then "historicize" them, allowing what was the object of their analysis to emerge as subjects; in the process they enter into a new history, different from that of the class from which they come. They place themselves outside of the logic of supply and demand whereby the demand is always subordinated to the kind of supply most conveniently available. They shatter the economic logic whereby every response to a need means an organization that lives and prospers on an expansion of the very needs it should be satisfying. Thus, in seeking to liberate others from oppression, technicians can free themselves from an alienated state, from an oppression of which they are both the objects and the subjects.

Bourgeois technicians live in an alienated state which

they can end by destroying the objectified condition of the oppressed. In the logic of capitalism technicians foster the movement from oppression to alienation; that is, they provide the ideology that enables the oppressed class to identify with bourgeois values. Real needs and the necessary kinds of responses will only arise from the search for a mutual space in which a new subjectivity can develop. When they share in the search for liberation, technicians betray the dominant class, but their role, their class origins, and their status will give them relative protection even as they reveal how ideologies are tools of manipulation and control. They reveal all the family secrets; those that only the father knows and hides from his children, for fear that they would lose respect for both him and their family.

The birth of the human sciences initially seemed to create new possibilities and outlooks in the struggle for human liberation. Psychiatry, psychology, and psychoanalysis seemed to offer new tools for research and help in alleviating human suffering. Criminology proclaimed that it wanted to protect both society and the criminal from his abnormal tendencies. Sociology seemed to offer a tool for analysis and knowledge of social phenomena which would help to transform reality and overcome the contradictions that were discovered. However once these sciences were imbued with the logic of class division and the logic of one class's oppression by another, they became tools used to strengthen this oppression.

This gave rise to a series of cultural institutions which classify and define behavior, silently ignoring primary needs while creating artificial ones, teaching people the meaning of their existence, who they are, what their life and their death will be, and what relationships to establish with one another. While religions functioned to manipulate and control through distinctions between good and evil, reward and punishment, guilt and innocence, the human sciences seem to have specialized in defining normalcy versus pathology, and correct versus deviant or criminal behavior. This no longer occurs in terms of an absolute value that unites people on different levels when faced with death and the responsibility for their "sins," but in terms of the interests of the dominant class. These disciplines, born in the name of mankind and its liberation, have functioned to define normal behavior and its boundaries, and to control deviations from the norm through therapy and confinement. This function was based not on human needs, the needs of all people including those who deviate, but as a response to economic demands and to the needs of the dominant group that counts on controlling most people to ensure its own survival. Intellectuals and technicians in the human sciences have legitimized this control.

Today as never before the role of the professional technician in capitalist society stands out clearly. He or she seems to have taken up once again, centuries later, the role of the intellectuals in the Royal court, where poets, painters, and musicians worked explicitly on commission. The distance between lord and servant was so great that the lord did not need intermediaries to hide his abuses. He commissioned works from the "artists" that attested to his prestige and power. The commission was clear. When the servant began to oppose the lord and social reality changed and became corrupted by notions of equality and democracy, ideologies then allowed the lord to proclaim those principles as real and undisputed, so that he could continue his domination and abuses. Obviously this discussion lacks historical precision, but its schematism helps us understand how a certain kind of technician and intellectual can be used as a functionary of consent, so that actions which might clash with the principles of the rights of man, which must be formally upheld, can be passed off as something else.

It is important to remember that over the last 200 years, torture has officially disappeared in "civilized" countries, as a legitimate tool of the state. The types of control used by deputies, functionaries, and creators of ideologies, have evidently been sufficient to ensure order. Torture is practiced today illegally and "barbarically" only in those countries lacking industrial development with its false liberation from want or in those countries unaware of the advantages offered by the human sciences and ideology as forms of social control.

Now, two hundred years later, "civilization and its discontents" seems to have caused the general reemergence of torture. What is most surprising is that the torture is solely preventive, the persons being tortured and killed having nothing to confess except their refusal to be slaughtered and killed. It is a torture carried out to obtain unconditional consent, positive acceptance, and adjustment to ever stricter rules that respond less and less to the needs of those obeying them. The logic and reason of the state prevails over the last vestiges of humanism, and violence is no longer afraid to reveal itself for what it is. Has control by the legitimators of the state proved quantitatively insufficient? Or is this the start of the apparatus of the state power—constituted for the whole of society in anticipation of moments of crisis in command and direction when spontaneous consent has failed?

In the wake of the great social struggles and movements demanding the rights of equality and nondiscrimination, it became more and more difficult for the class in power to obtain spontaneous consent. Where the contradictions are the most explicit and visible, it was necessary to reinforce the apparatus of state power. Through the most openly repressive institutions—the army and the judiciary—the political infrastructure could directly administer its power, and the technicians could be utilized to ensure the "legality" and the "scientific" nature of torture and crimes. An example of this is found in Latin American countries where psychologists and psychiatrists are appointed to provide technical aid to those who are tortured.[6]

Depending on a country's level of development and the strength of its opposition, it can have recourse to either the apparatus of state power or to an increase in the number of functionaries of consent. In the United States, the most technologically and industrially developed country, there is greater access to advanced technical and professional training as well as the creation of intermediate roles for these newly-trained professionals. This has contributed to the establishment of a single universal middle class and to destroying the working class forces that have generally supported the values and the ethic of the dominant class. All of this has been to the detriment of the American proletariat and the proletariat of less developed countries.

In Italy, although the educational structure is still highly discriminatory, the same process has begun, but the new jobs that the technicians in the human sciences are being trained for—psychologists, sociologists, social workers—do not exist and young people are already discontented. This gap has yet to be filled because the social reality in our country is bungled, concocted, and

temporary. What is more—and this is of fundamental importance—we have a working class which has not yet received the
"kiss of death;" it has not yet assimilated enough bourgeois values to see and defend them as their own.[7]

Beyond the abstract polemics about negating one's role,
or about the fears of being coopted to produce new ideologies, at
this point we need to analyze the technicians' function in a bourgeois society and to understand if technicians who are conscious
of their function can help the subordinate class appropriate this
knowledge. As was true in the area of health care, this is possible
only if the technician acts with the subordinate class to identify its
needs. There is a real danger that this negative worker, as Lourau
called him, will once again be drawn into producing new ideologies.[8] The more he or she is isolated from those needs that must be
identified, the greater that danger, but we cannot allow ourselves
to be paralyzed by those fears. Every contradiction that is revealed
calls for the end of an ideology that would define and classify it,
but it carries within itself a future contradiction. It is up to us to
identify contradictions and to continue our critical analysis of
what we do, what it means to be a functionary of consent and
what it might mean to refuse to be one. We must discover the
forms that this refusal can take, so that it can meaningfully influence the subordinate class, which is generally led to "spontaneous
consent" and support of the dominant values through our constant technical assistance.

We are aware that this involves cultural and political
problems that have been debated for years. What we are interested in is the attempt to confront this controversy from a more
practical perspective. The functionaries of consent are not only
the classical intellectuals who create ideologies. Today all ordinary technicians, even those coming from the working class or
the almost proletarian petit bourgeoisie, who have benefitted
from their greater access to bourgeois culture because of their identification with and defense of their role, represent and enforce
dominant values. Because of this, we must also analyze how the
dominant class incorporates a part of the dominated class into its
values. It expands the group of functionaries by increasing access
to jobs in the tertiary sector, giving them the illusion of sharing
power and thus ensuring their loyalty.

The purpose of our analysis is thus to answer the questions we have raised in the course of our denunciations in a way that can be used by the subordinate class for its liberation. Can the technicians' rejection of their delegated authority and the search for another relationship with those they normally manipulate facilitate their understanding of how their manipulation occurs? In the case of psychiatric treatment, can the technicians' refusal have more than symbolic value and help to stimulate the patient to take control of his or her illness? Can this refusal increase the consciousness of their role in society? To do this, intellectuals or professional technicians must renounce their identity, but their identity is also the class they belong to, and one cannot simply give up one's class and choose another one. Nonetheless, can they use the tools they possess to reveal the processes of manipulation and control inherent in their work? What are the limits of what they can reveal, and how can the manipulated classes come to possess this knowledge?

The professional technician is the conscious or unconscious functionary of the peacetime crimes perpetrated in our institutions, in the name of the ideology of health care, treatment, and patient protection or in the name of the ideology of punishment and rehabilitation. Therefore, wouldn't it help to publicize the violence and backwardness or our repressive institutions, as well as science's justification and legitimation of these institutions? Can the subordinate class take possession of this knowledge so that, aware of the ways that bourgeois science does not meet their needs, they can demand a science which does, and which they can control?

In our society, the different branches of science only plan solutions that seem to be universal for all citizens, but in fact they meet the needs of the dominant group, and control or restrain the needs of the dominated group. Every planned service is created more for the organization and its organizers than for the consumers of the service. Otherwise, there is no explanation for the overemphasis on health services rather than on the quality of the treatment provided. In the logic of capital every institution becomes a productive organism and the goal and justification for its existence (for example, the patient in the hospital) is secondary. However paradoxical it might seem, the hospital exists for the doctors and staff, not for the patients. Moreover, technical assistance is presented under the guise of neutrality, and there is supposed to be no social difference between the person offering the service and the client who needs it.

A public health service, usually planned without the participation of clients, tends to meet the needs of its planners. A clear example of this is found in a questionnaire circulated in 1972, with the theme "utopia and reality in the psychiatric organization of the future."[9] The questionnaire had been sent by Professor Christian Müller, director of the Cery Psychiatric Clinic in Lausanne, to us and to a few other psychiatrists who he felt represented the most advanced area of psychiatric science. We quote here only the introductory preface and excerpts from the answers we gave.

Suppose that you were living in a European or American-style Western society, organized according to your political ideas. You are asked to organize mental health and psychiatric services for a demographic group of up to 100,000 inhabitants in an urban area. You are free to choose your methods, within the limits of a budget that is reasonably proportional to the population's revenue.

We responded that the general premise had to be carefully defined. To ask respondents to make a theoretical hypothesis ("the organization is a psychiatric service for an abstract population of 100,000 inhabitants") while specifying the limits that restrict the theory ("a European or American-style Western society") means setting up a purely abstract discussion where the hypothesis, instead of serving to transform reality, is predetermined and neutralized. The Western world contains so many primary and secondary contradictions that any hypothetical service that does not take them into account or probe their meaning can only operate abstractly. Without this sort of knowledge one cannot identify the needs that the service should meet; without this knowledge the technical hypothesis can only meet the needs of the technicians and never the patients, since it results from an abstraction and not concrete needs.

How can anyone today think that psychiatric institutions should be closed worlds that maintain the scientific and technical ideology of those who run them? How can real needs be identified when needs are constantly defined and created in the form most suitable for the responses that are readily available? In our social context, the terms reality and utopia, proposed in the questionnaire, are not the terms of a contradiction which will then produce a reality incorporating part of the utopia. They are reduced to complementary terms with separate spheres of action, so that one can translate into the other without contradictions. Reality and utopia exist as two apparently different sides of ideology, that false utopia produced for the benefit of the dominant class. The reality in which we live is itself ideology, since it does not correspond to what is concrete but is the product of definitions, classifications, rules, and regulations created by the dominant class to construct reality in its own image, according to its own needs. The less these rules and regulations meet the needs of the whole community, the more they act as an instrument of domination over the subordinate class. All utopian hypotheses, which are contradictory aspects of realities unable to reveal their contradictions for fear of changing them, become ideologies of transformation; change is possible only as the ideology is used as a tool of domination.

Our social structure is determined by an economic logic that subordinates all relationships and all principles of life. It contains neither reality, or the practical truth which verifies whether hypotheses are real responses to needs, nor utopia, the hypothetical element that transcends reality in order to transform it. Utopia can exist only when mankind succeeds in liberating itself from the slavery of ideology and can express its needs in a constantly contradictory reality which contains the elements for its own transcendence and transformation. Only then will we be able to speak of reality as the practical truth and of utopia as foreshadowing the possibility of a real transformation of this practical truth. Then it will no longer be a utopia, but a constant search to meet needs and construct a life possible for all mankind.

How can anyone imagine organizing a hypothetical urban area according to their political and technical philosophy, if that area is already part of a well-defined political and economic reality that leaves no room for contradictions, unless they are first translated into ideologies? How can one hypothesize a service for psychiatric assistance without knowing the specific needs, as they occur in reality? How can one hypothesize the needs that must be answered except by turning the ideological knowledge we have into abstractions? What do we know about those needs, if they are prepackaged and if they result from the logic and culture that determines how they will emerge, which depends on the available responses?

When one organizes a psychiatric health service, the difficulty is to find concrete answers to the concrete questions that stem from the reality in which one works; they should both transcend that reality and transform it. In this sense, when hypothesizing a health institution, one runs the risk of falling into two opposite errors. One is to propose measures that go beyond a given level of reality and its needs, creating new needs through the production of new ideological realities. The other is to stick so close to reality that the measures proposed are locked inside the same logic that produced the problem. In both cases, the practice remains unchanged. There is still an ideological reality, and the measures are limited to defining and circumscribing the problems in each field.

In the health field, the first case corresponds to the creation of new services that do not cure the disease, but find new, undiscovered forms of it. The hypothesis under consideration will be the suitable ideological answer to these new forms. The plan does not arise as a direct response to specified needs, but out of the development of scientific thought, which proceeds according to its own logic and according to economic logic. So the plan ideologically anticipates its own reality, creating artificial needs and concealing real ones. Preventive psychiatric services, as they are planned and implemented today, are part of a scientific and economic logic that has reacted to mental illness by segregating it. The disease is incurable and incomprehensible; its chief symptom is dangerousness and obscenity and the only scientific answer is the asylum where it can be safeguarded and controlled. This axiom is consistent with another implicit one: rules represent efficiency and productivity and whoever does not obey them must be relegated to a space from which he or she cannot interfere with the rhythm of society.

Science and political economy proceed side by side, with the former upholding the limits of the norm that are most proper and useful to political economy. Carrying out its function of social control, science establishes a pathological difference that is exploited for the needs of public order and economic development. Preventive services, which do not change the segregation and exploitation of illness, show that treatment does not narrow the range of abnormal behavior, but expands it.

These services do not respond to the problem of the illness itself and the conditions that foster it. They only redefine behavior that was previously tolerated as normal—for example, the types of deviance that were previously acceptable but are now defined as sick abnormalities. The ideological utopia, in this case, merely transfers the definition of difference to another level, confirming its unequal nature and upholding the separation between health and sickness.

The second case, total adherence to reality, corresponds to the building of technically more efficient health units which maintain the identical definition and classification of mental illness, as well as maintaining the same measures to respond to it. Excessive realism produces answers that express the same skepticism inherent in the structure of asylums. Negative and reductionistic answers are given that merely confirm the negativity of a reality in which the utopian hypothesis cannot change the underlying logic and has no influence.

The relationship between citizen and society, and between health and sickness, must change in order to transform psychiatric institutions and services, and all social institutions. There must be a recognition that the strategy and purpose behind every action is the human being—not abstract humanity, but all human beings with their needs and their life within a collectivity that can satisfy those needs and achieve that life for all. This means that the value of the human being, healthy or sick, goes beyond the value of health or sickness and that illness, like every human contradiction, can be used as a tool for self-mastery or self-alienation, as a tool for liberation or domination. Depending on different concepts of the value and function of human beings, health and sickness can represent absolute positive and negative values, which express the normalcy of the healthy and the abnormality of the sick; or they can express relative values as experiences, contradictions, and events in life that unfold between sickness and health. When the value is the human being, health cannot represent the norm, since the human condition lies constantly between health and sickness.

When the social relations of production are the basis of every relationship between human beings, as they are in capitalist society, it is understandable that even illness can be used and exploited to support the exclusion of some, according to their social class and their economic and cultural power. This does not mean, as is sometimes misunderstood, that mental illness does not exist and that psychiatry or medicine should not take fundamental human processes into account. It means that illness, as a sign of a human contradiction, can be used within a system of exploitation and privilege. It can acquire another, social appearance which turns it into something that originally it was not.

When a health service is planned based on the social and political premises we have described, that which is included as part of the illness actually has nothing to do with it. Instead of responding to real needs, the service only contributes to expanding the boundaries of the illness, adding on social components and eventually identifying the illness with them. The technical hypothesis is an automatic translation of ideological reality; and therapeutic institutions never respond to the illness, but to its double, that is created to meet the needs of production and consumption.[10] For a health service to meet real needs and to reduce illness, there must be an awareness of how illness is used in terms of certain social groups.

It is therefore both impossible and futile to plan a service for a hypothetical abstract population. Impossible, if limited to an ideological utopia created to benefit a few, where the needs of the majority cannot be known or satisfied. Futile, if looked inside the boundaries of the present ideological reality without going beyond it and transforming it. Doctors and other professionals do not develop health services as a simple technical response to a human need. They carry out the authority of their role, which derives from their belonging to the dominant class. This allows them to use their technical knowledge as a tool of power and domination over the subordinate class, whose only alternative to exploitation when sick or disabled is segregation or total destruction.

Since this domination underlies relationships between human beings, how could the therapeutic relationship between doctor and patient be free from the class element present in every social relation? How can we speak about preventive psychiatry when one of the places most harmful to the health of all citizens is the health institution, permeated at all levels by the abusive relationships inherent in the structure of our society? If the institutions created for prevention produce illness, prevention only upholds their function, because they exercise control by means of the illness and promote illness rather than cure it. These institutions are ineffective as long as they support relations of domination through the relationship between the patient and the technician. Technicians, in offering the patient their technical knowledge, automatically act with the authority of their role, which derives from their social identity, class, and the status of their job. When they relate to a patient from the same social class, their power is offset by the patient's power; when they relate to a patient from the subordinate class, their power acts as a type of domination and distance that prevents the patient from having a social identity and rights.

The only alternative to the perpetuation of this domination is to separate knowledge from power, both of which are currently and inseparably linked in the role of the doctor. Technicians who have become conscious of this relation of domination are acting against medical power so that patients can insist on the kind of health service they are entitled to and that technicians have a duty to provide. As long as this power exists, human contradictions cannot be treated as if they were naturally caused. Illness in the subordinate class will continue to represent an absolute negative value, exploitable in every way, in contrast to health as the absolute positive value and the indispensable condition for staying in the productive cycle. As long as health services are planned by the dominant class, they will continue to meet the needs of the dominant class.[11] The institution meets the technician's needs more than the patient's, even if it appears that the doctor is really curing the patient and the patient is really being cured.

So much for our response to the questionnaire. The technician who has become conscious of these processes can play a role in identifying how they are concretely used on a daily basis by bourgeois science against the subordinate class. Through this analysis the subordinate class will know how its oppression occurs and this knowledge will become part of its struggles. The more technicians manage to differ from the intellectuals who "teach the oppressed the road of liberation," the more they will see that they are also oppressed by the same processes, since they are appointed to carry them out and legitimate them.

Perhaps putting an end to our eleven-year experience at the Psychiatric Hospital of Gorizia represented the technicians' ultimate refusal to be accomplices in veiling the process, legitimized by a science that purports to control psychological deviance, and that perpetuates the marginalization of a class.[12] The statements issued by the treatment staff during this period clarified their action and the position taken by the technicians in terms of problems that could not evolve any further without the risk of reestablishing the logic of the asylum in their isolation.

In addition to the symbolic value that "opening" the asylum and gradually rehabilitating patients might have had,[13] we were principally interested in focusing on a social problem rooted in a specific practice that suggested more general issues and comparisons. Even though we were conditioned and limited by the bureaucratic structures typical of hospital organizations, the strength of this kind of action lies in how it is used, since its expresses a new kind of contradiction. To speak of "using" an action does not mean, as the most vulgar and crude interpretations often have it, that patients are exploited in the name of "the revolution," or that if they cannot be used for the revolution they should not be helped. Using our action means that the patients, during the gradual rehabilitation process, represent a crucial point in terms of ideology and the social structure. These problems must be continually reintroduced so they can be confronted on a different level, and this is the task of the technician.

The following documents [from the end of the Gorizia experience in 1972] should be read in this sense as an indication of the political use of a repressive aspect of general social conditioning.[14]

Press Release
Eleven years ago, we began to transform the asylum at Gorizia. Today, I have handed over to the Attorney General the proposal to draw up commitment certificates for 130 persons in our institution, together

with a proposal, in keeping with Article 4 of Law 431 (1968) that makes 68 patients "voluntary"; that is, persons who voluntarily ask for psychiatric assistance, but who retain the right to be discharged at their own request. There remain 52 patients still covered by Law 1904,[15] in addition to the present "voluntary" patients.

I have handed over to the President of the Provincial Administration a detailed report on the current situation at the hospital and the proposal sent to the Attorney General. I have informed the Provincial Board of Health of this, and at the same time I have offered my resignation as director of the hospital, along with the resignations of the medical staff.

We started from the premise that the mental asylum, in addition to being a refuge for the mentally ill, was also a dumping ground for deviant people lacking economic and social resources. We proceeded to rehabilitate slowly these patients, who had been destroyed more by their long isolation than by the illness itself. Today we can no longer accept keeping the majority of the patients isolated in an institution that allows them no openings or outlets and would rapidly reduce them to the level of institutionalization and personal demoralization in which we found them. It's pointless to ask the Provincial Administrator why he refused to open community health centers, even though they have been proposed and planned since 1964; or to explain his negative attitude which has made cooperation between the hospital and local agencies so difficult. Such cooperation would have provided a protective net, in terms of prevention and after-care, and allowed many voluntary patients to be finally rehabilitated, instead of being forced to reinstitutionalize themselves.

In this situation, our presence in the asylum is not only useless, but we think it is harmful to the majority of the patients for whom, as psychiatrists, we continue to represent a justification for their being in the asylum. We personally cannot continue to keep people locked inside the label of "mental patient," with all the consequences such a label involves, simply because no solution could be found outside the asylum for these people, because they were poor, rejected, or alone.

At present we do not know what decision the Attorney General and the Provincial Administration will take. We only know that we leave the hospital at Gorizia with bitterness. Notwithstanding the controversies, the attacks, and the state of siege surrounding us, we were able to show in ten years of work how medicine can be honestly practiced, and how psychiatry can be made into an instrument of liberation, instead of oppression.

Publicizing what we have done will once more be interpreted as the desire for notoriety and success. If we put a clear end to
the enterprise we began over ten years ago, perhaps it will be easier to
make the public understand the meaning of what we have been saying about these issues. It hasn't been easy for us, but we believe that
we have shown in practice the meaning and function of the psychiatric label of mental patient.

In conclusion, the only thing we can say is that the patients
and former patients who have been with us for so many years have
shown that they fully understand what we have done. They have matured as we have matured, and they have expressed the need for a solution that goes beyond the limits of medicine. They have attested to
this need by the maturity and clarity they have shown at our general
meetings in the discussions on their future. For their sake, we hope
that none of our colleagues returns to this hospital to recreate, with a
stroke of the pen, their illness and their tragic "career."[16]

[*In response to the statement released to the local newspaper
by the President of the Provincial Administration, Franco Basaglia sent
the following letter*]:

Dear Mr. President:
After the statement that you released to *Il Piccolo* [Gorizia newspaper]
on the resignation of Domenico Casagrande, the director of the Psychiatric Hospital at Gorizia, I feel the need to make several clarifications. I
unconditionally agree with the action taken by Dr. Casagrande, which I
deem proper both professionally and morally. The decision he made is
the logical outcome of the work we began eleven years ago and attests
to its effectiveness. To define it as an "emotional" and therefore immature reaction means to view it as an isolated act, completely detached
from its context. This step could only be in reaction to the impossibility
of continuing our work, which had no future and which ran the risk of
once again setting up a model for "asylum administration." What sign
of immaturity is this, when for years we've waited for those general solutions which alone would have permitted the rehabilitation and gradual reintegration of patients who no longer have to stay in the asylum?
Isn't it a sign of professional seriousness to call the public's attention to
the limits the technician encounters when he carries out his work,
when those limits are the responsibility of the public welfare agencies?
Isn't it a sign of civil and social responsibility to point out their responsibilities to those in charge of administering public welfare?

If all of this is a sign of immaturity, we should hope for more immature people.

Moreover, your statements are contradictory. They recognize the effectiveness of what you define as the "Basaglia method," yet the Provincial Administration you preside over doesn't allow it to continue—you condemn it to death by suffocation. If you are willing to recognize that the changes occurring in the Psychiatric Hospital have been crucial for rejuvenating psychiatric issues in Italy, why do we have to wait for a study of the overall situation of Italian psychiatry in order to take further steps? What information can come from an abstract study of situations yet to be transformed, when we are faced with meeting concrete needs in an already transformed situation? Government commissions are just an excuse to obstruct bureaucratically actions which should be taken because they spring from real demands and needs. At Gorizia, we attempted to meet the patient's immediate needs, which matured and developed in a qualitative sense as their rehabilitation progressed. What can the treatment staff do now except halt their work and declare that the present needs of the majority of the patients are not within their jurisdiction?

The technician who wants to protect and defend those who request his help can use the tools that "science" offers only if he makes them into a means of liberation and not oppression. Science, like law, always starts from the need to protect and liberate mankind, but it can easily become a new tool of oppression. Technology can be used as a tool of liberation if we are able to understand the real needs to be met, and if we don't assume that science and law are there to meet the needs of either the technicians or the society that appoints them. Hospitals are created to cure patients and not to provide a job for the hospital staff, or to defend society from patients. When a patient in a hospital expresses needs that extend beyond his illness, the doctor no longer responds and the process of rehabilitation ceases. For this reason, Dr. Casagrande's position is perfectly consistent with everything we believe in, and his proposal, which stems from the patients' needs, is a practical one for an alternative to science and institutional violence. It points out everyone's responsibility to search for a mutual solution, so that there will no longer be a perpetual scapegoat who must pay in order for others to be protected and secure.[17]

[When the Administration did not respond positively, the "pro Basaglia" staff resigned *en masse,* sending this letter to the patients]:

Dear Friends:

After eleven years of work, today we are leaving the Hospital. You know what our state of mind is, since you share it. It is pointless to explain once again the decision we made; you know that it was made because it was no longer possible for us to meet your needs.

We had to show the public which is concerned with these issues what could be achieved in changing an institution, and what were the obstacles we encountered with each new change. The Hospital at Gorizia has shown in practice how to confront the problems and suffering of people who are ill. We have all faced difficulties, struggles, and lack of understanding, but until now we have been able to carry on our work, which had such an exemplary value that it revived our hope for a different relationship between human beings. At Gorizia and elsewhere, it is the citizens, potential patients, and potential consumers of health services, who have discussed the open hospital, the closed hospital, and the need for a health reform that meets patients' needs. It is the citizens who have taken on the issue of illness and its treatment.

This final decision to leave the hospital is consistent with our refusal to accept the limits imposed on us from outside, which interfere with our work and destroy it by postponing until tomorrow what could be done today. In the present situation, if you were to legitimately ask, "When can I go home?," we would have to answer with the old lie, "tomorrow," knowing full well that for you tomorrow would never come.

In our refusal to be accomplices, what unites us is all we have done together with you—the patients, nurses, and doctors. Perhaps the deepest meaning of what has happened at Gorizia is that it happened because of an effort to make every member of the institution take responsibility, so that everyone contributed to radically changing the institution.

One of you said that it is not the doctors who have transformed the hospital. They just put the key in the keyhole, and the patients turned the lock and opened the door. You showed that you understood what those running the hospital have not yet understood.

The hospital, because of its history and because it has become a landmark in the development of Italian psychiatry, had a responsibility to report on the obstacles it encountered to its continued progress. This wasn't an irresponsible game we played behind your backs—the entire hospital had achieved a high level of maturity and responsibility. We have struggled together and many times we have won and succeeded in proving something very important. If we leave

you now, it is not a defeat for either you or us. It is another stage in
our struggle that we must continue to wage, even if separately. The
new doctors replacing us will perhaps not immediately understand
what we have meant to each other, what it means to share in the creation of one's own liberation, and what we wanted to do and were
prevented from doing. Now it is up to you to prove that the Hospital
will not be able to change, because you will determine its course. The
roles have already been reversed. You will have to show the new doctors the needs to which they must adapt. You will have to take care of
their anxiety and soothe it, because their task will be even more difficult
than yours, because you already know what your needs are. You will
have to make them understand our years of work and show them how
those deprived of responsibilities can learn to become responsible.

As we leave you then, we are sad but calm, because we
know that what we have done together is yours, and no one can destroy it. We are certain that all of you, patients and nurses, are capable
of continuing the battle, knowing that we will be somewhere else, but
struggling for the same thing.[18]

[The final resignation letter was posted by Franco
Basaglia to the President of the Provincial Administration of
Gorizia on November 20, 1972]:

Dear Mr. President:
I write to you in your capacity as President of the nominating committee of the Psychiatric Hospital at Gorizia and as President of the Provincial Administration, to tell you that I have decided to resign as a member of the committee. . . .

The Provincial Administration is finally free to end the experience that, as you yourself have stated several times, had begun to
transform psychiatric services in Italy. Evidently it also caused too
many tensions and controversies, bringing to national attention a
problem that some would have preferred to cover up with ambiguities. Yet you know very well that if the issue of psychiatric treatment
is now familiar to the public, it is because of Gorizia and the way the
significance of Gorizia was publicized.

Now that its game is finally clear, the Provincial Administration can no longer claim that it is ready to continue the so-called
"Basaglia line." Its last chance to show that intention, in practice,
would have been to understand that the treatment staff, in its resignation, wanted a firm commitment [to community services and the con-
tinuation of the hospital's transformation] from the agencies responsi-

ble for the future of the institution, in light of the changing of the
guard that the Provincial Administration clearly desired. That commitment was bureaucratically avoided, and this clears up any misunderstanding about the Provincial Administration, which can no longer
hide behind the "Basaglia Line," supporting it officially but obstruct-
ing it in practice. This has been an important moment whose events
have made us understand that the situation at the hospital tests the
morality of the medical profession and the government administration. It is not coincidental that the last measures taken by the Provincial Administration were supported by the Italian Social Movement,[19]
and by the most reactionary and conservative forces. At the same
time, doctors have begun to end the corporativism that up to now has
kept the profession iron-tight. An internal split is now visible and is
based on a fundamental technical and political choice: the use of science as a tool of liberation or oppression. The way that the Provincial
Administration wanted to escape from the impasse, in which both the
hospital and its patients were placed, demonstrates once and for all
what they have chosen for the future. I therefore do not intend to support a decision that excludes those who have struggled to transform
not only the Gorizia asylum, but all Italian asylums, and to change
both the general attitude towards mental patients and the definition of
mental illness as irreversible and disgraceful.

　　For all that ties us to the patients at Gorizia, and for our long
and difficult experience together, I can only hope that the Provincial Administration, even with a more docile and less "rebellious" medical
team, will immediately be forced to confront patients' needs and that
this will push them to remedy an otherwise untenable situation.

　　In order not to disrupt patients' lives, we won't meddle any-
more, either with arguments or attacks on the Psychiatric Hospital,
and we hope that no patient will have to pay for the irresponsible, re-
vengeful action of its administrators.[20]

　　The doctors resigning from the Hospital at Gorizia refused to set up a model of hospital management which would
have inevitably turned into the traditional asylum administration,
allowing the technician to resume his old role as the manipulator
and functionary of consent. The therapeutic value of the first critical stage was inherent in the transformation of an institution, in
which all aspects were called into question, including the relationship of the institution to the social structure. This new approach
became acceptable [to the Provincial Administration] but only if it

was set up as a new technical model, ingrown and incapable of further development. The process of transformation ended, reduced to an adjustment to new rules which destroyed the therapeutic value of the new hospital organization by paralyzing the initial impetus. The technicians rejected this regressive process of adjustment, indicating possible further developments which were then blocked and prevented.

The contradictions that have been opened up will be again hidden away. And everyone who revealed those contradictions will continue to be called "immature," "emotional," and "irresponsible"—perhaps we should point out that these adjectives better describe our forerunners and those who work in other asylums. Order is reestablished with the repression and concealment of real problems.

The experience at Gorizia, therefore, had to be physically eliminated, no matter how, because it had not aimed to offer a new technical model, as might have been the case in England with Maxwell Jones' therapeutic community, or in France with the 13th Arrondissement—both psychiatric showcases for displaying the latest consumer products.[21] Our experience, which saw psychiatry and asylums as emblematic situations, pointed to fundamental political and social problems that could not be resolved through humanitarian changes in the hospital, although we implemented them. We saw our experience as an opportunity to discuss the nature and goals of asylums in terms of our social structure.

Once the contradictions could not be taken outside the asylum into the larger society, the resignation of the treatment staff, which had become imprisoned in the communitarian island they had created, became a way to reintroduce the issue of psychiatric treatment on a higher level of clarity and struggle.

A Conversation with Jean-Paul Sartre

It was on issues concerning [Gorizia and] the position of technicians of practical knowledge that we held a conversation with

Jean-Paul Sartre in the winter of 1972. Some of that discussion follows:

FRANCO BASAGLIA: The bourgeois technician, appointed to administer various professional fields, can be considered an intellectual in Gramsci's sense in that he both receives and produces ideas that maintain the institution where he works, and consequently maintains the survival of his own class and the social system.

In the light of the movements of technicians in recent years to reject the social authority of their role, how do you view the problem of the intellectual and the professional technician in terms of institutional practice? I pose the question both for institutions in general and psychiatric institutions in particular, where we work.

SARTRE: I am not well informed about psychiatry. I have followed your work and I'm in complete agreement with what you've said. However, I can talk about what I think of intellectuals in general. In my view, the intellectual is not simply a technician. For example, an American scholar who studies the atomic bomb is not an intellectual, but what I would call a "technician of practical knowledge." He becomes an intellectual when he begins to question the significance of the atomic bomb and ends up opposing the work he does; that is, when he realizes his own contradiction, which is to use his general universal skills for the particular goals of a specific group. He is then in total contradiction with himself because his skills serve the goals of a bourgeoisie that uses him for their own gain.

This is what I would call the old intellectual, typical of the period from 1930 to 1960. This individual had two faults. In the first place, he believed he had to reinstate the general or universal dimension whenever it was clearly being used for particular ends. Thus he had to get closer to the masses, who represent the true universal, and to their needs and necessities. At the same time, he was still an intellectual and was still satisfied to represent this "unhappy consciousness," this relationship between the universal and the particular that allowed him to be a sort of leader. He could continue to be the kind of intellectual who signed petitions, organized debates, and participated in certain political activities. All things considered, he was a leader. He didn't believe he had an innate gift for being one, but he considered his power to derive from his knowledge, and from the contradiction within himself. The second fault was that intellectuals constituted an especially self-enclosed group, because they were technicians unhappy with the work they did. They even managed to think that revolution was the dictatorship of the intellectuals.

In France, after 1968, it seemed clear to most young people that the intellectual was completely contradictory. On the one hand, he advocated actions with universal ends, yet at the same time the state and the privileged class asked him to play a particular role. The intellectual suffered from this contradiction but his suffering became noble, because he felt that his contradiction allowed him to reveal that the allegedly universal actions of governments or classes really had particular ends.

It was obvious to these young people that if the intellectual's contradiction had been a true, total one he would have had to abolish himself as an intellectual. He would have had to refuse to maintain this unnecessary contradiction so as to see the significance of classes as institutions created by civil society and the political system. Only by uniting with the masses can you discover their real goals. It isn't enough to criticize the ruling class. You must enter into the real and constant struggle that the masses wage against that class.

After '68, the intellectual who was conscious of his own contradictions no longer had to embody a tormented consciousness hovering over the masses. He did, however, have to abolish himself as an intellectual. He could be a technician, an engineer or a doctor, but to be able to unite with the masses he had to cease being an intellectual. He would become one amongst many—someone with his own profession who analyzes problems from the perspective of "universal needs," the needs of the masses. Today's intellectuals want to abolish themselves as such and don't perceive themselves in the same way. They understand that the fight must be simultaneously universal and particular. That is the fundamental change occurring in our country. Many young people, educated to become technicians of practical knowledge, have given it up and some have gone into the factories, *les etablis,* as we say in France. These intellectuals are now workers who are also doing political work at the same time. The skills they acquired in their studies can always be used, but they don't place those skills beyond the reach of the masses. Perhaps they are more skilled at writing something requested by other workers, but in their work together they are all equal.

A difficult problem arises because obviously society doesn't accept these people who automatically belong to the other side and who oppose all institutions as pursuing particular ends. These young people are outlaws, since they challenge all the institutions created by a society that uses the universal as a means to satisfy particular needs.

Originally, the intellectual was a product of bourgeois institutions, but when he finally forceably grasps his own contradictions, there is only one solution—the leap into illegality to challenge and reject the society that has shaped him. This presupposes that he fights for a society in which intellectuals no longer exist, in which everyone will be a technician of both practical and manual knowledge, as in China, where everyone works with the peasants, in addition to their own work. I believe that this is the desire of intellectuals who want to return to the masses.

It goes without saying that all of this makes the intellectual challenge what society does to people who are on the margins of society, and this includes those who are usually called crazy. What happens to those whom society rejects? They are put into prison, some for longer than others. The society that we want to create is one in which no one will be marginal. In reality, people on the margins of society are like intellectuals. They are people who, given present reality, react in a solitary fashion and are called crazy. The reality is that they have been placed in a solitary situation, and in their isolated way they are challenging the entire society and challenging reason itself.

Our problem is not so much the psychiatric institution which creates crazy people. It is knowing how to help people who are isolated and fighting in muddled, uncertain, and complicated ways to struggle in a more clearcut way. Is this possible? It's very difficult. We know that psychiatry is exactly the opposite of what it should be in order to help these people. The very idea of recovery seems absurd to me. To be cured in this society means to adjust people to goals that they reject; it means teaching them not to fight, and it means adapting them to society. This has been one of the great faults of psychoanalysis. The goal of psychoanalysis has been to take an individual who is more or less on the periphery of society, and make him conform. If he becomes a nice executive, or something else, then he's cured. But actually he's not cured at all—he has been slaughtered. It's important to understand his opposition, what he was trying to say.

When we negate the intellectual, we also consider it fundamental to abolish psychiatric institutions because they are based on completely incorrect principles. They never approach people as individuals in their own right. They see people schematically—this one is healthy, this one's sick—and this has no meaning for us. Meanwhile, we are struggling against all kinds of prisons. Our Information Group on Prisons is a group of intellectuals working on changes in prison administration, with a view to largely abolishing them in the future.[22] In France there are also what we call "antipsychiatrists," who try to approach individuals in their individuality, which constitutes a kind of universality. They try to give them a more social form for their opposition, without changing them as individuals. Those who criticize the antipsychiatrists think this is individualism, but it's really a kind of universalism.

BASAGLIA: The bourgeois technician automatically accepts the way the institution is administered, as if it were not possible to question it or as if he didn't also define the institution. According to you, what are the technician's theoretical and practical problems when dealing with reality, given that our reality is a completely ideological one?

SARTRE: The technician is surrounded by an ideology that contradicts itself. For example, a practicing psychiatrist has direct contact with those marginal people that society calls crazy. He's surrounded not only by ideology, but by an institution, both of which create definitions of madness. The practicing technician who sees and treats people has nothing to do with the technician who is a theoretician. For the practicing technician, until he learns to reject this kind of institution, he will have to enforce it. As a doctor in a psychiatric hospital, he will be told that what must be done, must be done—those are the rules. It is a question of both institution and ideology, since ideology is nothing more than the institution carried to another level.

Since he is a practitioner, he finds himself in conflict with the ideas of the dominant class, but these ideas are also present in the oppositional classes. They, too, are used to thinking that a crazy person is truly crazy, because the dominant class has passed on its ideology to them.

Similar difficulties are encountered in the prisons. There is the ideology of punishment, and then there's the reality that prisoners' sentences are different than the real punishment they suffer. Issues about the right to punish them or the form it should take aren't even posed. If a man is condemned to four years in prison, to the judge this means four years of isolation in a room with food and nothing else. In reality, it means sending him into a hell, because there are people who fear him, who beat and torture him. It means a constant temptation to commit suicide—have you noticed that there are one or two suicides a day in [French] prisons? You could never imagine that a judge sentencing a guilty man to four years was condemning him to four years of being beaten, tortured, and perhaps driven to suicide. There's a profound contradiction here. On the one hand there are those with power; on the other, those who exercise power, like the prison warden and the guards. They ally themselves with the technicians and this leads to the suicides, the uprisings, and the torture.

Once again, it's clear that practical reality differs from ideological reality. An ideology emerges from practice, and that is what we must clarify. All of us, not just intellectuals, have to clarify this.

BASAGLIA: That's the problem. We have to create a practical alternative in these institutions that meets the needs of those using them and not those creating them. Working with the patients, prisoners, and all those oppressed by the dominant class, we have to create a realistic way of meeting needs that reverses the use of science as a method of class oppression.

SARTRE: I think that in the bourgeois world, science is also ideology. It contains universal aspects, but it contains particular propositions that are presented as universal ones. We find these erroneous propositions especially at the point where theoretical science turns into technical and practical science. In certain specific fields like psychiatry, it is up to the masses to demand a different conception of science. The human sciences are bourgeois sciences; they can manage even to justify the massacre of Indians.

In *Les Temps Modernes* we published several issues on anthropology.[23] Ethnologists maintain that since we are tied to imperialism, we look upon Indians as savages. If we didn't use soldiers against them, they wouldn't obey us. So what should be done? We discussed this issue at length.

There is a very precise point where science and imperialism become intertwined. We need to analyze how much bourgeois ideology there is in science in terms of practical concepts. I believe that psychoanalysis is completely bourgeois. It can't spread to the masses because it would be meaningless to them. Group therapy is practiced but it is sheer madness even from a Freudian perspective. I remember the case of a 27-year-old friend who was part of a leftist movement. He had many problems, he had lived alone, he had taken LSD, so he went to a psychoanalyst, who wasn't able to understand the impulses and the experiences of a young militant. He maintained that this young man had a certain influence on his comrades because he wanted to play the role of their father. That's absurd. It was something quite different. Psychoanalysts don't realize what happened to the young people who were involved in the struggles of '68.

BASAGLIA: Faced with the task of transforming both institutions (i.e., schools, hospitals, prisons, etc.) and the ideologies underlying them, the technician has two alternatives. There can be an ideological radical change which just sets up a new model of administration, or a real radical change with utopian elements that anticipates a reversal in the direction of science and bourgeois technology. The danger of the second alternative is falling into another ideology, since we are still walking on the minefield of bourgeois ideological reality.

SARTRE: That would mean proposing changes that aren't yet feasible. I understand your position but I don't totally agree. It seems to me that if we examine the masses' inherent negation of these institutions, and we try to reinforce it, there won't be any need to proceed by means of a utopia. We latch onto science and institutions without defining what will follow. What we want is not offered, and what we want is never exactly what we get. Do you understand what I mean? I don't disagree with you so much; it's just that I don't like utopias. You negate what exists, you negate it both globally and individually and then you try to destroy it. I believe that is the path to take to accomplish something.

BASAGLIA: In our reality, for us to create a science along with the people who will use it is already utopian, even if I understand that my way of using the term isn't philosophically correct. I don't mean detaching myself from reality, but trying to answer people's real needs, the needs that science claims it is dedicated to fulfilling. To achieve this in our reality becomes "utopian."

SARTRE: Many people would agree with this, but for me the word utopia is too charged with nonbeing, with the imaginary. On the other hand, utopias arise from the system, as a negation of its institutions. I think that positive issues like this will necessarily emerge from the institutional destruction that we want, because we aren't talking about totally negating or rejecting the present system, but gradually struggling against it.

     In our practice we will find elements that can soon become new ideological signs. We don't know whether we can do away with all ideologies. When the general ideology is no longer science, can there be a valid ideology? This poses the problem of philosophy, which I don't want to raise right now. The issue for me is whether there can be a universal ideology, a good philosophy, that differs from science, or do we have to do away with all ideology? The answer is difficult, and will partly depend on the nature of the new science. It could replace philosophy if its procedures are different from the old analytic methods that establish the *law y=f (x)*. If another different science were to emerge from the dialectic, then philosophy would perhaps be unnecessary. We will only learn this through negation. If human beings change through the negation of their role as psychiatrists and patients, and if we can achieve something like a new conception of mankind and social being, then perhaps there will be no need for philosophy. If this doesn't happen, and if science is still *y=f (x)*, then it will be necessary to have a dialectic conception, which would be philosophy, the only possible ideology. All of this remains to be seen.

BASAGLIA: Years ago you wrote a sentence which struck me. "Ideologies are always liberating while being created; oppressive once created." I don't know whether this is a projection, but I think this means having to experience slowly contradictions as they emerge, even if this means turning to an ideology originally created as a rejection or a negation, without clinging to the same ideology to survive. The problem in this society is how to survive without having to resort to defensive weapons and succumbing to the very thing we are struggling against.

SARTRE: I think I understand what I meant. There's an element of creativity in every ideology, even in a bourgeois ideology. Once created, they are alienating. If another ideology must be created, let it be one that doesn't alienate us but lets us all be a part of it.

BASAGLIA: Going back to the situation at Gorizia, which you are familiar with, we might say that after the first stage, when we denounced the function of psychiatric ideology, we ran the risk of becoming fixed in a new ideology. The ideology of a "good" administration of the institution, and a new model translated into a new therapeutic technique, would have reintroduced the same oppressive logic which we were fighting against. The second step we took was to bring the problems of institutions to another level. Gradually, we were able to make the issue of health services more real, ending up with the well-known resignations of the doctors. We made clear that it was above all an issue of public welfare that had been evaded by the responsible agencies, with the cooperation of psychiatrists and psychiatric institutions. Do you consider the resignations as an abandonment of institutional work, or as an effective part of a strategy of institutional struggle?

SARTRE: It's hard to know. I could predict what the French government would do in such a situation, but I'm not familiar enough with the Italian situation. Italian politicians and administrators seem more flexible to me than the French. Perhaps because they are more flexible, they will try to avoid a total breakdown in the institution because of the resignations. In France, the current government would have accepted the resignations and replaced them with Fascist doctors. There have been examples like this in France, although not as important as this one.

BASAGLIA: Then the important thing is to avoid thinking in terms of victory and defeat. The only possibility is to continue to struggle because it is only while struggling that new contradictions emerge, and we create new relationships with people.

SARTRE: Right now, that's what I believe. I'd like to know what a revolution would lead to, since there is always someone who wants to take power. Wouldn't it just be a change in power from one group to another? That would be no improvement. Or would it mean, in spite of everything, greater opportunities for us? In any event, I'm certainly on the side of those who hope to take power with a revolutionary struggle. I hope that institutions and the ideology inherent in science and everywhere else, will be abolished. I hope that human beings will try to establish different relationships with each other. We cannot fail because everything we do remains and everything we accomplish continues.

For Sartre, intellectuals become aware of both their contradictions and those of their social reality and negate themselves as intellectuals through a specific, yet total confrontation. We were using the term "intellectual" as Gramsci meant it, as the "functionary in charge of consent," which led to a certain ambiguity in the discussion. When we now refer to a technician of practical knowledge who becomes aware of his own role in the game of social power and who acts from that awareness, the meaning is similar, so long as both technician and intellectual wrestle with their own contradictions and with those of social reality. Sartre himself speaks elsewhere of the need to separate knowledge from power, indivisibly linked in the repositories of traditional culture. For technicians, this would mean rejecting the power of their social role, and using knowledge to no longer defend the interests of the dominant class and its values, but those of the dominated class. The problem is to examine what it means, practically speaking, for intellectuals to negate themselves as intellectuals, or for technicians, who negate their power while implicitly maintaining it, to separate knowledge from power.

For example, a medical student's political choice to give up medicine and become a worker may serve his purpose more than the worker's. Wouldn't it be more useful for a doctor to defend worker's interests, with all the ambiguities involved, than for him to choose to be "on the other side of the barricades?" Isn't that still a purist choice, a personal solution to resolve one's "unhappy consciousness?" A member of the bourgeoisie is still bourgeois, even if he becomes a worker, precisely because he is able to make that choice instead of being compelled by necessity or the impossibility of doing otherwise. Doesn't he continue to possess the whole package of cultural tools that will always make him a different worker, even if he does not use those tools to become a foreman? These are problems that have become increasingly clear in recent years, and we will return to them later. For the moment, we would like to reexamine an issue raised in the conversation with Sartre, which points to the main thrust of our argument. Since, as he puts it, "the masses are used to thinking a crazy person is truly crazy because the dominant class has passed on to them its ideology," they must be enabled to appropriate the knowledge held by those technicians who refuse to be "functionaries in charge of consent."

This, then, is the direction towards which we are moving: to bring to light, along with the oppressed class, the necessity of identifying and unmasking the processes by which one is manipulated, in order to facilitate the expression of real needs. These processes compound the exploitation and oppression of people, imposing an unconscious, spontaneous consent upon values that are implicitly destructive.

NURSES AND THE ANTI-INSTITUTIONAL MOVEMENT

One of the central problems in breaking the logic of the asylum concerns the attitude of the nurses and other personnel, who come from the same social class as the patients. We have all internalized a positivist conception of mental illness, seeing it as a biological mutation, for which nothing can be done other than isolating the sick, protecting them through institutionalization. In other words, all of us think that if people are crazy, they are simply crazy and should be put away. This, then, is the area where we must intervene and take action.

The central problem is to render ever more explicit in our practice what psychiatry serves as a science, how asylums and other punitive institutions function in our social system, and how these exclusionary institutions survive by also providing jobs for nurses, guards, doctors, and social workers. In terms of the economic logic that determines our lives, every move that apparently fulfills people's social needs really fulfills the needs of the dominant class by limiting the possibility of social disturbances, creating jobs that guarantee immediate consensus, and by offering people an identification with their social role. The dominant class openly plays on the divisions within the same class: between those who are crazy, ill or marginal, belonging to the proletariat or underclass; and nurses, paramedics, and attendants, who are also proletarians, but who play an active role in the productive cycle (that is, in the hospital organization). This they defend for their own survival, and each in his or her own way serves as a functionary in charge of consent.

Every attempt to transform that reality comes up against this division, which makes it so difficult for the nurses and hospital staff to develop a class consciousness. The logic of the asylum thus operates on two levels: the pervasive internalization of a certain concept of mental illness, and the division between personnel and patients.

In the psychiatric field, the positivist school's absolute, rigid scientific ideology that is descended from Lombroso sees criminals and mental patients as possessing an innate biological condition. There is only an extreme solution: confinement. Medical ideology provides the justification for locking away those biologically different. Thus, in Italy the 1904 law on psychiatric treatment sanctioned both patient care and the protection of society from the dangerously insane.[24] This law was based on the incurable contradiction between the concepts of custody and cure, between the individual patient's interests and the safety of society. In other words, the collectivity had to be defended from the danger posed by the illness. This contradiction has meant that custody has prevailed over cure, obviously to the patient's detriment and to bourgeois society's favor. From the beginning of this century until the present, the acceptance of this logic has guaranteed social control over behavior deemed biologically different and incurable, thereby ensuring the safety of "civil" society.

But the changes taking place in psychiatric institutions in recent years have demonstrated how often this biological diversity, labeled as mental illness, actually has quite another character. It is the original sin of belonging to the dominated class, whose presence in society is acceptable only if it conforms to the rules created for its subordination.

If we examine the working class movements of this century, it is disconcerting to see how, until very recently, the issue of health has been largely neglected. It is considered only in an explicit, direct relationship to occupational hazards. The explanation for this lack lies again in the universal acceptance of a positivist conception of illness, which placed the issue on an objective, scientific level, completely separate from the sphere of political action. Up until now, we have all accepted the definition of illness handed down to us, and the consequences of such definitions: the clear separation of illness, which involves medical skills, from health, which could involve issues of political struggle. Since we now know that the progression of a disease, like its medical codification, can vary according to the patient's social class, we can no longer accept the division between science and politics, and the fact that doctors and nurses have become the guardians of this division.

It is here that we situate the transformation of health institutions, which carry out political goals and therefore must be changed through political struggle from within. In psychiatric institutions, the nursing staff, for example, which carries out the most immediate control and domination over the patients, is only just now beginning to stray from the path of pure corporatist demands in their struggles. But if they ignore the relationship of domination between nurses and patients in a psychiatric institution (or for that matter, medical hospitals), they will only buttress the relation of domination existing between nurses and doctors. Wage demands, even though legitimate, especially now that the doctors' salary increases have created an enormous wage differential, cannot be disconnected from demands for a redefinition of nursing. This would involve a different relationship to both the patient population *and* the medical corps, which functions in the hospital to maintain the dominant ideology. But, even in this sphere, the targets of political struggle are very unclear. The hospital nursing staff sees its demand for a new professional dignity and for skilled technical training as moving the staff closer to the medical model. However, the nurse's subordination to the doctor, which could be maintained intact even with the new skills, recreates the existing model of domination. If this model continues to function between doctors and nurses, it will also be reproduced between nurses and patients, so that patients can only hope to reappropriate their health through a dependency on the nurses and staff—which is exactly the current logic of the asylum.

In the current nurses' struggle to control their own work place, a fundamental element has not yet emerged, at least not in a generalizable form, and that is the solidarity of the nurses with the patients who are both of the same class and who need to liberate themselves from their mutual subordination to the doctors' power. The struggle which has begun in recent years in psychiatric institutions has correctly suggested the connection between technical issues and political issues. Everyone in the hospital fulfills a precise role in controlling patients, by the delegation of power, of which we are all accomplices. Yet we cannot automatically halt this delegation, but rather must proceed through a series of steps, given that the institution exists and survives in its particular form precisely because it offers individuals powerful positions which are hard to refuse. Privileges become strengthened, bureaucratic hierarchies reinforce the privileges, an undergrowth of power and blackmail compounds the aggression, which is then vented on the weakest link in the institutional hierarchy, the patient.

The struggle to change psychiatric institutions has also

shown us how difficult it is to break this circle of power. For example, the nursing staff has always taken on and internalized the doctor's aggression and domination as their way of relating. The nurses have then turned it into aggression against the patients. The maintenance of the asylum and the logic of internment has been carried out by passing on this aggression to the nurses because they have the direct contact with the patients. The asylum can continue to exist, then, because it also allows those involved in these power contests, whether doctors, administrators, or bureaucrats to vent against the patients the aggression it has instilled. The asylum's function of control can thus be guaranteed by everyone, at all levels.

The possibilities open to treatment staffs for struggling in a different way, by involving unions and political organizations, have evolved from the liberating practices at several psychiatric hospitals.[25] Our work there over the years allows us to discuss its nature and to make comparisons with other types of workplace struggles.

In the factory and in most places where working people are exploited, the forms of struggle are easy to identify. The object of the work clearly shows how the worker is alienated, noxious conditions in the factories have an obvious effect on health, and workers' demands are made at the direct expense of their employers. But when the object of one's work is a person and not a machine, the issue is more complicated. The workers in a health or psychiatric institution are able to unload the aggression that they experience, and which should be directed at the employers, onto the sick people who are at their mercy. The workers in a factory have only their chains to lose, but the nurses in a hospital stand to lose the right to put the chains on the patients. The ideology of custody and cure, then, has the advantage of masking everything so that the person carrying out the aggression is not even conscious of what he or she is doing. Although doctors, nurses, and psychiatric workers must come up against this medical ideology that justifies everything they do, it is not immediately clear to them how to struggle to destroy this logic.

When the movement for change in psychiatric institutions begins to perceive the patient as the principal protagonist in the transformation, then the functions of the treatment staff become clearer. Only when they stand face to face, the helper and the helped, can they begin to see that the institution creates two opposing, antagonistic sides which are really the two contradictory terms of a single problem, with health being represented by the treatment staff and sickness by the patients. However, health and sickness are not so distinctly separate. Just as the patients' "illnesses" are also due to the violence and segregation they endure, the nurses and treatment staff are "sick" because of the violence and isolation they inflict. From this a new strategy can arise, based on the common goal of struggling against suffering, that goes beyond workers' economic demands. Those claims are legitimate, but without the enrichment of new goals and themes, they would only continue to keep patients and their keepers locked in the same cycle of violence.

Thus, the recent struggles have caused a crisis in both the scientific ideology which legitimizes violence in the asylum, and in the relationship between different levels of administrators of this violence. We have learned that what allows our social system to maintain these institutions is not just the doctor, who is its direct representative, but also the nurses. They are oppressed by the doctor's authority, by the threat of losing their jobs, and by the responsibility that the hierarchical structure loads on them. They are also corrupted by the opportunity to act as jailers as an alternative to the oppression they experience. In these conditions, they identify totally with their role to the extent that the class configuration of the situation is obscured. A complete confusion reigns between custody and cure; between legal responsibilities and personal risk; between subordination to the doctor and an illness which the nurses and doctors see only in terms of behavior that is acceptable or is not to the hospital administration.

In this situation, the nurses' choice is not easy, nor is it easy to bring the solution to fruition together with them. The more it is based on the contradictions emerging in several psychiatric institutions, the more the medical profession, in crisis because of these discoveries, defends itself and covers over the contradictions. In the best of cases, the doctors defend themselves by means of a sort of enlightened corporativism which eliminates the custodial ideology and adopts another—the sociological one, whose most current, modern passwords are preventive medicine, health maintenance, and community struggles. But in practice, when the hierarchical model of authority and power remains unchanged, as is too often the case in psychiatric institutions, these passwords are reduced to pretexts, useful for concealing reality.

These passwords will only be meaningful when we have broken the institutional cycle, that is, when we manage to end the doctor's power, which serves as the model for the power of the nurses. We still move in a divided camp, where technology and politics operate in separate spheres and not as two complementary aspects of the same problem. But by becoming aware of our complicity, we will be able to take responsibility for our work with all the consequences, thus ending the division between science and the sociopolitical structure. The petit bourgeois corporatist struggles that go on in nearly every asylum, which we discussed above, attest to this division. The nurses rarely fight in an organized way to change their work and their relationship to the patients, to free themselves from an internalized ideology with which they defend themselves, but which was actually created to prevent them from becoming conscious of their place in society and of the repressive power they wield in their position. They continue to separate their awareness of the meaning of their work from the political or union struggles that they carry on outside the institution, thus perpetuating the division upon which the asylum is based.

When a crisis has been brought about in a hospital, two possibilities exist. First, the institution can become rationalized and absorbed within the ideology of social psychiatry, creating a new type of control which contains the emerging contradictions at the level of ideas and discourse—an alternative which we rejected at Gorizia. Or else the hospital workers can take charge of the crisis. To be consistent in terms of the political consciousness of their roles and their jobs, they must participate directly in changing their relationship with the patients. In the latter case, the burden of the crisis can be shared with the doctors who originally caused it, but the principal protagonists must be the nurses, who join with the patients to remove the crisis from the hands of the bosses, and use it politically for the benefit of their own class.

Unless they intend to call a halt to this process, political and union organizations can also become protagonists in these changes. They can begin a new kind of health struggle—a unified struggle that includes both the healthy and the sick. If this does not happen, then the divisions within the class will be maintained, unconsciously contributing to the oppression of healthy workers, like the nurses who feel justified by their political commitment to the union and at the same time live under the illusion of possessing some power, which they exercise as violence against patients. They contribute as well to the oppression of marginalized people, such as the patient who is subjected to this violence.

In recent years, many leftist parties and groups have considered the movement in the health field to be equivocal. Separate groups have competed in an intellectual game, where patients' suffering and nurses' dissatisfaction with their work offered the opportunity for new power games to appear. Technicians, because of their cultural background and class, can easily revert to their classic role, reestablishing their domination and recreating a division in the struggle. This is why the working class movement and the unions are needed, to check and control this process. Yet only now has a unified position begun to develop in the struggle against institutions and their ideologies. Up to now they have not taken clear steps to break the institutional cycle that locks nurses and patients in the same vise-like grip. The working class movement and the unions often seek a direct relationship with the consumers of health services, and ignore the institution.

This direct relationship, however, can only occur when the political organization is ready to confront the problem and when the workers are the ones to change the administration of health services, demanding services that meet their needs and which they can control. It will not happen by claiming, as they often do, that such a situation already exists. The limits of the anti-institutional psychiatric movements, which have been rightly regarded with suspicion by the unions, are that they have emerged from an avant-garde of doctors, followed by a tiny avant-garde of nurses. This maintains the separate groups where rivalries, psychological tensions, and intellectual pretensions have the upper hand. We have tried to overcome such obstacles by creating groups [such as Democratic Psychiatry] that try to end corporativism for both doctors and nurses, as well as the nurse's identification with petit bourgeois ideology, which is fostered by their identification with the doctors. We have proposed a unified struggle where the technician's work can serve to keep in check psychiatric, health, and other political demands.[26]

THE STUDENT MOVEMENT REFLECTIONS ON ANTONIO GRAMSCI
    The prospects for our struggle are not easy. In addition to all the difficulties of battling against medical power and the dominant ideology, the new ideologies that develop among health workers who are struggling must also be surmounted. Young technicians are in a state of permanent crisis with the institutions which would be an ideal situation if the nature of the crisis were clear. Having just come from the student revolts [of 1968], they have behind them an experience in which they were also to keep the contradictions of their situation alive by totally rejecting the future that the social system had planned for them. As students, their refusal can be a global one, for they have by definition a passive role in the learning process which does not require compromises. Their only weapon is this refusal which, when shared by all students, becomes the only means of power they possess.
    One has the impression that since the events of '68, students have experienced a sort of omnipotence, which reaches fruition as they become aware of their strength. However, the effectiveness of their refusal is diminished during moments of retrenchment like the present one. Because of the impossibility of real action, it turns into slogans which express a sort of institutionalization of the struggle, where the correctness of one group's political position is weighed against another's, and groups split off and form around these positions. It can also turn into irony, as a sign of impotence (the other nondialectic side of omnipotence) when faced with a reality that should be changed. At the height of political struggles, their sense of omnipotence corresponded to an awareness of their strength and a recognition of their social importance in a given historical moment when action was possible. For this strength to be well grounded in times of political inactivity, however, requires unity so that we can oppose all those who want to destroy us. To do this we must know the methods they use to destroy us; if we do not, we can always escape, but only into a new form of oppression.
    Students' professed ties to the working class are rarely

true in practice. The students falsely believed that they had caused the explosion of the workers' movements. This is not dissimilar to those intellectuals who stand on the sidelines, giving instructions on how and when the struggle should take place. In the students' eyes, their movement has taken on an ideological value, which justifies their disunity and internal dissension. Aware of this, they are trying to find more concrete ways of working within it, perhaps in response to the threat of a new kind of fascism and repression which looms over the country.[27]

There is another important issue. Students have their own specific territory upon which they have yet to leave their mark, because it has been easier to escape into a broader form of political activity that allowed them to feel politically correct while they endured the effects of archaic educational policies. Each student tended to react in a solitary fashion with his or her own psychological suffering, but despite denunciations there was no overall action taken against the educational ideology with which all of them had to contend.

For example, in order for a doctor to gain a permanent position in a hospital, three to four years of attendance is required at a school for specialization. The number of applications for admission is higher than the available slots. No organized opposition to the admissions process has arisen; instead there is a race for the few places available, using all the traditional methods, including high-level recommendations, favoritism, and patronage. Nor is there an organized protest demanding that everyone be admitted to these schools, assuming that they are useful given their present structure, or rejecting totally the institution of specialized schools. Rather, whoever is admitted accepts the privilege unquestioningly, and whoever is rejected accepts this as an act of fate. Students in these schools of higher education spend three or four years absorbing a number of ideas, accepting them as noncritically as they are dispensed. Any critique takes place only outside the bounds of scientific ideology and the elite roles that it produces. This split between political activity and professional work in one's own field, like the split between theory and practice, resembles the traditional training of the intellectual as a functionary of consent.

Once they have surpassed the stage of rejecting the class

nature of the school system, how do these students and college graduates become further politicized? How can they affect the institution and the ideology aimed at them? The omnipotence they experienced during the moments of intense political struggle can easily turn into a real impotence in a period of decreased political activity like the present, especially in terms of their own specific reality. If they move on to a more generalized political level, without the mediation of their own reality, they may escape into a new ideology that justifies and hides their own impotence. Although the struggle could be shifted onto this larger, yet vaguer level, linking them to the primary contradiction between the working class and capitalism, the students would only be able to borrow the working classes' motivation and issues, at the expense of issues arising from their own reality. Yet if a dent could be made in their own reality as well, the span of areas in crisis would be stretched further, establishing real links with the workers' movement.

Once again, Gramsci has provided us with a key for interpreting the period we are living through in his essay on the issue of young people:

There are many "youth questions." Two seem especially important to me:

1) The "old" generation educates the young. There will be conflict, disagreement, etc., but these are superficial phenomena inherent in any educational work, unless there is class interference when the young people of the ruling class (understood both in the economic, political and moral sense) rebel and go over to the progressive class that is historically ready to take power. In this case, the young people go from being managed by the old of one class to being led by the old of another class. The real subordination of the young to the old generation continues, even in face of the conflicts mentioned above.

2) When the phenomenon assumes a so-called "national" character, and is not openly a case of class interference, then the issue is more complicated and chaotic. *Young people are in a state of permanent rebellion with persistent, deep causes, but there is no possibility of an analysis or critique of it, nor can they overcome it in an historically real and not in an abstract, theoretical way.* The old people really dominate but . . . *après moi, le deluge.* They can't manage to educate the young, to prepare them to take power. Why? Because the existent conditions call for the old people from another class to lead these young people, without doing it for extra-

neous reasons of political or military pressure. Although its normal outer signs have been suppressed, the struggle spreads like gangrene to the structure of the old class, weakening it and rotting it. It takes on sickly forms of mysticism, sensualism, moral apathy, pathological, psychological and physical degeneration, etc. The old structure cannot satisfy the new needs, and the permanent or semi-permanent unemployment of the so-called intellectuals is typical of this inadequacy. It is particularly harsh for most young people in that it leaves no open horizons. On the other hand, this leads to a closed, feudal, military-type situation that exacerbates problems it doesn't know how to resolve.[28]

Only an awareness of the nature of this permanent rebellion [see emphasis above] will allow it to be transformed into a movement that really supports the workers' movement. Only then will it avoid the danger of mystifying a new sort of interclass collaboration, in which each party's motivations to struggle are inevitably different. Through an analysis and awareness of the full range of motivations, we can avoid the chaos that Gramsci speaks of and recognize the national, and not class, character of the movement. We can also apply the analysis that we have outlined here for the rebellion of the technicians of practical knowledge to the student rebellion. Just as the technicians bring about a crisis in the relationship between their professional roles and the social structure, thus linking up with the larger struggles, so must the students act from their own reality, if they are to avoid falling into some sort of vague discontent.

Once students can identify the contradictions in their own specific terrain, they can move beyond that area, making the connections between their issues and those of the oppressed classes. It is working people who, with their labor, finance the schools, universities, and other learning institutions. But in order to appropriate them, they must possess knowledge of how these institutions perpetuate social divisions. And it is the student, as well as the technician, who can bring this knowledge to the more general political struggle.

Unless we eliminate the ambiguity of this situation, we run the risk of remaining entangled in our own specific fields, simply playing the part of the oppressed worker, and perpetuating the separation between the higher sphere of political struggle and a specific field of study or work. Or else we limit ourselves, within our respective fields, to sterile, dead-end disputes over our professions' internal contradictions. Here the only outlet is as a source of knowledge for the workers' movement, which can make it the grounds for their own revolt.

We cannot struggle *for* the oppressed class or *in the name of* the oppressed class, or else we will continue to maintain the same distance as the traditional intellectual. We have to struggle *with* the oppressed class but in order for this not to be limited to a verbal declaration, we must bring our own motivations to the struggle, enlarging its scope and depth. If, as technicians and middle-class students, we borrow the motivations of others, they sound empty, ring false, and arouse the just suspicions of the very people with whom we want to struggle. With their own motivations, the student rebellion can find real links with the workers' struggles.

The ambiguity becomes clear when students graduate and face the reality of a professional role that they theoretically reject; that is, the technician of practical knowledge. This role is the first defensive weapon they possess, and in moments of crisis they may use it, perplexed by the contradictions they experience, and which their professional activity helps to create. We can illustrate this phenomenon, even if only schematically, with the example of what happens in a psychiatric hospital undergoing the process of being transformed.

When patients are liberated and alternatives are created to free them from the institutional context that imprisoned them, the contradiction that emerges inevitably distresses the medical staff and the nurses. This anguish is greatest when only a low level of participation and involvement has been created in the hospital. The crisis itself provokes a break with the past, since their medical roles are called into question with a new awareness of the authority of those roles. Once the rigidity of the roles is broken, the organizational crisis must be dealt with as a constant contradiction, since the treatment staff is responsible for liberating the asylum and for letting patients gradually reclaim their freedom.

The freedom [for example, from restraints] that the patients acquire inherently limits the freedom that the staff has traditionally enjoyed, one which corresponds to the freedom of society, which its technicians and laws ensure. A total commitment to the patients is the sign of a true recognition of them, which will enable everyone—patients, nurses, and doctors—to become autonomous subjects. This commitment, inherent in the mutual task of changing the hospital, is sometimes experienced by young technicians as an authoritarian demand that limits their own autonomy and the sense of omnipotence they acquired during the student rebellions. The open asylum is easily experienced as if it were already a liberated territory, as if the commitment did not carry with it the necessity for compromising with social, administrative, and bureaucratic structures, and as if action were directly linked to the general political struggle, without being affected by the specific situation of the hospital.

The contradiction between negating the institution while administrating it is the first one that must be confronted. To the young technicians and veterans of the student revolt, this seems like a compromise with those in power. They tend to concentrate on radicalizing only one pole of the contradiction—the negation—and do not see that it takes place within a scientific ideology whose logic we must break. Instead of acting on the basis of the contradiction that has emerged, they tend to take extremist positions—a luxury of those who have no concrete reality to challenge them. Having been used to situations of noncompromise and limited for the first time by the ideological rules and bureaucracy they face, they experience great difficulty in challenging an all-engulfing immobility.

Additionally, they are used to thinking in terms of a clear, all-encompassing enemy—the social system and capitalism. This makes it difficult for them to pinpoint a target against which to struggle as they work towards a negation of the traditional institution and the simultaneous creation of new relationships. Usually, it is easy to choose an enemy in their midst, who changes from moment to moment and from situation to situation. In this explosive setting, however, the construction of a common goal is shattered by antagonistic groups which promote the same divisiveness that they originally fought against.

With three years of practical experience behind them, younger health workers are changing their views, as they have had to constantly measure up against and adjust their goals to the reality of the hospital. Nonetheless, in the beginning there was frustration with the fact that "work in a psychiatric hospital isn't that revolutionary after all," and involves more compromise than the need and desire for total purity would allow. There were two ways out of this frustration:

1. Searching for a "revolutionary agent" who, belonging to the proletariat, would ensure the "politically correct" line of action. Here the political interest shifted from the patients, who are also proletarians, to the nurses and a struggle to develop their political consciousness. The patients tended to be abandoned as a secondary issue, as was the relationship of the nurses to the patients. Yet since this relationship corresponds to the relation of abuse that underlies our social system, they abandoned the issue of breaking the logic of the institution and ending that abuse.

This approach ran the risk of promoting the nurses' identification with the doctors and bourgeois values instead of a consciousness of belonging to the same class as the patients. That might have caused them to identify the fight for their own liberation with that to liberate the patients. The nurses would thus assume a new authority, promoted by the activist doctors, through an identification with their values and their mediated relationship to the proletarian struggle, to be the agent of the abstract, all-encompassing "revolution." For the nurses, this revolution is not based on the real motivation of their own class and takes on the character of a bourgeois revolution that the doctors have proposed. This can only result in the weakening of the nurses' strength, as they assimilate the speech and opinions typical of doctors and their class.

2. Defending the autonomy of one's work to the bitter end. This is possible in an institution that is undergoing change, but when separated from the responsibility toward a shared strategy in the struggle, it can easily turn into a defense of one's own privileges and power, disguised by anti-authoritarian and antitheoretical slogans. And common goals vanish as the game of group dynamics, resistance, and counter resistance is reestablished, leaving behind an ambiguous situation where individuals are easily drawn into a vortex of psychodynamic interpretations and paranoid tendencies.

At the same time, the general hippie ideology of individual liberation was also present in the culture of those engaged in anti-institutional struggles. The now, or "everything at once" ideology contrasts with the dead weight of the situation and of the society at large. "Everything at once" makes sense if the popular and working class movements demand it, but when proclaimed by students or technicians it sounds like an empty slogan or a rationalization of our own impotence, or yet another demand for our privileges. The everything that students and technicians want for themselves should be included in the struggle for "everything—but we don't know when," waged by the oppressed class. When students and technicians learn how ideologies produce what they do, they have to communicate their needs in such a way that the oppressed class appropriates it as part of the everything that is their goal.

The uncertainties that will arise out of this situation must be carefully analyzed so that the permanent rebellion of young people turns into a tool of positive struggle. Our level of understanding our reality varies according to our experience and culture. When genuine action is possible and its meaning is clear to everyone, the goals of struggle can be shared. During more restricted periods, when fewer actions are possible, diversity and individual needs reemerge. In moving ahead, the same problems exist always, the same obstacles are collided with, the climate of violence that we live in promotes divisiveness and psychological tactics as a defense against the fear of succumbing. We must be aware of this and not fall into the trap of divisiveness, for we are both its victims and its perpetuators.

We must proceed with the uncertain search for new forms of struggle that will express themselves in our practice. But in order to survive the uncertainty, we have all internalized the necessity of living only one side of the contradictions that are slowly emerging, a side that changes depending on need. If we are to transform reality we still have the problem of simultaneously transforming ourselves. The transformation of human beings is the most difficult one, for we are imbued with a culture that makes us deny even our own contradictions, by rationalizations and escapes into an ideology that exaggerates only one side of all contradictions.

A Dialogue with R. D. Laing

In the last few years, our work has moved along paths that were both similar to and different from those of Ronald Laing. Even though our methods differed, we have both been committed to a concrete struggle to transform reality. Laing's theory and practice tend to focus and concentrate on individual subjective change; instead we tend to concentrate on social transformation, while keeping in mind other levels of the problems. Laing tries to shake the individual out of his inertia from within; we try to shake the society out of its inertia through working in a particular field. Concentrating on something does not mean reifying it, and these two aspects, the subjective and the social, are two sides of a single reality. They coexist within us and they both define us. In 1972, we held a conversation with R. D. Laing in which we sought to find the common denominator in these two experiences taking place in psychiatry:

FRANCO BASAGLIA: In recent years, political and cultural movements have established new methods and new perspectives for struggle. It might be useful, in a moment of political inactivity like the present one, to analyze how the social, political and cultural context has been changed by groups that have acted to reject current values in various fields. As an immediate response to needs emerging from a given situation, these groups have each worked in a specific area of expertise. In the psychiatric field, or in the student, prison, or working class movements, when our attempts to meet real needs are blocked, the importance that follows can easily turn into an absolute choice of one group's specific area or method in opposition to others. Once again, an attempt to meet real needs ends up meeting the needs of a given group. Because of the limited possibility of action and of achieving what we want for ourselves and for our lives, we experience our positions and our work ideologically in self-defense, as the only choices. This is not the way to create interdependencies between our various areas of activity, since we remain locked inside a logic that reproduces permanent antagonisms within every group, even as they try to combat it.

Given this, it might be useful to examine different theoretical and practical experiences in the same field, with a mutual willingness to learn from each other's experiences. The debate about whether to work inside or outside institutions, inside the system or outside, pre-supposes that inside and outside exist as clearly separate and antago-nistic positions. Inside and outside are created as opposite and com-pletely separate poles by a social system that is based on divisions at all levels. If we accept this premise, we are already playing into the hands of administrators. Perhaps we should try to work on uniting the inside and the outside, since in reality they are constantly linked and it is only the ideology of the inside and the ideology of the outside that separates them.

There are those who work inside institutions and those who work outside them, but this is just a formal definition of where you work, the nature of the bureaucratic restraints and the legal responsi-bilities, more often present in one field than another. In reality there is no total outside; it is assumed because it confirms the existence of a to-tal inside. If the outside is completely separate from institutions and from the system, then the inside is truly impregnable. It is important to know what work to do inside as an excuse for the outside, and the outside as an excuse for the inside. You've worked for many years in psychiatric institutions, and for many years outside of them. What do you think are the limits of each kind of work?

LAING: There is endless talk about the limits of working in institutions—the institutionalized roles, the economic control from the top, the com-plex bureaucratic organization where everything is dominated by po-litical forces. Top appointments are always made on a political basis. In other words, everything is controlled by forces that have nothing to do with medicine. Even control by the doctors, who constitute a reac-tionary corporation, would be better than this nonmedical control.

You discover the limits whenever any radical action is ob-structed, because no one except the bureaucrats has any control over the bureaucratic apparatus. Even when you analyze the system, the analysis can go only so far and then it's meaningless. I don't know whether this is true in Italy, but I think everyone should know and un-derstand what the system is and then decide whether to spend the rest of their life inside it. If Franco [Basaglia] thinks he can significantly change things in the direction he wants by remaining inside institu-tions, and he thinks that is possible, I respect his opinion and hope he succeeds with his intentions. I made enormous efforts to do what I in-tended inside the system ten years ago, but there was no room to do it. I had a choice either to stay in the system and try to accomplish what I wanted, without succeeding, or to get out. I got out. Obviously, I didn't completely leave, because I still hoped to influence the system from the outside. I think I've had more effect in my present situation than I could have had as a consultant to some psychiatric hospital in Inverness, or if I'd been on the Board of Directors of the North-West regional hospital.

BASAGLIA: In reality, outside the system doesn't exist, and there is a continuum between outside and inside. It is a question of a different angle or perspective.

LAING: We've arrived at a sort of negotiation with those in the "system." Our activities haven't been swept away and ignored because we've kept the channels of communication open. Nonetheless, the system has in some way been undermined by our work. There is a real alternative being created which hasn't been and won't be destroyed or lost, and will keep developing. We survived the first stage, where it could easily have been crushed by the Establishment's heavy hand, and now it can't be destroyed. In terms of the Establishment, nothing succeeds like success, as Jack Sutherland, the director of the Tavistock Clinic, used to say. What we've done has been successful in the only terms that these people understand, as an established social phenomenon.

In the psychiatric hospital, you can proceed ad infinitum without changing anything, because the bureaucratic apparatus has at its disposal infinite resources. They can simply remove someone from a position, shift personnel, create a scandal, finance one department rather than another, obstruct a research project, or cut off its funds and end it. Every time something real and different occurs, it can be stopped. Even if you stay half in and half out, something can be accomplished. There are no laws against living in a house together with patients. Why not do it?

BASAGLIA: Aren't there laws in terms of responsibilities towards patients? In this sort of case, who has responsibility?

LAING: Certainly, there are strict laws about such things. It's just that there are no laws against a doctor living with a nondoctor, who happens to be the patient of another doctor. Many people are married to schizophrenics. There are no laws against that. There are no laws against someone diagnosed as schizophrenic living somewhere, and no laws against a doctor living with him or her, as long as no inhabitant of a building is a patient of someone living in the same building.

It's not even necessary that they be doctors—they can be medical students or anyone else. There's nothing to object to in all of this, if you state that you're not giving medical treatment. If matters were to be carried to extremes, an unusual legal case might emerge that might resolve many interesting issues.

We've had to contact municipal agencies, speak with the police, and handle any interrogations by Parliament and the Ministry of Health. No legal action was taken against us. No member of our community was a patient of mine. When one of the American doctors who had come to work with us in London requested a license from the General Medical Council, he had to explain what he planned to do. He explained what we were doing—no medication, no prescriptions, no form of treatment. He explained this to the BMC [British Medical Center] and they responded that for what we were doing, no medical license was required. You can work with the Philadelphia Association in London without having a medical degree,* because they are not engaged in medical work. Students at Bristol who were fed up with psychiatry as they saw it practiced, bought a house and went to live there with patients, as in a commune. Similarly, in America, there are mental health communities where the staff consists of anthropologists, sociologists, psychologists, and many medical students, who run everything themselves. It isn't the easiest thing in the world to live with people who are disturbed, who suffer a great deal. Being able to endure their agony is a difficult thing. I couldn't do something like that right now, but there are people willing to do it. I would have been able to do it ten or twenty years ago.

BASAGLIA: There's also the anguish that you have to face every day in the institutions and perhaps that's why it's hard to work "inside." This is the difficult problem we come up against: why put up with this increasingly oppressive anguish?

LAING: I think that as you get older and have done this kind of work for a certain number of years, you become like an aging boxer; after a while, you have to retire and devote yourself to coaching. The people who are best suited for this kind of work now will already be too old in a few years. It's like athletes; the best years are your youth when you can cope with making a great effort. When you get older, you've

*The Philadelphia Association was a charitable trust organized by Laing with his associates including Cooper and Esterson. In 1965 the Association leased Kingsley Hall, Laing's radical therapeutic community in the East End of London.—Ed.

had enough so the oldest can turn to training the youngest. The young can do this kind of work—they have the vitality and the endurance. They can cope with not sleeping for nights on end, being completely exhausted and then sleeping it off. It's very demanding work and both physically and emotionally strenuous. It's all right for someone twenty to thirty years old, before having a family or after their children are grown, but not while they have small children.

BASAGLIA: The issue of training is the focus of our work within institutions, but the picture in Italy is still very confused. In the field of psychiatry, university training still avoids any real contradictions. The patient being treated in a university hospital must offer some special pedagogic, scientific interest in terms of the professor's notion of pedagogy and science. It is a somewhat artificial reality. The young students know nothing about real patients in asylums, where "true psychiatry" is practiced. They need a practical training that puts them in direct contact with the psychiatric field, but instead they are required to take academic courses. The educational authorities once again manage to destroy a great deal of potential.

    At Gorizia, we tried to explain the function of psychiatric ideology as it masks social contradictions, and to point out the political nature of definitions of the norm that are increasingly being established outside of psychiatry, and which psychiatry merely validates. A problem we found is that many young people coming from the student movement often make the typical error of focusing on the political aspect of their work and abandoning the patient, who is still the central problem of the psychiatric hospital. They tend to direct their political interest toward the nurses, believing this is a more political choice. In practice, they experience their relationship with the patient in an ideological and humanitarian light, and their relationship with the nurses as political, because the nurses belong to the working class and represent a further step in the fight against the institution.

    What was originally a movement aimed at understanding how an ideology develops and is maintained in a specific situation, in order to enlarge our practical understanding of how ideologies function in our social system, is presently in danger of becoming part of the general political ideology, incapable of affecting the specific institution. This would mean returning from the specific to the general, regressing to the stage of institutional politics that we had before we learned the political meaning of our specific technical interventions.

    This is the situation in terms of training in Italy, and I imagine in other countries as well. The phenomenon is occurring in various fields, not just in psychiatry, as students encounter the reality of their professional roles. This is why it is worth trying to understand so that we don't continue to make apparent changes without really making any progress.

LAING: And what do Franco and his group do? What do they tell young people who come to them? Do they just give them a political interpretation of the situation in Italy, that they can get elsewhere? If young people want to collaborate with the nurses, then they are forced to take an interest in the patients and have less fear of them than the nurses have. Anything else is just an excuse not to deal with the patients. Their task is to provide an example for the nurses through their way of dealing with the patients.

BASAGLIA: That's what happened at Gorizia, but now the politicized young people are afraid of falling into the trap of making Gorizia, and what it represents, into an ideology.

LAING: Someone has to overcome this fear, this flight from the pain of others that reminds us of our own unhappiness, our own limits and desperation. Someone has to manage to stay with someone whom they realize they absolutely cannot help, without experiencing a sense of failure. This negative capacity is fundamental and important for our analysis. To face uncertainty and doubt when it comes, and to be totally disoriented by it, constitutes a falsely positive ideological position. It is a defensive escape from exercising that negative capacity I spoke of before, and it is completely nondialectical. The young psychiatrist who possesses a new language, internalized as ideology, develops a kind of agitation syndrome. His sense of guilt and personal fear means he can be dishonest with himself, often resulting in the adoption of an air of purity and superiority simply because he belongs to the New Left or the post New Left, and that he isn't a fascist. In practice, however, he may not be better or worse than some idealistic bourgeois psychotherapist who makes his patients pay for their sessions, but perhaps does a serious job.

     I think the best solution is that experienced psychiatrists who haven't chosen one of these false solutions teach young students by their example, and not with words or seminars. . . .

BASAGLIA: That is what we're trying to do and if we succeed, the institution should be therapeutic at all levels, even for the therapists. This is what constitutes training. However, it's also necessary to understand the real constraints on our work. In terms of young students, is there an analogous problem in England, since the phenomenon is happening in many other European countries?

LAING: It isn't a problem for us because whoever comes to us for training lives with the patients. They don't just spend a part of their time there—they all live together.

BASAGLIA: In a psychiatric institution, however, there might be a thousand patients and seven hundred nurses, and the body of rules governing the organization of the hospital complicates matters.

LAING: Exactly. But what prevents you from using a house where ten or fifteen people can live, half of them medical students and the other half schizophrenics? This house could be part of everyone's training, for a period of time, and could be a part of every psychiatric hospital. It's a simple thing to do. No nurses are needed. Everyone is responsible for themselves, without a need for rules and everyone does what they can to manage to live together. If you want to overcome the dilemma of institutions, then why not simply leave them?

BASAGLIA: To continue to work inside institutions can have both a real and symbolic value; whatever one's role, one can show the majority of inmates that in spite of everything, institutions can be fought. Acting outside the institution could become an alternative, but one not available to everybody. The exemplary value of these alternatives would diminish whenever they involve privileges, in comparison to work in the public institution. There would still be the problem that everything can become institutionalized and as you say, at a certain point you can only go "outside" so far and not further.

LAING: If you were to go to the psychiatry section of a bookstore and read the major texts published worldwide, you wouldn't know that I existed or that this approach to mental health existed. If you then look at the beginning of the inaugural speech of the newly-formed Royal College of Psychiatrists, here, too, this new approach to mental illness scarcely exists. Yet there are two paragraphs later in the speech which defend the system against a position about which it pretends to know nothing. Or else a psychiatry professor contacts me and tells me somewhat ironically that his attacks on me seem to cause the opposite effect on his students. Both his students and staff have asked that I come speak to them. Since he doesn't want me to meet his students, he would be happy if I were to meet with older staff members privately, as if we were beginning some sort of negotiation.

There's a kind of grumbling, especially among older psychiatrists, who feel that the earth is giving way beneath them. I don't know how significant this is. I have the impression that the same thing is happening in America. I don't think many young medical students believe in the psychiatric texts the way we had believed in them twenty-five years ago. They still have to finish college; they still have to acquire the jargon, but many are deeply dissatisfied. Many realize that everything is heavily institutionalized. They know where the money comes from, how jobs and careers are controlled, and that all of this offers them very limited and circumscribed futures. There is a genuine change of consciousness within the psychiatric profession. It is something very subtle, and in certain fields it is stronger than in others, but even when weak it is still there.

BASAGLIA: What are your current plans?

LAING: I am trying to find money for the Philadelphia Association. Real estate values in London are increasing rapidly, so it seems a good time to buy a house and have a permanent place, without always worrying about not being able to pay the rent or having to move from house to house.* We already have a secretary, a library, and a place to hold seminars. We want to have room for all our activities and funds for scholarships. In short, we need all the things that money can provide, and it's good to have the money to buy them. We could use a place in the country with easy access to the city, not that there are any specific advantages to the country-side. I hope that a similar place will be opened soon in New York, which will have close ties to us and I hope we'll soon establish a kind of central headquarters for training therapists. As I tried to say the other evening, we want to relate physical, emotional, psychological, and social factors to the mental sciences; in other words, a type of training that doesn't fragment these things as is now done, and that doesn't compensate with words for an empty practice. I know of no training center for therapists that works on the

*The Association ran a total of seven therapeutic group households in London. In 1977, the Association took over an estate in Somerset in order to found a farming, craft, and study center with both "disturbed" and undisturbed people living collectively. —ED.

body, and on sensations and emotions, as well as with so-called psy-chotherapy, with dyads, triads, family systems, networks, etc. We want a therapy that combines theory and practice and includes all fields, without devoting itself to the exclusive study of any single one. It can be done, not only by theoretical seminars and study groups, but by working with families and living in the community. I hope we suc-ceed in creating this center. It would be a training center where people from all over the world could come, and it doesn't matter whether it is located in the United States or England.

Laing, sometimes incorrectly associated with Cooper's antipsychiatry,[29] suggested the creation of an asylum which would meet the need for protection and shelter for those who are different, a place where they could express themselves without limitations and where others could learn to live with them. Just as Laing hopes that we persist in our struggles within institutions, we hope that his asylum manages not to become an institution. It is inevitably part of the social and economic logic of psychiatric in-stitutions, even if not bureaucratically defined by them. Although Laing's approach probes more deeply than ours into the subjec-tive dimensions, it does not have the same incisiveness about the political and social reality in which subjects become objectified. Nonetheless, we have to learn to see the experiences of others not as antagonistic, but as complementary, so that we can avoid the logic of divisiveness and not be isolated, each in our own little fields like traditional intellectuals who defend their own ideas and their own trifling inventions.

Science and the Criminalization of Need

In recent years, two kinds of war have increasingly taken shape: a worldwide imperialist one alongside anti-imperialist movements; and the constant everyday one with no promise of armistice—the war of peace, with its own instruments of torture and its own crimes. War inures us to accepting its disorder, violence, and cru-elty as the criterion for a peaceful existence.

Hospitals, prisons, asylums, factories, and schools are the places where these peace crimes are carried out in the name of order and in the defense of mankind. The people who are supposed to be defended are not people as they really are; they are people as they should be, after treatment, indoctrination, destruction of their potential, and after recovery. They are people who are divided, separate, and split, and this kind of manipulation is ideal for adjusting them totally to the social order that breeds on criminalization and crimes.

Hospitals and drugs kill more people than they cure. (American statistics acknowledge that eighty percent of medicine is used to cure illnesses caused by medicine itself.)[30] Prisons produce more criminals than they imprison. Asylums produce custom-made illness by creating the passivity, apathy, and total annihilation necessary to control and manage the institution. In factories, workers are exploited, forced into dangerous work conditions where so-called "white deaths" are calculated as a necessary evil.

Schools continue to not teach and not carry out an educational role by weeding out those who have not learned or been educated. Students who demand a reorganization of teaching and some guarantee of future work are accused of subverting public order. University studies degenerate increasingly and do not teach necessary skills. While there will be jobs for those who have studied abroad or who have learned a specialization in industrial schools, there will also be a new flood of underemployed or unemployed university graduates. Seas and rivers are polluted because their waters carry the chemical death produced by industry, but only when it becomes widespread are millions set aside or spent for purifying and filtering plants that could have prevented the damage beforehand, rather than remedied after the funeral.

All of this is accomplished in the name of the good of the community, in the name of progress which will presumably give people well-being and happiness. But which people? Every time there is a real crisis, the abstract concepts of mankind and humanity resurface with the progress of science and civilization existing for their sake. In order to meet the needs of this nonexistent mankind, progress continues to mean the progress of technology, of industry, and big capital that can only deal with people by exploiting them and reducing them to its own design as surreptitiously as possible. Progress is human when industry and capital are expanding. When these are in crisis, what becomes human is austerity, an economic rule that brings people back to the old and lost values, as happened in the recent energy crisis. It is economic logic, whether in favorable or unfavorable conditions, that decides what is human or not, what is healthy or not, what is beautiful or ugly, and what is proper or worthy of blame.

These are such obvious points that it is almost embarrassing to make them. It is the time-worn tale of the child who sees the emperor with no clothes standing amidst a frightened and cowardly crowd who fears him because they have been duped. But emperors are always naked and we are the ones who give them clothes when we accept, rather than reject, their manipulations as they constantly create new rules for our lives. Scientific and institutional ideologies guarantee this manipulation by bringing together the manipulators and the manipulated, the controllers and the controlled, so that the former identify with their seemingly active and autonomous role and the latter endure what they are not in a position to reject.

Yet there are those who still maintain that in the last century giant steps have been taken by mankind in achieving its own freedom and control over its destiny. Science declares that it is always searching for new tools to liberate mankind from its own contradictions and those of nature. If you examine or work inside the institutions created by our science and by our civilization, you become aware of how technologically innovative tools have really only given a new appearance to essentially unchanged conditions.

Ever since the time of the ship of fools—which according to medieval legend sailed the seas and rivers with its bizarre, undesirable cargo—science and civilization have only managed to maroon more firmly these "islands of isolation" where both sick deviants and healthy (but guilty and therefore criminal) deviants are sent. For the morally corrupt, prison; for the spiritually sick, the asylum. This has been science's great achievement.

For centuries, criminals, prostitutes, homosexuals, alcoholics, thieves, and eccentrics have shared the same place where differences in their "abnormality" are leveled by an element common to them all—deviation from the norm and from its rules. The walls of the asylum have limited, controlled, and hidden the possessed and the crazy, who express an unintentional spiritual evil, along with the criminals who express a deliberate, intentional evil. Madness and criminality have together represented a part of human beings that have had to be controlled, hidden, and eliminated, until science has sanctioned their strict separation, according to their different characteristics.

According to Enlightenment rationality, the prison was to be the punitive institution for all those who deliberately disobeyed the rules embodied in the laws protecting property and defining proper public behavior, structures of authority, power, and the degree of exploitation. The spiritually sick, disordered person, the crazy person who didn't live according to dominant rationality, or the eccentric who lived according to the rules created by his or her reason or madness, began to be defined as "sick." An institution was needed where the boundaries between reason and madness would be clearly defined and where those infringing on public order could be relegated and labeled as outrageous and dangerous.

Once prisons and asylums were separated, they continued to maintain the same function of protecting and defending the norm, and abnormality became the norm only where it was hemmed in by walls which defined its difference and its distance.

Science has therefore separated crime from madness, giving each a new dignity. For madness it is the dignity of being translated into an abstraction and defined in terms of illness; for crime it is the dignity of becoming the subject of research by criminologists and scientists, who have continued to find the biological factors responsible for abnormal behavior, including the discovery of the extra Y-chromosome. Notwithstanding the formal separation into two abstract entities, each with its own institution, in reality the function of each institution remains unchanged. Despite abstract recognition of their new dignity, neither the criminal, who must atone for the offense done to society, nor the madman, who must pay for his maladjusted and rude behavior, have ever been considered human beings.

The institutions created for both their reeducation and redemption, and for their treatment and rehabilitation have not changed as they continue their separate development along parallel lines. Legal reformers on the one hand, phrenologists and specialists on the other, have at times established new regulations,

categories, theories, and subdivisions, yet the relationship between civil society and those it excludes always remains the same.
None of them have changed the nature of that exclusion that is
based on violence, humiliation, and the total destruction of institutionalized individuals. This demonstrates that the actual goals of
these rehabilitating and curing institutions are the suppression of
those who should be cured and reeducated.

An analysis of the various institutions for deviants, at different levels of industrial, technological, and economic development, might explain their unchanging function of controlling and
eliminating their populations.

In countries where the economic and social situation
does not demand a kind of divided institutional super-structure,
deviance is still subjected to undifferentiated, open violence without coverups. Science has not yet been asked to justify theoretically a kind of discrimination between deviants. It has not yet
been asked to perform its colonizing job of dividing up abnormal
behavior. This division, useful at a later stage of development, is
not yet known, and violence or the threat of violence is still
enough to guarantee public order. When a division based on scientific principles does exist, it is an imported institution that
does not correspond at all to the local reality. For example, in a
city like Rio de Janeiro, there is an attempt to import a Yankee-
style psychiatric institution because in an area that is industrializ-
ing, a different kind of control is needed. In general, however, in
Brazil, especially the Brazilian Northeast, open violence and undifferentiated imprisonment remain the only means of control.
There is no need to mystify repressive measures towards deviants by a scientific approach that divides up deviant behavior. A
clear example of this is the Kleinian psychoanalytic organization
in Porto Alegre [Brazil], which only helps the psychoanalysts
who run it, while the unmet needs and suffering of many people
are controlled by an overt, [militarist] violence that has no need
to hide itself behind sophisticated scientific masks.

In this perspective, the horror of torture in South American countries and elsewhere takes on an organized form, turning
into an institution. Torture is the super-structure that really corresponds to the structural level of these countries. Torture as an institution is the only method that politicians (that is, the military)

know for controlling a situation so potentially explosive that only the constant threat of violence maintains stability. For a people that have no hope of changing their unbearable conditions, or who have hope but have not turned that into a concrete struggle, the threat of being thrown into prison, or into an asylum as the punishment for deviant behavior has no effect. For example, those who are starving or homeless can actually see imprisonment as a way *to* survive. In such a context, torture becomes the only effective means of elimination, the only real threat of destruction, and therefore the only social control that corresponds to a more "primitive" level of [capitalist] development.

Economic structures and institutional organizations correspond at every level of development; it is not coincidental that asylums develop with the beginning of the Industrial Revolution. Like all kinds of public welfare, they take on their broadest institutional form when what is productive must be separated from what is unproductive. With the birth of the industrial age, the relationship is no longer between people and society, but between people and production, which creates a new criterion of discrimination for anything—deviance, abnormality, illness—that might stand in the way of productive rhythms.

At the level of technological development typical of Western countries, the organization of control is no longer clear. It is both masked and legitimized by different scientific ideologies. For the asylum there is the medical ideology that justifies the institutional violence and isolation by defining the disease as incurable. The prisoners pay for the offense they committed against society. The patients pay for an offense they did not commit, and the price they pay is so disproportionate to the guilt, that they experience a double alienation because of their total incomprehension and the total incomprehensibility of their situation. The ideology of punishment underlying the prisons, and the medical ideology of incurable disease, which is the basis of the asylum, have no bearing on the problems of criminality or of illness. Their function is simply to repress and control deviant behavior. Ideology conceals the repression by justifying and legitimizing it, but legitimized violence is still violence.

If the rehabilitation goals of both institutions were genuine, one would find rehabilitated patients and prisoners reinte-

grated into society. This rarely happens because entering one of
these institutions marks the beginning of a career with familiar
patterns and outcome.[31] The formal similarity between these institutions seems to be only a negative one. While new interpretations tend to justify both criminality and mental illness in terms of
psychosocial dynamics, the institution is still based on the concept
of atonement for guilt through punishment.

The madmen that Pinel separated from criminals in
chains are still symbolically and really in chains. Both categories
are in separate institutions, based on the same destructive principles, and they are both defined by the same value judgment that
sees them as dangerously different. For both, the reality and the
violence remain the same. It does not matter whether the torture
is sophisticated or not, whether the chains are real or symbolic, as
in more technically developed countries. The goal is always to protect the dominant group by destroying whatever interferes with
social order. The logic of subordination and repression is the same
whenever it tries to create submissive, noncritical people who totally identify with the laws. At the same time, separating and isolating human contradictions like illness or crime means treating
people affected by them as if they were permanently branded.

The paradoxical effect of this stigma is that precisely
those people who have exhibited a tendency to behave strangely
are asked in institutions to lead an exemplary, perfect life. Whoever is stigmatized is recognizable and can be immediately singled
out; generally they are weaker, more vulnerable, and their situation is unstable. They have no economic, social, or cultural power
with which to fight the cruel campaign that calls for them to behave perfectly. The inmate or patient embodies a contradiction
which must be covered over. Because it constitutes a threat to public order, the contradiction must be immediately defined, classified, and neutralized and must not call into question the absolute
rules that ensure this order.

Criminality and mental illness are human contradic-
tions. They can also be natural [i.e., biological] facts but most often they are socially and historically produced. Yet the afflicted
continue to suffer the consequences as if it were a matter of individual guilt. It is always the people without cultural or economic
power, those playing no positive social role who have no private

place for their deviant behavior, who suffer the stiffest penalties. The dominant group protects public order, production, and organizational efficiency and thus protects itself and whoever works for it from the potential threat of the nonproductive people by threatening them with possible isolation. In the name of efficiency and exploitation, the dominant group recreates the master/slave dialectic wherein the master protects the slave from the threat of those who might disturb his work by creating institutions to isolate and neutralize the threat. Yet the existence of these institutions threatens the servant who could be subject to the same penalties as well. These so-called rehabilitational institutions therefore have a double function: violence as a concrete system for elimination and destruction, and violence as a symbolic threat to eliminate and destroy.

At our level of technological development, every contradiction must be isolated in separate spaces where individuals pay for the very contradiction they represent. People who are different must be singled out immediately and isolated to demonstrate that we (the sane, normal, good citizens) are not them; it is not the structure of our social organization that produces contradictions. It's always the others—the foreigners, the strangers, the corrupters, the bad company—who produce the contamination which must be prevented and counteracted. The noncontradictory nature of social norms, the boundaries defining moral and public order, must be protected. The preventive character of ideologies and the violent nature of institutions is based on the early identification of diversity and the confirmation of its inequality.

The complicity of science with the law means that one can define the criminal as psychopathic, weak, or crazy, but not permanently if the label is less prejudicial than that of a criminal. Psychiatric evaluations are merely a tool that permits one to cross over from one field to another by measuring quantitatively the abnormal features of the subject under examination.

Whoever crosses the threshold of a prison, penitentiary, or mental asylum enters a world where everything contributes to destroying people, even if it is apparently organized to save them. Yet criminologists continue to see the reality of the prisons as the most direct and glaring proof of the prisoner's essential criminality, just as psychiatrists continue to see the nature of the asylum as a sign of the psychological and moral degeneration produced by the illness.

The efficiency of institutional organization is maintained with this destructive logic, because the institution as an organization cannot take risks. The missed opportunities turn into negative realities for those held within, since the institution does not have to respond to their demands. Being classified mentally ill or criminal robs these people of all basic rights, even when the institutions continue to define themselves as therapeutic and rehabilitational. Ultimately, rehabilitative institutions, to which individuals are relegated when they do not participate in production and do not or cannot accept the rules of the game, share the same function as the "positive" institutions—family, school, workplace. These institutions are interchangeable, communicating vessels marked by changing definitions and labels. A young boy sent to reform school will later go on to prison or to the asylum, depending on whether it is his healthy or sick deviance that is stressed. Once he has been stigmatized by the first experience, he can only manage with great difficulty to avoid the last two alternatives.

These are the kinds of institutions that correspond to the level of development in most European countries. When the country is more industrially advanced, as is the United States, the usual control of deviance through isolation and segregation is no longer enough. In the more industrially advanced countries, the capitalist system, in addition to producing more consumer goods that signal the well-being achieved by the population, also produces more contradictions, that is, more deviations from the rule. Control no longer occurs exclusively through the institutions that segregate deviants, although they do continue to exist. They may even be reorganized, modernized, and made less openly repressive because control now occurs primarily elsewhere. New, subtler, more pervasive ways identify diversity through early diagnosis, prevention, health services, and welfare, and through medicalizing behaviors that have little to do with psychology as psychological conflicts.[32]

This way of controlling deviance, which places most social conflicts under the domain of psychology, medicine, and health services, is a new model ready for export [from the United States] to less developed countries. In areas where this kind of control is not yet needed to protect public order and industrial development, artificial needs must be created for the new model to meet. Precisely because the needs are artificial and foreign to the new concrete situation, they offer a new opportunity for domination.

The imposition of a foreign culture is one of the classic methods of domination and colonization, a method well-tested by missionaries whose faith and morality was followed by conquering armies. Domination always occurs by destruction and annihilation of the indigenous culture. Only when the dominated population is robbed not only of its economy but of its values, can it accept the conqueror's values. In fact, it is enslaved and conquered in direct relation to the distance between its values and those of the foreign culture. An example is the proletariat's lack of access to bourgeois culture, which reinforces their own inferiority in terms of a distant and incomprehensible culture.

Oppression always occurs on two levels—either outright murder and massacre, or the imposition of new values and ideologies which manipulate and mask the violence, murder, and massacre. Exporting ideologies and institutions like the therapeutic community or community mental health centers to underdeveloped countries provides a cover for the open violence that continues to correspond to their level of development. When a population becomes aware that it must meet its own needs itself, the strategy of domination is revealed for what it is—a primitive system for colonization and a return to open violence and murder. The Popular Unity movement in Chile is a clear example of this. If a population took control of meeting its own needs, the imperialist system would blow up rather than run risks. In such a situation when violence *within* institutions is no longer useful, the hegemonic forces revert to violence as *an institution* with no need for scientific cover-ups and deceptions. They kill, torture, and eliminate those who have discovered their game and who look for tools to escape.

These different kinds of violence, whether legitimated by scientific ideologies, hidden behind welfare institutions, or simply openly practiced, are the methods of control that correspond to different levels of development. They are all simultaneously present at any given moment. When there is a crisis the most suitable method is chosen, whether the form of control is based on the psychological analysis of conflicts or on mass murder. Those with power always find a way to legitimate violence, simply by imposing it. They combine the various methods at their disposal until they manage to humanize torture, at which point they provide those who are tortured the aid of doctors, psychologists, and social workers.

The socioeconomic level of most European countries is still tied to institutional control as a form of repression. Reforms have only recently begun to be planned to create more permissive institutions where illness, deviance, and criminality can be controlled without overt recourse to violence. But within the logic of capitalism, the construction of new prisons signifies the creation of new prisoners. If the goal remains the control rather than the satisfaction of needs, building new hospitals will only create new patients. Controlling needs means creating new institutions that offer new jobs and services and which automatically become part of the same productive cycle. This process is typical of all organizations whose justification is their own maintenance and survival.

In Italy, no one would dare say that locked institutions are worthy of a civilized country. No one is unaware of the inhuman conditions in which patients live, but the transformation of these institutions only leads to formal changes. Even when there are partial benefits in terms of the patients' lives, the changes are new technical and organizational rationalizations that become a new system of control. If the overall logic is unaltered, transformation, rationalization, and control are merely stages in a self-perpetuating process that creates constant changes in the forms without ever altering the structure of things. The transformation occurs as a technical answer to an economic demand: every level of economic development requires a different form of control. It is always economic laws that then necessitate a new technical rationalization which can keep the transformation under control.

Emotional indignation against the violence in our repressive institutions should lead to the demand for changes that might adequately meet the needs that are expressed by illness and deviance. Prisons, asylums, and torture will remain the same as long as our economic system sees the present institutions are useful to its further growth. Stanley Cohen correctly maintains that ever since prisons have been in existence, people have talked about prison reform.[33] Prisons, asylums, and torture can change only if the fundamental structure that these institutions uphold is changed. This is supported by the fact that while there is much theoretical talk about the need to change them, every practical attempt to change the status quo is obstructed and violently repressed. This response shows us that when transformations do occur, they are not simply technical responses to specialized problems.

In order to work within these institutions of violence, and to reject our authority as functionaries of public order, we must reveal the nature of these institutions and give those who live inside them the chance to understand how they operate. From this perspective, the technicians' job in these institutions must be a political one—to link their specific professional work to the larger social structure and reveal the connections and implications. Their work and analysis of violence should be limited to demystifying the contradiction between custody and rehabilitation so basic to asylums and prisons. Above all, they must try to clarify the goals and the methods of this violence in terms of the social structure in which it occurs. We need to develop an analysis of the social structure and to emerge from the separate, specialized fields that imprison us, while still preserving our specific perspectives and our work.

The bourgeois state is founded on an artificial, historically created division which is assumed to be a natural division into classes. Once this division is accepted as a natural phenomenon, a series of regulations and institutions—apparently aimed at resolving those natural contradictions—in reality work to maintain the original division that supports the socioeconomic structure. The more unnatural the regulations and the social structure, the more violent and repressive the control mechanisms. They do not resolve the natural contradiction they were established to resolve, but instead maintain the artifice that the regulation tries to conceal.

This process is neither so simple nor so obvious as it first appears. There are various ways in which our social system manages to maintain the class divisions necessary for its survival. There is a common denominator between them—the tendency to isolate phenomena, as if they did not arise and exist in a network of reciprocal relationships, so that they are separated from their context and can take on an absolute, natural character. Scientific theories try explicitly to isolate phenomena into deceptive, specialized fields while institutions try to prove that phenomena are fixed and unchanging. In reality, both attempt to identify and establish natural differences with the same process used for the original division into classes, the model for all later divisions.

With the ideologies and institutions that attempt to control deviance—asylums and prisons—the negative, abnormal behavior is isolated in such a way that the individual is totally subsumed as if the history, environment, values, relationships, and social forces present in every individual's life had ceased to exist. The patient's negative behavior is one aspect of a complex of biological, social, and psychological factors, but it is isolated and turned into something absolute and unchangeable. The criminal is irreducibly criminal and prison is the only place to control his or her madness. Yet criminality and madness are occurrences that are part of human life; they are expressions of what human beings are and what they can become through the world of relationships. Criminals and madmen (and we will not go into the complicated matter of how these definitions are made) retain, in their criminality and madness, all the other aspects of their humanity—their oppression, impotence, and suffering, and their vitality and need for a life which would be neither criminal nor sick.

But delinquents automatically become the jurisdiction of criminology, a science whose research object is criminality and not the total human being. Similarly, madmen and the sick as deviants become the jurisdiction of psychiatry, a science which conducts research on psychological deviance and not on total human beings. Scientific ideologies thus function to establish absolute definitions for phenomena in their field, and turn them into natural events, just as institutions act to prove concretely that these natural phenomena are irreversible. If mental illness and criminality, are caused by biological abnormalities, and not historical and social phenomena, then locking people up is the only logical and responsible solution. The repressive institution and segregation are the only alternative when society must be protected and secured. As in the face of natural disasters, no one is responsible, no one is guilty. The individual becomes totally crazy or totally criminal. Even though this negative totality is artificially based on reifying one or another aspect of the individual, nonetheless it will be the basis of his or her social exclusion and of his engulfing social identity.

Hence, individuals are being dissected, their diversity isolated, and their differences magnified and strengthened. To what end? From the results, one certainly cannot say that the process serves to rehabilitate deviants or restore the patient's health. If that were the case, the majority of inmates in both asylums and prisons would end up rehabilitated and cured. The general failure of these institutions is not explained by the limitations of science. The one very obvious element in this process that is never taken into account by psychiatrists and criminologists is the economic class of the people in these institutions, who, not coincidentally, are almost all of working class origins, as are those in many other reeducational or welfare institutions such as orphanages, correctional facilities, and penal establishments. Except for those rare cases of middle-class criminals with means, who in any event always manage to find the instruments for avoiding or reducing their sentence, it seems that incurable criminality and madness are the privilege of only one class. For despite new sociological theories and interpretations, science continues to confirm in its practice that madness and criminality are natural events. Are they really part of the nature of the proletariat or is their madness and criminality made natural and unchangeable by reifying their diversity?

If mental illness and crime are natural events, the almost total absence of members of the dominant class in prisons and asylums seems to prove that outside these institutions there is a different concept of recovery, and illness and criminality lose the natural, unchanging character they have in the prisons and asylums. Recovery is dependent on the tools available and the will to recover. The bourgeoisie provides itself with those tools and that will. In terms of mental illness, psychotherapy and psychoanalysis are available to those who agree to search for the unconscious causes of the abnormal behavior. The behavior is not interpreted as natural or unchanging. Sometimes it may turn out to be, but its history and development are investigated, and the various aspects of its process are probed whenever possible.

The analysis of the unconscious and the elaborations on complexes and conflicts are part of a culture and a set of values that have nothing to do with the proletariat. What is more, a new code language would have to be mastered, completely unknown to them. In Italy, the petit bourgeoisie and the proletarians who aspire to bourgeois values are just beginning to be affected, but assimilation of this culture, foreign to them and their needs, can only act as a further element of domination and not as an instrument of liberation. Whether or not a proletarian patient in a mental hospital has an unresolved Oedipal complex will seem ridiculous even to the layman. Yet is any other research conducted into the causes of abnormal behavior in patients in our asylums? Why are the symptoms of the bourgeois patient explained and justified? Why are their unconscious motivations investigated and explained while the proletarian patient continues to be seen as having a natural, unchangeable illness and to be completely identified with his or her symptoms? How can we understand the deep causes of the illness when asylum psychiatry is based on robbing individuals of their history?

The same description holds for criminality. A wealthy bourgeois criminal has no problems being rehabilitated and reintegrated into society. The crime committed is accepted as historically and socially produced, and this justifies the criminal act. It is an event which will not determine the entire future of the criminal, nor is his past read totally in terms of the crime that, in a given moment, he committed. In the environment and in the life of these people, there is room to recover that is provided by their class affiliation. The problem of rehabilitation is nonexistent because these criminals have a history that, for their peers, explains their crimes. Economically and culturally they do not need to commit crimes again. Furthermore, crimes committed on a vast scale—corruption, political crimes—receive only minor sentences, immunity, or pardons. The respectability of the perpetrators remains unharmed. With this type of crime, corruption is considered a natural act inherent in politics, which always being dirty makes it difficult to keep one's hands clean once one plays the game. Corruption is so deeply ingrained in politics that it grants immunity to those committing the crimes and reaping benefits. Individual corruption is seen as an historical and social occurrence, justified by the number of unavoidable circumstances that influence the individual.

This never happens with the oppressed class that commits a crime. Their kind of criminal has no history, or rather his or her history is only the history of his or her offenses and criminal record. These are criminals by nature, just as the unemployed are lazy and do-nothings by nature. There are no social, psychological, or economic causes that justify or explain their acts—only their criminality, which is seen as biological, ingrained in their character, race, or somatic characteristics. Any attempt to trace the history of a proletarian criminal is doomed to failure because it would be a history of privation, abuse, and violence, all traces of which must be eliminated.

Even Lombroso, who can be credited with historicizing the delinquent by recognizing the social factors present in abnormal behavior, in his practical conclusions ended up confirming the natural differences that required the isolation of the proletarian criminal.

Who investigates why crimes are committed? The widow of a farm laborer killed by the police twenty years ago during the occupation of uncultivated fields in a large landed property stated on a recent television program: "If people had work, they wouldn't have to occupy land in order to live." That seems elementary, yet those who occupy land are punished and killed, without the understanding that unemployed farm workers do not decide to occupy land either on a whim or because of innate criminality. The obvious consequence, however, is that the laborer is punished as a criminal, and the land remains untilled if the owner wishes it.

Our social system cannot rehabilitate these criminals and these madmen. Otherwise it would be another social system. When transformations and reforms are planned without changing the overall structure, nothing changes. There is talk of a new criminality and yet no search for its causes in the decline of values, in the broken promises, in frustrated expectations, or in the dissatisfaction with a life that is more and more impossible, devoid of meaning, violent, and repressive, and in which the struggle for survival becomes harder and harder. If this is not taken into account, every time new distinctions between more or less serious forms of criminality are formulated, new regulations and institutions identical to the preceding ones will be realized. Confronted with new forms of deviance and abnormal behavior, which might be symptoms of an unbearable, abnormal life, lists and technical terms are found to categorize them. This may be brought up to date with a vague reference to a hypothetical "social" factor, which supposedly guarantees that the problems will be confronted in contemporary, modern terms. In the meantime, prisons and asylums continue to preserve their marginal, class character.

In this social context, the problem of criminality or mental illness is not even touched. Either it is not known what it is or it is known a priori and the definition is applied that is most suited to eliciting a repressive response. The functionaries focus only on that aspect which implies social disturbance, but mental illness and deviance exist not only for the society that defends itself against them, but also for the individuals who must defend themselves or who experience the madness and illness as their rejection of an unendurable existence. What do we know about these people and their suffering? We are bourgeois technicians and the limits on our knowledge, treatment, and rehabilitation are the limits that we created to meet our own needs and protect our own survival. Our technical answers always meet the needs of our class, and this is why they turn into the segregation of others. Mental illness and deviance are only opportunities to carry out this segregation with the approval of science, and with a technical justification for an act of social exclusion.

If we want to confront the issue of deviance and illness, we have to do so in terms of social structure, and the basic division underlying that structure, and not as isolated phenomena passed off as individual abnormalities typical of an unfortunate percentage of the population.

Once again, the institutions that should respond to these problems start from the formal presumption of treatment, rehabilitation, and reeducation for the inmate's eventual recovery. However, if these goals were not just formal ones but were actually achievable, the problem would already be resolved. A formal function is one thing, and a real practice is something else. Truth lies in the institutional practice which shows us that inmates in our asylums and prisons rarely emerge rehabilitated because the real goal of these institutions is still the destruction and elimination of their populations. In countries with a high percentage of unemployed and underemployed, what interest is there in the rehabilitation and cure of this human refuse? This is where the technician's work can be crucial in clarifying the contradiction between ideology and practice, as well as the social goals of this ideological practice.

Technicians who work in these institutions must show how their specialized skills are utilized and the ever-changing but always identical ways that contribute to this utilization. The problem of rehabilitation and cure is neither technical nor organizational. It is a political problem linked to the original division on which our society is based. What would they do with those who are rehabilitated? Is there a place for them in our society? Once they are rehabilitated, will they find a job able to meet their family's needs? Are not these institutions based on rules that make rehabilitation impossible because these individuals, even if rehabilitated, would remain on the margins of society, constantly exposed to the danger of breaking the rules again? The possibility of rehabilitation is directly proportional to the availability of manpower, to the jobs that exist in the so-called free society which depends on the stages of economic concentration and expansion. Fluctuations in the number of patients cured and released from our asylums is directly linked to general economic trends, and depending on whether there is inflation or recession, there can be broader or narrower definitions of abnormal behavior and greater or lesser tolerance for that behavior. These trends are presumably similar for incarceration, since the same process of segregation and control is being used.

There is another phenomenon related to this, which is always ignored. Inmates in asylums and prisons completely lack a sense of belonging to society. It is clear why. If asylums and prisons are established to meet the needs of a "free" society, then inmates do not see themselves reflected in this society which punishes, segregates, and destroys them and gives them no possible alternative. Nor can they identify with rules that do not meet their needs. They cannot experience their confinement as something that helps them to become rehabilitated. Rehabilitation requires a subjective participation from the individual, but in order for them to participate in this process, they would have to see the institutions that segregate them as rehabilitative and therapeutic. Making amends and acknowledging deviation makes no sense unless the deviant feels she is a participant in society and unless she believes in its laws, because she has contributed to determining them.

These individuals, with their history of a marginalization constantly perpetuated as that of a class, cannot feel like participating members of this society or its laws and regulations. There is no law in our society which answers to their needs and their rights. It is only through struggle that this class will be able to assert their rights, but not everyone manages to channel the struggle in a positive, organized direction. And so some react with sporadic, isolated, criminal acts or with abnormal behavior that is automatically punished.

It is significant that in countries where there is an ongoing struggle to change the social order, where everyone feels themselves to be actors in this transformation, criminality and certain forms of deviant behavior undergo a tremendous decline. In the few short years of the Allende regime, the rate of alcoholism in Chile, which had been the highest in South America, was reduced in half, and the same was true for the phenomenon of drug abuse. We know what position was taken by the doctors (and the lawyers and judges who were partly responsible for the fall of the Popular Unity government) in this struggle, because with a victory they stood to lose every privilege and all power to discriminate and dominate.

This does not mean, let us repeat, that mental illness and deviance do not exist, that diversity as a human phenomenon does not exist, or that changing the social order would be enough to wipe them out. The problem lies precisely in this concept—the necessity to wipe out diversity as if it were not a part of life, to eliminate everything that might undermine the false harmony of this facade.

While the diversity of the dominant class is accepted as a

human phenomenon that needs specific "different" answers, the diversity of the oppressed class is never accepted, and responses only serve to eliminate them and prove their inequality. In a class-divided society, illness and criminality in the subordinate class become something other than what they are. The only response is concealed repression, because what determines the nature of the response is not the nature of the need, but the class of the person expressing it. If a social system is based on an economic logic that does not satisfy the needs of all, if reforms and transformations are demanded in the name of an abstract humanity that does not correspond to all human beings, then the handicapped, the weak, and the incompetent will be eliminated, because for them rehabilitation and cure are not possible.

The answers to these problems can only be repressive, and never dialectical. Increasing the personnel employed in repression and control, providing more specialized training for the technicians of repression, and increasing the severity of police institutions are the only preventive measures that a social system like ours knows how to plan. They can only respond to the rise in crime and deviance by increasing the number of police and psychiatrists. These measures, as an answer to the criticism implied in every deviant act, allow them not to call their institutions or their values into question.

Someone might object that our analysis has only examined the violence perpetuated by the dominant class against the dominated class, while we have not examined the nature of the violence inherent in deviance, except as the violence of the dominated. We have no intention of undialectically reversing the situation and arguing that mental illness and deviance are the only sane responses to a sick world or by suggesting that they are positive values, opposed to the negative values of our social system.

We only want to focus on how the criminalization of mental illness and deviance is scientifically carried out, and on how the needs expressed by them turn into crimes to be punished in order to justify the criminality of the punishment. Political dissent is also undergoing this same process of criminalization in a more explicit way, because science has not yet found the right pathology for characterizing this behavior. For dissent, the response is direct and needs no mediation—it can be murder or torture.

Our analysis gives us an understanding of how all the institutions in our social system function only to respond to needs once they have been criminalized, reduced to what they are not, or reduced to a symptom. The criminalization of need is in reality its artificially created nature, so that two forms of violence and criminality must be confronted, one in response to the other, without knowing how to recognize the real need any longer. Deviance and abnormal behavior are crimes because they carry a dangerous potential; but the institutions for their treatment and rehabilitation commit crimes in the name of preventing this danger. For these institutions, there are no needs and therefore no answers to needs. In such a situation it is difficult, if not impossible, to know the nature of deviance and mental illness. It is also difficult to really interpret these social phenomena.

In Italy, for example, we have lived for years with the threat of violence. Right now, we no longer know if the paranoid climate in which we live is real or created artificially as a new system of control in which every citizen mistrusts every other. We are therefore both the subjects and the objects of this control that the violent institutions can no longer handle. Social imbalances and social contradictions in our country are stronger than in other European bourgeois democracies, as is the opposition. In Italy, because of the intensity of the imbalances and our awareness of them, there is resistance to the creation of a single middle class, which would identify with the values of an extremely small center of power that would control it. Nonetheless, the expansion of the middle strata which identify more readily with dominant values is a sign of this process. There is still a working class numerically strong enough to prevent this kind of conspiratorial maneuver. The paranoid atmosphere, whether real or artificially created, weakens the forces of opposition which live in a constant state of threatened violence. The processes we have analyzed here also contribute to this weakness because there is not a clear awareness of the functions of these institutions and ideologies.

The assimilation of ideologies and values created by our social system is not always seen as a part of the passive acceptance of domination. If the oppressed class does not become conscious of all the ways in which this domination—which extends beyond exploitation and workplace hazards—is accomplished, we might easily find ourselves in a universal asylum, where we were defined by symptoms that we would perceive as real.

We are at a very dangerous turning point. Even in Italy, the threat of violence as a form of control can easily turn into open violence. This might happen if the ruling class thinks that traditional institutions no longer suffice and that the new ideologies of control, already being imported, need time to take root and acquire the scientific credibility to reinforce their domination. Right now, the strength and vigilance of the class that opposes this process can be crucial in exposing and preventing it. The alternative to the threat of violence that we now live with is violence without masks and coverups; it is massacre and torture.

There are already indications that this new use of science and technology is beginning. The French General, Massu, in his book *La vrai bataille d'Alger* explains that if circumstances require it, you can practice a "healthy" torture that will ensure success.[34] From a clandestine Brazilian newspaper, we learn that a psychoanalyst, while awaiting entry into the psychoanalytic society, is employed to give psychological assistance to torture victims. In Uruguay, therapists of patients who are political suspects are released from professional secrecy and are required to tell what they know about their patients, under threat of torture. If science and its institutions cannot adequately answer or control needs, then torture is established as an institution with its own rules, codes, and morals, opening up new fields of activity for technicians in the human sciences.

Faced with this reality, we can no longer assume that if we accept the authority of our role, we will not be asked to provide technical assistance for mass killings. We must turn our work into a service for the consumers that will also make them aware of how the service is usually used. This means that we must refuse to be functionaries of consent and become instead technicians of practical knowledge. Going beyond the privileges which we inevitably enjoy because we are bourgeois and are agents of the domination inherent in our role, we will try to identify the needs of the oppressed class, and reveal the processes that transform their needs into something other than what they are, even in their own eyes.

Part Four ON THE NATURE OF MADNESS

Introduction

Anne M. Lovell

I don't know what madness is. It can be everything and nothing. It is a human condition. Madness is present in each of us as is reason. The problem is that society, in order to call itself civil, should accept reason as well as madness. . . . When someone who is mad enters the asylum, he stops being mad and is transformed into a sick person. The problem is how to undo the knot, how to overcome institutional madness and to recognize madness where it originates, that is, in life.[1]

Originally written as an entry for a major Italian encyclopedia,[2] "Madness/Delirium" intended to question the neutrality of science, especially medicine and psychiatry. The Basaglias, however, go further than the intellectual concerns of their time by connecting the role of science to social organization and the social control functions of society. The theoretical and historical nature of this essay departs from their earlier writings, which had primarily documented Basaglia's work. In fact, Basaglia considered this piece a summary of the evolution of his thought and practice to date.[3]

For years Basaglia had been concerned with the problem of exclusion, whether that of the mentally ill, minorities, women, Jews, or other marginalized groups. In this essay the Basaglias are also concerned with madness as an historical object of exclusion. Michel Foucault,[4] and that branch of the Frankfurt School represented by Max Horkheimer and T.W. Adorno,[5] shared the Basaglias interest in the idea of madness as "other." By tracing the history of madness and its relationship to Reason, the Basaglias uncover the ideologies that justify and mechanisms that produce and perpetuate the exclusion of all that is different in society. It is a difference that, since the beginning of the Enlightenment (which the Basaglias, like Horkheimer and Adorno, consider the crucible of the modern bourgeois world) is measured against reason. Later, with industrialization and capitalism, it will be measured against norms defined in terms of production and efficiency, or, in the language of critical theory, of their rationality. With the progressive rationalization of society—the reduction of all that comprises it, whether things or people, to quantifiable, mutually exchangeable abstractions—all that does not fit the goals of capitalist production must be excluded.

Interpreting Foucault, the essay begins with the historical moment during the Middle Ages when madness is undifferentiated and unfettered, when it belongs to another world. It traces the way madness is seen through psychiatry's establishment as a means of mastering madness, not of knowing it. The Basaglias read Foucault with a Marxist key: madness at the zero point, or beginning, is undifferentiated needs, and the transformations it undergoes, from the Enlightenment on, are ways of organizing not true responses to these needs, but responses that exclude and control those persons who express them.

In this genealogy of the concept of madness is a concern with the individual as subject and as body. This is not the Marxist subject (class consciousness), but rather the concrete human being: "the body (heaviness, inertia and passivity, a subject that seeks to appropriate them) and the coercion of which it is an object (institutions, ideologies, and social organization.)"[6] In his earlier writings, Basaglia had demonstrated how the body becomes the institution when the individual's needs are totally subsumed under the goals and logic of the asylum.[7] Here the expropriation of the individual body is traced in two, closely-linked directions. With Western biomedicine, the individual is objectified into the "ill" body (sickness), a passive, dead weight. And the body social subordinates the individual to its socioeconomic tasks. For the Basaglias, medicine's objectification of the body, accomplished by the end of the eighteenth century, allows it to be dominated and exploited. With this achievement, the human being has been rationalized.

In the essay's historical outline, the relationships of reason and madness, subject and object, constantly shift, so as to question the possibility that madness can be defined as preexisting entity. The juxtaposition in the title of madness and delirium calls for an explanation of the reality they supposedly define, as well as of their antithetical relationship. Madness suggests the unfettered otherness, the irrational in life, that which cannot be encompassed by our rational way of seeing. In fact, we do not really know what it is. Once delirium is constructed as a medical concept, madness become objectified. Yet madness is converted into a disease without ever questioning the validity of that from which it derives.

Although the Basaglias hold delirium before its medicalization to be the subjective voice of madness, the true expression of what it is, they never present its message but only the language imposed upon it, the way in which it is classified. Each subsequent transformation in the definition of madness as delirium accomplishes the same end of classification and measurement, of objectification into frozen diagnostic concepts. With psychoanalysis, the "unreason" at the root of the deviation inherent in madness will again be restored to the "normal" person, as the boundaries between normal and pathological are blurred. But the Basaglias point out that this process of reuniting the rational with the irrational (unconscious) takes place outside the real realm of social conflict (e.g., in the analyst's office). Hence the roots of this separation are not affected.

What is madness for the Basaglias? Once they have deconstructed the concept, we are left only with a definition of its "negativity," what it is not. The aim here is the possibility of a radical alternative to our way of seeing and treating it. In the essay itself, the mad do not speak—for that would require a new history, an underside of psychiatry or a minor history. We know only that expressions of madness can be covert forms of protest and resistance when survival needs are unmet. This interpretation has led some to identify Basaglia's anti-institutional work with the theory of radical needs, prevalent in the Italy of the seventies.[8] However, Basaglia's analysis of needs preceded its diffusion in Italy.[9]

Like Walter Benjamin and T.W. Adorno, philosophers of the critical theory that so influenced him, Basaglia refuses to describe (name) the other—in this case, the madman. Elsewhere, Basaglia comes close to his phenomenological beginnings when he states that the subjectivity of madness is expressed as an existential suffering. However, those who are imprisoned by material conditions "do not know existential suffering but only the suffering of survival."[10]

The negative definition of madness also creates dangers present today as consequences of questioning all types of knowledge after the social and intellectual upheaval of 1968. Basaglia's way of working and seeing madness was never codified; it was really a form of tacit knowledge, continuously evolving and changing. Today, even in Italy, there is a desperate return to techniques, therapies, medical models, in part because they fill a void for which a new body of knowledge was never defined. Nor did the results of the anti-institutional experiences find their way into the university and medical curricula.[11] Yet the refusal, exemplified in this essay, to define madness, can still spur us to consider what it might be under different conditions.

6. Madness/Delirium

Not existence but knowledge is without hope for in the
pictoral or mathematical symbols it appropriates and perpetuates existence as a schema.

Horkheimer and Adorno

Reason and Madness

No history of madness exists that is not also a history of reason. Foucault's attempt to trace the itinerary of the madman's silence and speech throughout the centuries is the search for an interpretation of what is ultimately "the monologue of reason about
madness."[1] But implied in such a monologue is an act that will
prove to be essential to the evolution of madness, by inscribing it
on the language of those who listen and judge, and by confining
its expression within the framework of an alien logic. The history
of madness is that of the gradual evolution of values, rules, beliefs
and systems of power; the latter constitute judgments upon
which the social group is based and which bear the imprint of all
phenomena that affect the process of organizing social life.

Over the centuries, the rational and the irrational come
to coexist, while remaining separate. Yet they are drawn closer
once reason is in a position to neutralize madness by recognizing
it as a part of itself, as well as by defining a separate space for its existence. Such a process does not merely represent the evolution of
science and knowledge. Nor does it only signify the transition of
madness from tragic experience in the world to sin, guilt, scandal,
condemnation, and objectification of unreason—elements which,
in our critical view, are still fused and present in madness. Nor
does it simply represent the signs of an animality that surfaces or

With Franca Ongaro Basaglia. Translated by Anne M. Lovell.

flares up as long as reason is able to view it critically, differentiate it, sort it out. Nor is it merely a measure of the extent to which people's fears and miseries are obliterated by torture, repression, authority, science, and power.

A common denominator is assumed in these transitions. It is the quantity and quality of space available to a person for expressing the needs of his or her body and subjectivity (defined as the relationship of one's body to other bodies and subjectivities) through reason and unreason, health and illness, truth and error.

The concern here is not with problems of compassion, justice, tolerance, consciousness, and knowledge in the face of suffering, defeat, or fall. It is with all of this, but at the same time with something more global and extensive which comprehends the person in the totality of his or her needs and desires. It also has to do with the attitudes assumed by both the social group in which one is placed and by the organization which must respond to such needs and desires in the face of this totality.

Until the collectivity acquires the strength to express its needs as demands requiring responses, madness, delirium,[2] violence, precariousness, religious beliefs, and rites are mingled and confused in the penury of an existence constantly under the threat of a cruel death. All this while, value judgments, such as those of bestiality, error, sin, guilt, degeneracy, disorder, and vice remain common to the forms of unreason. But they are common as well to the many ways in which misery, oppression, filth, illness, and indigency can be expressed. The face of hunger is not far from that of madness; their voices become confounded if no one listens to them or if they are denied the right to speech.

In a period of tolerance, madness is confounded with life. If, during the Middle Ages, madness gave birth to monsters, life itself could not be far from the monsters born of it. Famines, epidemics, plagues, religious beliefs, rites, cruelty, oppression, and domination were molded from the same violence that shaped monsters. Does not religion produce the same terror from which it is hewn?

During this period, in keeping with a spirit of charity and piety, lazar houses and almshouses shelter not illness, but an indigency which is ill. Similarly, prisons shelter that destitution which is expressed through unreason and threatens civil society and common beliefs, and that until now have been imbued with the mingled elements of reason and unreason. Delirium, as the subjective expression of the mad person—its etymologyical origins mean "to move out of the furrow"*—is still the mediation between a transcendence that encompasses and explains everything and the world of destitution and harshness, justified by transcendence and with which it is confounded. Madness does not yet have an autonomous voice, because the needs of the healthy/ill person are deprived of a voice, and the response to these needs is entrusted to charity and punishment. As long as destitution is silenced, madness can be confounded with the common language of needs, as of yet unvindicated, while the few who have the means for survival find ways of coping by themselves. The definitions given for madness are inscribed in the magic, religious, ritual world which impregnates culture, and which encompasses madness and misery, in the same way, within the totality of natural/supernatural human phenomena.

The moment that the destitute begin to reclaim their rights, an operation is set in motion that individuates and separates the various voices among them in order to avoid responding to the global nature of their cry. It is not by chance, then, that in this historical moment, the voice of madness is first singled out.

When Pinel—within the logic of the Enlightenment and under the impulse of the liberating tendencies of the French Revolution—frees the insane from the chains that have linked them with delinquency, deluding himself into thinking that he has given them a voice by conferring upon them the dignity of sickness, he in fact begins to separate the world of misery and unreason. He thus gives madness, once confused with human misery, a qualitatively different meaning. This involves fragmenting increasingly urgent and global demands of the masses, and structuring a new logic that, by focusing on particular technical responses, such as phrenology, allows them to be thwarted. When the silent multitudes, deprived of a voice until now, are about to speak up, reason, which is already identified with power, begins

*Literally, to go awry in plowing, to deviate from the straight line.—Tranlator.

to determine for everyone the ways, times, and places they may speak; and it always does so in terms of language and logic that, by parcelling human needs, implicitly denies that they are global.

The transition from prison to asylum—beyond the humanitarian meaning implied in this operation which took for granted that criminals and delinquents belonged to a subspecies deserving of prisons, dungeons, torment, and tortures—in fact begins to invalidate the voice of madness, while at the same time recognizing in illness its right to speech. Criminality and madness, understood as phenomena of the natural and the unnatural, possess an indomitable character; prison segregates and punishes alleged criminals, with no intention or possibility of modifying or correcting them. The existence in humans of both possibilities, punished when they represent a threat to the collectivity or to its values, is implicitly recognized in this shared segregation. Thus criminality and madness are couched in terms of a judgement that, like the objectified act that segregates them, has only a punitive meaning.

The removal of madness from this confused amalgam of unreason and guilt overlayed with misery, and the dignity conferred upon it as illness, imply a process of judgement. Reason begins to separate out what resembles it from what it either does not recognize or acknowledge as its own only when it circumscribes or dominates it, putting brackets around the misery that informs it. What was originally accepted as one of the many possibilities available to human beings, and later punished harshly when it threatened collective life, now becomes an object of compassion and understanding. Accordingly, the responsibility for every act is now attributed to unreason, and no longer to the individual, whom reason appropriates in the very moment that he is stripped of all responsibility. Assuming the responsibility for unreason, reason, in this humanitarian and scientific act, holds the unreasonable person under its sway. Since reason cannot punish individuals for their reprehensible acts, it will inflict punishment on the individual as a whole by extending its sanctions to all behaviors, thus setting in motion the processes of control and behavioral change around which treatment and therapy will develop. Delirium, as the subjective expression of madness, thus becomes objectified as the potential nucleus of asocial behavior.

Delirium is now considered a threat, that while no longer punishable, must be controlled, prevented, corrected, modified, that is, treated. Madness disappears in the objectification of delirium as illness.

Such an operation will have major consequences in the evolution of madness; what it will become after this separation renders the analysis of this historical moment crucial. When Reason begins to judge madness, the distance between reason and unreason is already fixed: it is the distance created between the subject of the judgement and the object that is judged. The objectification of unreason is the indispensible premise for domination; unreason will be allowed to exist as a part of reason only to the extent that it has already been objectified by it. But one must emphasize that the Age of Reason, during which time these processes of diversifying needs began in the name of man's triumph over nature, corresponds to the birth of the rationality of a new power, and to the establishment of bourgeois reason as the only acknowledged one. This operation of sorting and separating reason and unreason allows the dissociation of the new rationality from that which, following the logic of one's own needs and desires, is expressed with its own language, and thus implicitly undermines the rational bases of the new power. Giving a name to this confounded language, then, means protecting the rationality of power, thus forcing madness to be expressed in terms of a deciphering code which has been prepared by the new rationality.

When reason, on these bases, lends a voice to madness or begins to listen, the incommunicability of the two languages becomes insurmountable. Whoever allows the other to speak also determines the modes through which madness must express itself, at the risk of being forever excluded from the domains of human intelligibility, dominant reason having become Human Reason. The rupture is irreparable; by imposing its own language on madness, reason prevents it from ever speaking in its own voice and expressing what it is, even if, throughout the centuries, it will continue to allow madness [an alien] voice.

The history of psychiatry consists essentially of continually lending a voice to something which cannot be expressed in an imposed language. If the true language of madness—delirium—is the subjective expression of needs and desires that can only be expressed through irrationality and unreason, it can never become the language of the rationality of power. The impossibility of communication between reason and madness is therefore implied in the definitions reason gives to itself and to unreason. The new rationality recognizes unreason as part of itself—as part of the person whom it claims the right to represent—the moment it finds the means of controlling and dominating it. The relationship it establishes is, from the beginning and by its own objective nature, one of domination, given that it attempts to harness unreason within a rigid and closed interpretative scheme, which will become that of mental illness. Madness—circumscribed and defined by reason— will have to express itself according to this interpretative scheme that is foreign to it; that is, in the language of disease, which is the language of the rationality of power. Here the subjective experience of the insane, expressed in delirium, will be definitively objectified.

What was once merely the harsh punishment of unreason in prisons, jails, and with tortures acquires, due to the medical intervention that recognizes it as illness, the connotations of charity, solicitude, and treatment. Charity, solicitude, and treatment which, through implicit, but final confirmation of the incommunicability of the language of madness compared to the rationality of power, are translated back again into punishment. Thus they affect the same segregative modes and the identical value judgments involved in all phenomena of unreason contained and controlled by reason. That madness becomes "mental illness" and is accorded a dignity and status of its own does not change the fact that in order to assert its domination and diversity, reason continues to separate it, segregating it behind the very walls and with the very chains from which it was freed. The pity that leads to the recognition that illness has the right to a space of its own is translated into treatment/punishment that consists of the obligation to enter a foreign space which is separated and different from that of rational humanity. In fact, the relationship of psychiatric intervention and science (reason) to mental illness remains one of punishment, exactly like the relationship that earlier assured the continual confusion of madness with criminality and delinquency. This is a relationship of punishment, softened by a medical ideology that under the guise of justice or compassion, veils what is from the first a victorious contest between an abstract rationality and the rational/irrational humanity that the new reason and new power ready themselves to organize.

But the newly recognized right conferred upon illness to a space of its own is accompanied by the expanded obligation that all behavior must enter this foreign space when, in the eyes of reason, it reveals the presence of unreason. This means that the gradual engulfment under the control of Reason—and hence under the reign of punishment—of all that is potentially, though not yet explicitly, a-social and threatening, is facilitated by the identification of mental illness and the scientific attitude toward it. This in turn will bring about dire consequences in terms of the control of human behavior, and explains how we reached the rigid definitions of normality and abnormality as we know them in the modern era.

If prison punished the actual crime of whoever had "lost their senses," the asylum will punish, above all, the presumed menace, intention, and danger of behavior that does not clearly present the characteristics of rationality. The expansion of the rule or reason over what "could happen" and what "is presumed can happen" is the basis for what will become medicine's gradual invasion of the territory of human behavior. It is also the phantom of the transfer of the insane from the prison to the asylum, which will haunt the concept of mental illness itself, because the transferred disease has been identified above all in the criminal acts carried out by the "senseless" whom the new rationality no longer holds responsible, but considers ill. This phantom will be projected onto disease, penetrating its deepest zones, determining what will later become its essential nature: danger to society.

The character of the new rationality of power therefore presupposes, in and of itself, a proportionate and corresponding rationality in human behavior; otherwise it would be excluded from human rationality. To this enlightened reason, madness is part of the nature against which reason struggles and which it wishes to dominate. The "sack full of air" (*follis*),[4] which was formerly used to represent the concept of madness and back to which the word can be traced, does not find a place in this new rationality that wishes to explain and dominate everything. A head cannot be full of air, nor senses pushed by the wind, nor souls nor bodies possessed by spirits and demons. There must be a rational, scientific explanation. But the only explanation this abstract reason is able to provide is that it has to do with disease; and the word "disease"—a more scientific and dignified metaphor than air that blows in an empty sack—will definitely replace that gust of wind. Now the sack will be swollen with disease, whose different modes or expression and degrees of closeness to, or distance from, human normality will be minutely described.

The connections between the rationality of power and the normality which it imposes as the only possibility, preventing whatever does not resemble it from expression, are obscured. But this rationality, which does not coincide with everyday life where reason and unreason are inextricably mingled, will have to be denied. Mental illness and the medical science that begins to deal with it are translated into one of the essential instruments through which bourgeois reason, having become the dominant ideology, manages to face the contradictions which belie it. Thus begins the slow separation between normal behavior, which corresponds to the rationality of power, and abnormal behavior, which is endowed with a rationality of its own that is not subject to the rules so foreign to it. Thus must these behaviors, as such, find a separate space in which they will be repressed.

Reason and Misery

The historical moment in which madness, having now acquired a dignity through the concept of delirium, is first transformed into mental illness, marks the consolidation of the foundations for the empire of reason. It is now possibile to understand another essential aspect of that rational, humanitarian, scientific process through which illness becomes the mediation between dominant reason and misery.

If bourgeois reason has become Human Reason, the relationship between reason and "segregated" madness is essentially that between power and misery. Madness without misery is explained elsewhere, beyond the territory where the response to needs are either collective or nonexistent. One confronts madness, tolerates or eliminates it, transforming it into misery. (The nobility and moneyed gentry used judicial interdictions to reduce the mad to a state of penury to assume guardianship over their assets). With power and money, madness takes on extravagant and bizarre overtones, but it is safe so long as it leaves the patrimony intact. The concern here is not with a problem requiring legal measures, laws, and interventions (except interdiction). Madness without misery is always beyond the law, as it is beyond everything else that involves conventional power: rules and provisions are made for others. Reason, then, does not address *this* madness, but rather the segregated, institutional, incarcerated one that is always the madness of poverty—essentially misery itself—while the other madness continues to be expressed elsewhere, beyond segregative control. The relationship between reason and this madness is therefore the relationship between reason and misery, but a misery which, in this particular historical moment, is protesting loudly, and which must be answered if the newly proclaimed rights founded on liberty, equality, and fraternity are truly those of all people.

Granting this madness with misery the dignity of disease is one way of not responding to the totality of misery, of carving up its various aspects, and thus maintaining the status quo. This hypothesis will be confirmed by the successive evolutions, through institutional recycling, of the asylum, whose major relationship will always be to poverty and indigency through the mediation of disease. Madness, once wrenched from the whole of undifferentiated needs comprising the panorama of the vague, segregated a-sociality with which it had been confounded, assumes sounds, inflections, and gestures—to the ears of those who listen and in the eyes of those who observe—that are no longer easily connected to that indistinct world of needs. These are needs which are no longer answered but which become deciphered and read as an ensemble of signs, devoid of explanation and defined abstractly. Illness, which medical intervention singles out from the tangle of guilt and unreason, is transferred from the sphere of punishment to treatment which continues to be punishment. For what remains unchanged in this transfer is the misery that constitutes illness and that determines the essential character of the relationship maintained with it. Illness therefore becomes the mediation between the new rationality of power and misery which must be organized, classified, and fragmented into as many sectors as there are technical responses already waiting, so that the delicate balance between destitution and abundance, and especially the way these are distributed, is not altered.

What would madness have become had psychiatry begun to respond to that world of confused and undifferentiated needs that were becoming articulated? What would psychiatry have become had its actions been consistent with its proclamations? If, rather than being mediated by an "institutionalized" illness it had "cured" the suffering that arises from oppression, from the repressions of subjectivity and of the body? What if psychiatry had responded to the needs of this subjectivity and this body before naming the suffering that arises when it cannot be expressed, physically or psychologically? Or if Pinel, instead of freeing the insane from their chains, had classified the relationship that was being forged between reason and power, and hence had determined the nature of unreason and madness? What if psychiatry had been a "science" in the sense of a knowledge that is structured dialectically in its relationship to power? What if, beyond charity and the scientific and humanitarian attitude with which it had tried to restore subjectivity to the mad, psychiatry had searched in the world of needs and desires for the moment when inattention, oppression, and violence can set off the explosion of a reaction and violence that take the name of insanity? What if it had not been involved in rearranging definitions so as to single out an illness, which, to be defined in the very way it was, took reason as its master and unreason as its servant?

The crucial part is to comprehend the moments in this process by grasping the passages of this mediation that have been constituted from illness and the role that science has played in organizing each phenomenon separately. Only then can one understand what madness will become once it is contained in the strait jacket of a mental illness that is objectifiable, quantifiable, and definable in the scientific terms of the rationality of power. For the break between reason and madness is implicit in the very nature of this new rationality that presupposes the domination and production of a norm in which it is mirrored. From it, all that does not resemble this rationality is excluded, from the moment that "the awakening of the self is paid for by the acknowledgement of power as the principle of all relations."[5]

Illness is power's rational discourse about madness which it dominates by encompassing it in a space that in the same gesture both excludes and acknowledges it. Such a process continues as long as madness is not expressed in the language of a rationality which power imposes on it as Human Rationality. Similarly, these procedures are extended to whatever else does not express itself in such a language. Madness thus enters this sphere of rationality; dominated, excluded, confined, and segregated, it can be silenced by the language of illness. So, too, does misery, if it accepts defeat, remain misery and resign itself to silence.

On the basis of this ambiguous, gradual manufacturing of a norm that responds to the requirements of bourgeois rationality, psychiatry begins to erect the labyrinth of classifications: the subdivision into different clinical pictures, the nuances of analogies and differences, the defining of the quality of deliriums, and the different specifications of their content. Now it is concerned less and less or not at all with what madness really is, expresses, and represents. In the same way, the erection of its institutions—with their practices of punishment, control, and torture, now accepted by science—is begun. Psychiatry refuses to see the close connection between, on the one hand, the ideology of the norm that constitutes it, governing its practice and theory; and on the other hand, the social organization that begins to be structured through the division of labor and the various disciplines, so that it can appropriate the individual who must therefore adhere to that norm.

Science finally is concerned with an illness (about which it is totally ignorant, except for the nominalistic specifications it has given it), contained in custodial and treatment institutions. But the nature of this illness and of these institutions, and hence the nature of the treatment and the custodial care that will be carried out inside them, will remain closely tied to the relationship that bourgeois rationality continues to maintain with misery. For it is the obligation of the institutions, through the mediation of illness, to contain and control this misery.

Reason, State, and Norm

In the first half of the nineteenth century, a new organizational phase was actualized in Europe. With the gradual structuring and centralization of its apparatuses, the various states established and reinforced the institutions from which emanated the positive rules and orders for "civil society." In 1883, the French Parliament approved the first European law on the insane; from this moment on, psychiatry acquired a judicial and institutional body that would be decisive in the evolution of the theory and practice of the discipline.

The legislative definition put an end to the ambiguity of a doctrine that, while proclaiming involvement with an illness, was always engaged in problems foreign to it: dangerousness and public order, but also misery and indigency. This ambiguity was nevertheless resolved by the medico-legal normative standard thus tipping the balance in favor of the dangerousness and public order side. It also put brackets around indigency, forgetting the element that had brought about the distinction between madness and criminality. For the individual's subjective suffering—expressed in irrational terms—had required measures other than the punishment which linked it to delinquency. Under the new set of norms, this suffering was considered only when called an illness or entrusted by law to the medical body and to an institution that claimed to be curative. Medicine's and institutions' task nevertheless remained the control and containment of dangerousness to society and potential subversion of the social order.

The medical body and its science, relieved of this institutional function, found itself justifying in scientific terms measures adopted in the legal area. The latter, strengthened by this medical backing, shed an ever more sinister light on illness and on the scientific responses that need to be deployed. Illness, psychiatry, and the hospital were reduced to pure nominalism; illness became the dangerousness that presumably has to be contained; psychiatry became a branch of law that punishes anyone suspected of dangerousness; and the hospital became a prison in which this presumed dangerousness is segregated. Psychiatry became a science that is born and dies the very moment the contract between medicine and law is actualized. From that moment on, psychiatry sided definitively with law, hence with power, forgetting the subject for whom it exists and whose suffering justified its very birth.

Bourgeois rational thought had managed to confine within institutional rationality (the asylum) the madness that had by now lost its particular characteristics, reduced purely to one element of disturbance to civil society. Impoverished, emptied of all tragic and subjective meaning, defrauded of the historicity of personal experience, split off from life to which it belonged and of which it was an expression, objectified by a reason that, to better invalidate its voice, defines it as an illness to be treated, madness could once again enter the logic of social order and scientific thought. It is now welcomed in a space "natural" to it, prepared by a state concerned with the organization of its citizens' needs and by a science concerned with an illness whose essential element, notwithstanding, consists of dangerousness to society.

Reason has reached the height of its triumph: evil (nature) is always domitable; it need only be individualized and circumscribed. That all of human society has within itself the characteristics of unpredictability and dangerousness is a fact that reason only theoretically accepts; otherwise it would have to acknowledge these insidious elements within itself. Danger and threat are inherent to human nature, but specifically to certain people in whom nonreason becomes personified. It is enough to individualize and isolate them before they produce contagion and destroy rational order.

But what comprises this rational order that is imposing its rules on all sectors of social life? Does it still have to do with an abstract, "enlightened" reason that subscribes to the vision of a world of happy people, freed from the slavery of a nature that is by now domesticated, and guided by the intelligence and science that have contributed to this domination and happiness? Reason, which appeared so bright and full of hope, was speaking about itself because it spoke of a man, a reality that do not yet exist. Assuming that the Reasonable Man could overcome and vanquish all contradictions, it had played the new power game that was then being structured and has now become its order, its rational base. The rationality of the liberal state is the concrete outcome of the Age of Enlightenment, the rationality that allows for and upholds the development of industry, of capital, of the exploitation of people, and the division of labor that guarantees this process. It is this rationality that will give the new, more rigid and precise connotations to the norm according to which one is either encircled by or excluded from the social consortium: the norm from which every suspicion of madness will be rigorously banished.

The organization of capitalist relations of production determines a reality in which the degree of efficiency required to gain access to the world of production rises continuously. The distance between who succeeds and who does not widens, and those who fail—or who cannot find a place in the organization of labor which has become the only socially recognized value—remain severed from the world, deprived of identity and rights. In this new dimension, the productive person is formally a "free" actor in the social contract; the unproductive person remains at its fringes, and the only identity offered to him or her is to be part of the unproductive marginality. But the unproductive marginality includes not just the incapacitated, the retarded, the feeble, the handicapped, women, and the elderly, but also the unemployed—all of those whom production does not need. In other words, they belong to the world of unfortunates who, in Malthus' words, "have a losing ticket in the great lottery of life."[6] It cannot circulate unleashed, and civil society is forced to defend itself against them so that the effective functioning of work and "free" exchange is not hindered.

To respond to such requirements, once the norm has become identified with efficiency and productivity, all that is outside this logic falls under the censure of invalidation. For this process appropriate institutions and specific scientific ideologies exist: institutions and ideologies with the duty of protecting and safeguarding the freedom of those who participate in the contract by totally controlling the existence of those who do not. The social organization, therefore, defends the principles of freedom upon which it is built by delegating to its institutions the management of citizens' needs according to whether they belong to the contractual world or to the realm of invalidation. The latter coincides with social unproductivity, which must be included in the rationality, through a system of institutional apparatuses, aimed a precluding every possible autonomous expression by the subjects they manage.

Under the tutelage and protection of this organization,

freedom is thus the prerogative of those who work; that is, those who work as long as they are able at the required level of efficiency have the freedom to work in order that the product be protected. Those who are deprived of this guarantee, however, always risk becoming an object of the process of invalidation by aggravating any aspect of life that might arouse the suspicion of an abnormality, a defect, a lack, or an error that can justify being enclosed by an institution.

The relationship of reason and misery, which the contract between medicine and law places within brackets (consequently tending to identify misery with dangerousness), is reproposed here in all its crudeness: abnormality, defect, deficit, error, unreason, dangerousness, and menace that can characterize the behavior of individuals not included in the "contract". This list can now easily be individualized in what is rarely a "private" space in which social improprieties (these have for the most part become manifestations of a segregated madness) are part of the marginalized person's life and improper by definition. The rules of social life make sense for those who are part of this life, who find in it at least a partial response to their own needs. But for those who find only a confirmation of their exclusion, these rules represent the language of violence and oppression. The rationality implicit in these norms is foreign to that of the marginal person, simply because his or her rationality operated at the level of needs that the other rationality does not consider. All of the marginal person's behavior is foreign to the values, beliefs, and rules from which he or she is excluded, and the ease with which such behavior can be invalidated is obvious. So obvious that it is clear that the same rigid rules and the sanctions that apply to those who deviate from them are constructed essentially with the purpose of controlling, through invalidation, the types of individuals whom the organization of work excludes. If these persons who are excluded from the banquet are actually sick, the diners can continue to eat calmly, given that the social organization is "liberal" enough in concern to have contained their "illnesses" within the institution created for that purpose.

The illness that enters these institutions is, therefore, more and more distant from madness as the tragic experience of the world, as the relationship of a self that transcends it, or from madness as a monstrosity and a crime. More and more, it concerns the tragic experience of a body and the misery of a life it cannot live and a margin of subjective participation it cannot express. Could Lombroso, upon entering the asylum at the beginning of the twentieth century, where he found vagabonds, derelicts, peasants who had migrated to the city, and victims of pellagra, all locked up together under the label of mental illness, have sorted out illness from misery the way Pinel did with delinquency? Backed by the thought of the Enlightenment, Pinel had the possibility of creating an institution for illness that left delinquency intact, because that scientific, humanitarian gesture did not disturb the relationship with misery that a separate segregation continued to guarantee.

But suppose Lombroso, spurred on by the social movements of the beginning of the century, instead of recognizing pellagra as an illness, had denounced it as having to do with hunger. Where could he have put this misery that was confused with illness? Would he have brought it back to the streets where it had been banished so as not to be visible? Who would have listened to him, if this process of sorting out presupposes a social and political response to misery? The liberal state is not inclined to give such a response, and misery remains confused with illness, whose face it takes on so that it can save the face of the liberal state.

Economic Order and the Body

The history of psychiatry and its institutions, the history of a set of norms that has regulated its existence, can be read as a dialectic between individual and group, subjectivity and collectivity, and hence person and organization. Social life is founded on the institution of rules that allow the group's members to coexist. Norm is the limit imposed on the individual by the collectivity and the organization. If the individual participates in the definition of this norm as the expression of one's own and others' needs, one's subjectivity will be limited only in the existence of the Other, of other subjectivities. And for the individual it is burdensome enough to have to accept this limit. But if the norm is a rule imposed by a dominant group for its defense, it hinders any subjective expression in the dominated, reducing the individual to a dominated body, a body alienated and exploited by that which organizes it.

The dialectic between individual and organization should be expressed as the dialectic between an organic body (which the subject has appropriated in its organic relationship to the group, hence an organic body in relation to the construction of responses to its own needs and to those of the group), and a social body that represents the sum of the subjects who participate in their own organization, and in the organization of responses to their own needs and to those of the group. Organic body and social body would in this case be expressions of an individual subjectivity contained in a collective subjectivity.

But the system of production that has asserted itself is founded on the appropriation of the person's subjectivity; hence, of the reduction of the organic body to body, and of the tendential identification between social body and economic [order] body. In fact, the social body is merely the ensemble of systems that is dependent on the economic body, and hence upon the system of production that organizes the masses, who are reduced to so many bodies deprived of subjectivity. The dialectic between person and organization is reduced to the attempt to identify body with economic order, to facilitate the absorption of one by the other. Only in this dimension of gradual expropriation of the person's subjectivity will it be possible to sort it out from the institutions of production and of exploitation—or of invalidation and internment— thus reducing the expropriated body to the image of the logic that expropriates it.

The scientific apparatus has a crucial role in this operation, given that the objectivity of research and technical intervention are guaranteed by the objectivity of whoever is doing the research; just as the exploitation of people by the system of production had already carried out this process that will continue in the objectification of madness by reason. Both the clinic and reason need an object to work on so that their intervention will be aseptic and objective. And just as the clinic imposes upon the body the model produced in the image of its knowledge, so reason imposes upon madness the body of its language, "illness." Medical investigations are never concerned with men and women, their experiences, but with their own images imposed

upon the person as body. In the same way, the organization of labor does not produce for people, but for itself, and to do so, it
needs a person reduced to the body that produces.

The boundaries of the organic body, which medicine
identifies with the physical limitations of the *soma,* coincide, then,
with that which exploitation and the process of alienation tend to
reduce to the dominated and expropriated body. Medicine, in reducing man to *soma,* seems to precede the identification that the
economic body tends to create with the body. The positivist ma-
trix after which psychiatric knowledge is modeled will facilitate
this identification because the objectification of men and women
is already implicit in the scientific method. The concept of a causal
connection between the phenomena, mechanistically determined
by the natural sciences, flattens and confounds the biological, psychological, and social elements of which every human experience
is constituted, by placing within parentheses the contradictions,
present at every level, that arise from the dialectic between individual and organization.

Once this dialectic has been reduced to the coincidence
of body and economic order, the needs of one are absorbed in
those of the other, and the antagonism between such differing
needs is no longer understood in terms of what is ultimately a
class struggle between two artifically identified poles. When the
epiphenomena of this struggle are separated from the economic
order and one from the other, it becomes possible to inquire into
each of their causes. These are traced in a "social" space already
assumed, in a positivist sense, as nature, as a "given", and never
recognized as a historical-social product, hence never considered
an economic body. Confronting the illness of *soma* means, then,
confronting what might constitute the illness of the economic order and what could upset its equilibrium. And treatment is reduced to the healing of this equilibrium through the confirmation of invalidation.

In this way, the new lunacy laws began to delegate tasks
to the various disciplines, with a neutrality based on an apparent
division of competencies: the social body is placed under the tutelage of the justice system; the individual body under the tutelage
of medicine. But under the tutelage of both falls that threshold between spheres which consists of what explicitly belongs to the eco-

nomic sphere. What guarantees the operation is the fact that the economic order is disguised as a social body, in which each individual—hence each body, in an organic relationship to the various individualities which constitute the group—should recognize himself or herself. In a formal sense, the social body is structured to respond to the needs of the individual and the collectivity, but if the result is the ensemble of systems and institutions that constitute and sustain the economic body—the system of production based on profit—the social body will only be able to respond to its own demands, without taking into consideration individual and collective needs that are implicitly subordinated to the demands of the logic that determines it.

The gap between a body that refuses to be one and an economic order whose needs can only be antagonistic to those of the individual and of the collectivity, produces the conflicts and the suffering. The presence of suffering is the telltale sign of the missed identification between the body and economic body, hence the sign of a subjectivity that reacts and refuses to be an object of containment. When this suffering—forced to express itself in the language of illness, reduced to a language of social dangerousness—is confronted with medical-judicial terms and instruments, the technical intervention is determined not by the scientific attitude, but by the function it performs as the guarantor of the economic order. The game between suffering and treatment and dangerousness and custody protects both medicine and justice, by affirming the norm that both are obligated to protect, inasmuch as both are founded upon it. But this game becomes resolved when suffering and treatment disappear, engulfed by the dangerousness and custody that, alone, could provide these guarantees.

Is Madness Lent a Voice?

A voice confused with misery, indigency, and delinquency; a voice silenced by the rational language of illness; a message curtailed by imprisonment and rendered undecipherable by the definition of dangerousness and the socially necessary invalidation of which it is the object; madness is never heard for what it says or would like to say. Psychiatry has merely been the sign of dominant rationality's mastery of the word that escaped its grip, and the affirmation—intrinsic to this rationality—of an impossible communication. From the rationalism of the Enlightenment to postivism, rationality always involves defining, classifying, and controlling what it does not and cannot understand, because it has objectified madness in the language of illness, which is the language of a rationality that observes.

How are deliriums defined if not by ascertaining the diverse forms they take and by confirming the total incommunicability of what they express? Reason begins to individualize in the body the alterations responsible for delirium so as to distinguish and define the various forms of behavior through which it expresses itself. It is always linked to deviation from the straight and narrow path—dominant reason—which is considered an absolute fact.

When Diderot and d'Alembert confronted the problem of delirium in their *Encyclopédie,* the analysis of its causes, perfectly coherent with the phrenology of the period, was essentially physical (fevers, tensions, or relaxation of the fibers):

The most probable etymology of this name derives, according to several authors, from the word *lira,* which means a ditch in a straight line that is made in the fields and serves the purpose of draining the furrows; so that from the expression *aberrare de lira,* to deviate from the main furrow, is born the word *delirus,* which means, through allusion, a man who deviates from the path of reason, because delirium is nothing other than the bewilderment, the error of the spirit during its waking state, which makes erroneous judgements about things known to everyone. The soul is always in the same state, because it is not susceptible to any alteration; thus it is not to it that one must attribute this error, this defect of judgement that constitute delirium, but to the disposition of the body's organs, to which the creator wanted to unite the soul; this is beyond doubt.[7]

That the delirious person deviates from the rule of reason is for Enlightenment faith an absolute rule that does not allow deviations and that obviously is never questioned. If the soul cannot be responsible for abnormal behavior, research continues to be centered upon a body that does not reveal alterations and for which no ideal scheme (the model created in the image of scientific knowledge) can be manufactured for framing the validity of interpretations that are proposed about it.

More than one hundred years after the publication of the *Encyclopédie*, the *Enciclopedia Italiana Trecciani*—an expression of the cultural colonialism to which Italy has been subjected, it can be considered the summary of the evolution of French and German psychiatric thought—shows how this research on the alterations of the body has been toned down. Even if always implicitly, the research is overwhelmed by a mechanical description of the different qualities of the delirium; any reference to the "furrow" from which it deviates continues to be missing. But if in the presence of presumed physical causes, the exclusion of this essential element could be justified, the issue becomes more complex when the definition of delirium focuses on a behavior that can only be relative to the rules imposed by organized reason. Delirium essentially becomes an "error of judgment," expressed in varied behavior, that psychiatry limits itself to ascertaining and describing without ever putting into play, as a dialectical pole of the contradiction it represents, the rule from which it deviates and even less so the reason that formulates the judgment:

Delirium is the name given to those aberrations of judgment suggested by a state of passion or by affective disorders of morbid origin. Under the influence of affective deviations, criticial facilities become one-sided, relentlessly attack anything that might undermine the delirium, and allow all the errors that reinforce it to go unobserved. Experience is dominated by preconceptions: subjective images, springing from fantasy, pollute one's perception with delusional elements and bring about hallucinations, which confirm the delirium. Originating as suspicions, delirious judgments are soon affirmed as convictions that defy any criticism and become the ideal guide, often undisputed by action.

Just as the oscillations of affective experience take place in two opposite senses, depression and over-excitement, so can deliriums be divided into those that are depressive, about dejection, pessimistic delusions of ruin, misery, persecution, lack of worth, guilt, damnation; and deliriums that are expansive, over-excited, optimistic (delusions of vanity, grandeur, power, social reform). More specifically, deliriums are arranged around the instincts and basic passions of human nature: the survival instinct (delusions of persecution, hypochondria, and ruin); the passion for possession (delusions of pretense, revenge, jealousy); the sentiment of one's worth (delusions of grandeur, social and political reform, scientific delusions); the sexual instinct (erotic or jealous delusions); and religious feelings (messianic or prophetic delusions). The most complete expression of the delirious conviction is found in the systematized delusions of paranoiacs: because in these individuals the anomaly of passion and critical defect are constitutional and permanent, the delirium undergoes continual elaboration, nourished by the most common of events, which are interpreted in the sense of the delirium (delusion of interpretation), and so is consolidated even more, becoming a coherent system of obdurate convictions. In the affective psychoses, the deliriums follow the vicissitudes of the affective disturbances, and so during crises of melancholia, ideas of ruin, misery, guilt, and damnation arise, only to fade away with treatment or to become replaced by expansive deliriums during phases of manic excitement.[8]

If we take this description as a summary of the evolution of psychiatry up until the beginning of this century, it is evident that reason—through the definition of the various qualities of deliriums that maintain the characteristic of a value judgment—is limited to the establishment of a given (the delusion's mode of expression and its content), with which it is not able to establish any relationship. Necessarily distancing itself so that it can formulate a judgment, it finds itself too far away to understand and can only describe and state.

A prisoner of this impossible communication, Freud broke the certainty of reason and introduced doubt into the discourse: one must look again in the world objectified by reason to find the speech of madness, the meaning of its message, the deep zones from which it emerges, and where it must be made to flower. Unreason is inside us, it is part of our nature, not in the sense understood by an enlightened reason that would recognize it only in the moment in which it restrained and disarmed it; but in the sense that man is tragically harnessed by his own unreason. We must understand the profound reasons: "The self is no longer master of its own house." It is the assertion of this original split within the self that places the human experience, which critical reason had sterilized through its domination over unreason, back into the tragic dimension. A voice must be lent to this tragic experience, and it is this experience that must be deciphered and interpreted.

But who lends madness its voice? Who deciphers and interprets the message and on the basis of which code? And who decides to whom speech should be given? Is the neutral attention which Freud talks about possible, and is the message heard really neutral? How can we be sure that speech is not determined by the interpretation to which it lends itself? Who listens, what is his or her position of power in relation to who speaks, and to what degree does this power determine the meaning of the word? And above all, what is the language of the interpreter, and how can we be certain that we will avoid imposing the language of illness on madness? How do analysts confront the original split of the self, the self that is no longer master of its own house? Do they leave the wound uncovered, the doors open to invasions, or do they close them with the scientific certainty of their interpretation? When and where does madness speak its own language? Are we not again concerned with the concession of a dialogue that can take place only in the code of the listener? Does not the unconscious, in this operation, become the mirror image of reason; that is, of the interpretation, objectified in its eyes, just as madness was objectified in illness?

Freud recognized a self that was no longer master of its own house, but the practical conclusion arrived at by psychoanalysis is a different, subtler, and deeper form of mastery of the self, split between reason and unreason, dominated by whatever interpretation is made about this division. The circle closes: the door opened on subjectivity is now shut by the objectification of the self. Reason has acknowledged unreason within itself, but still dominates so as to define the boundaries of the game, to explain its meaning, objectifying the subjective experience naturalistically. And it is still about bourgeois reason. Even if Freud discusses and criticizes it at its roots, the language of interpretation remains within the rationality of its class and expresses its values, impregnating its culture through the discovery of a more tragic face of madness. It is a madness that lives between us and within us, and that we cannot ignore without altogether altering the madness and misery that reason continues to keep segregated, without altering the rationality that produces and controls this invalidation.

The game repeats itself and is implicit in that gesture of "lending a voice" that psychiatry continues to fulfill, keeping itself within a rationality predisposed to criticism and self-criticism, but only if they stem from those to whom the word has been conceded, and not from those who speak up because they recognize their right to speak and to be heard. This gesture, this listening, remains within the logic that distributes the parts, categories, possibilities of existence, roles, and functions even if it realizes that it is tragically compromised by unreason, by instinct, libido, aggressivity, madness, and the death wish. What surfaces from this consciousness is the tragic dimension, brought back to the life of the person, but as tragic individual, the subject, the self who recognizes itself as prisoner of that original split without being able to trace it back to all that the rationality that dominates and organizes makes of the self.

And it is the explosion of the irrational that, from time to time, will be experienced like a threat or proposed like a value, forever present in modern thought but controlled by it more and more. The madness of the artist, the unreason of the genius—like the insanity of the sick person—will find a place in this rationality that has understood that it need only lend them a voice and a separate space in which to express it to avoid being damaged by what they say. The response to the threat of irrationality that has been learnt is the terrorism of reason that organizes, divides, distributes, and separates the parts, punishing or rewarding whoever does not play the game. Just as the split of the self is resolved in the analyst's office and madness and misery disappear when locked away, the mad gesture of whoever breaks down the barrier of this rationality will be quieted by applause, in the museums and emporiums of Art in which its voice will be harnessed and neutralized.

The irrational continues to surface and, simultaneously, to be contained in modern thought, conditioned by this sometimes subterranean sometimes intrusive presence, and reposed as the sole possibility of subjective expression in a world of repression and violence. Until madness itself—stripped of the illness mask through which it has been forced to speak—is reappropriated as the only process of disalienation in a world alienated by technological-industrial rationality, it remains powerless. The task is to liberate madness as the only "experience" that vindicates the right of irrationality against the madness of dominant rationality.

But how does this liberated madness that vindicates the right to its own existence, opposing itself to alienated reality, penetrate the dominant rationality, unless it is limited to proposing itself as its opposite?

The Organized Conflict

Freud's contribution to the social and political problem of the relationship of reason and madness is extraneous. Although the relationship has been transformed into that between organization and invalidation, it maintains the same characteristics for around 150 years. Despite the vindication of the rights of the unconscious, from the moment the medical-legal definition of psychiatry is introduced, the economic body is emphasized while the body proper is annulled through the sanction of internment. The recognition of a fractured self has not corroded the mechanism that produces illness, because this mechanism is reproduced elsewhere, outside that space in which reason analyzes itself critically and scientifically.

The fact that the relationship between organization and invalidation was first questioned in the territory where this mechanism was produced can once again clarify the nature of the bond between reason and madness. The crisis of European legislation concerning psychiatric services and the questioning of the nature of the treatment of mental illness began to manifest themselves around the 1950s in several countries in which the restructuring of the organization of production and its consequent transformations induced the new labor-power, thus widening the sphere of those who participate in the contract.

The case of England is emblematic. When the expansion of production forced more to participate in the contract, the state used the Mental Health (England and Wales) Act of 1959 that sanctioned nationalization of medicine to push for the reconstruction of psychiatric services as well, thus cutting into the logic of internment for the first time. Rehabilitation and treatment of the mentally ill appeared possible once they became socially useful, that is, economically necessary, and psychiatry was once again used as the key element around which the new order gravitated.

The segregated body can and must be restored to the economic order; indeed its continuity, seemingly different in nature from the earlier identification between repair of the economic order (the eradication of infection and the containment of the infected) and repair of the individual body (treatment), must be restored. The custodial aspect, while continuing to exist, weakens, as rehabilitation and recovery are emphasized.

The apparent difference in this continuity is found in the fact that, while norm is defined in terms of efficiency and productivity, these terms never turn out to be rigid, but rather are subordinated to the oscillations and requirements of production. What shifts is the boundary between contract and invalidation, in the sense that the social organization can need to absorb those elements closest (or considered closest) to the norm—those that can be recuperated most easily—for the same system of production that expelled them may later need to reabsorb them.

A piece of legislation such as the Mental Health Act of 1959, that established the nationalization of medicine in a capitalist country, cannot in fact sever the roots of the relationship between organization and invalidation. This is what reduced a political intervention (a bill passed by a Labor government) to a simple technical intervention (rehabilitation, community psychiatry) within the same logic and goals that supported invalidation and exclusion.

Rehabilitation and recovery are not in fact antagonistic to this logic and to these goals when labor-power, even a rehabilitated one, is needed. What is interesting is that the possibility of shifting the boundaries between the contract and invalidation confirms the relative nature of the relationship between reason and madness, because those who were once locked up as mad are now rehabilitated as mentally healthy. The paradox is that if Pinel's era witnessed the transfer of illness from the prison to the asylum, now the tendency is to remove from the asylum a health extracted from this illness. It is the very concepts of illness and of recovery that are relativized in this shift. The fact that such an operation remains within the same logic, and thus cannot help but reproduce the same control outside the asylum, does not minimize its profound significance as far as the concept and definition of illness are concerned.

The community psychiatry experiences born during these years were founded on the conviction that it is sufficient to broaden the treatment of the individual to include the context in which he or she lives, to rectify at the same time the conflicts of a psychological nature as well as the social conflicts that produce them. Psychiatry found itself acquiring a new centrality. No longer was it limited to managing the world of invalidation and internment that it continued to treat; it now had to enter the social realm to control disturbances directly where they are manifested, singling out all the elements of which they are composed, including the social conflicts that can determine them. The services shaped by new legislation in the various countries (after the British Mental Health Act there was the 1960 *politique de secteur* in France, and the 1963 Community Mental Health Centers Act in the United States) continue to place a value on the medical aspect of psychiatry. Through its absorption of the new social sciences, medicine expanded the possibility for such interventions and innovations as catchment areas, preventive policies, mental health centers, brief hospitalization, and psychiatric wards in general hospitals. But simultaneously new technicians were introduced at an enormous rate: psychologists, social workers, sociologists, and counselors. Such an organization rotated around psychiatrists who, with the multidisiplinary nature of their interventions, could now face the simultaneous presence of the most diverse types of disturbances that the old psychiatry had flattened in the concept of *soma*.

The separation of body and economic order represented in the separation between asylum and community is resolved by diffusing, through this army of new workers, the technician's or the doctor's culture, definition, and treatment of the illness in the community. With the former inmate forced into the community and potential psychiatric commitment now prevented, a new form of control is facilitated; it no longer allows internment to be played out through judicial sanction, but rather encompasses ever vaster numbers of people to be helped. The new sphere to be controlled is no longer segregated, even if the old form of segregation continues to exist and to guarantee the efficiency of new apparatuses. But the person who guarantees good functioning from the welfare apparatus to medical-psychiatric treatment to commitment is always the psychiatrist. Community participation, in this phase emphasized as direct action and control over the technician, is instead constantly mediated and organized through the institutional filters and medical culture. In this way it is possible to guarantee that the subjective expression of the demand—of the need, of suffering, of the disturbance, hence of the contradiction between individual and organization—is directed through pre-established channels that are not antagonistic to the general equilibrium. This means guaranteeing that the demand is always for a therapeutic treatment that in turn has the task of attenuating conflict and organizing it in medical terms. Moreover, what is assured through the creation of these new services is the amount of human labor-power they can absorb (and that can be identified automatically in the newly developed roles), such that the control exerted over the individual consumer, and through the identification of the worker in his or her own role, affects the entire context of production that supports it. The medical model continues to prevail over the global characteristics of the intervention. The necessity of treatment is never questioned, given that it is limited to extending the range of solutions with which it can discriminate between different levels of dangerousness and upon which it bases the quality of treatment.

Although formally they differ from one another, the reference models adopted by every piece of legislation in this phase move within this scheme: the restoration of the invalidated body (or the prevention of its possible invalidation) to the economic order. This is a necessary condition if the struggle between organization and invalidation is to vanish within an equilibrium that this time will translate segregated invalidation into a semi-invalidation, assisted by social services. This process is by now generalized in most of the Western countries where invalidation and welfare tend to cover every nonorganized form of dissent. But it is present—even if articulated differently—in the Soviet Union as well, where the identification between State and institutions allows the use of illness as a form of mediation that justifies an analogous form of control.

Within this panorama, the case of Italy, where the problem exploded many years later than in other countries, deserves special mention. With respect to other European legislation, the

Italian law (Law 180) approved in May 1978 and subsequently incorporated into the health reform law, stated very explicitly the need for halting construction of further psychiatric hospitals and for organizing the elimination of existing ones. The formula that justified involuntary commitment—"dangerous to oneself and to others and of public scandal"—was replaced by a normative one that, while still allowing the entire responsibility for determining social dangerousness to fall on the doctor, introduced, even if in a confused manner, a new element. The judgment of severity [of the illness] remained, reinforced in cases where the patient refused involuntary commitment; but authorized treatment is compulsory only when alternative solutions to commitment are deemed impossible. The misinterpretation and exploitation that can derive from this subjective interpretation of a single case (who has the responsibility for determining that other solutions are nonexistent?) can put brakes on the new legislation, leading to a generic reconversion of psychiatric services into general medicine, as has happened in other countries. The fact that in Italy, asylums to back up the new services are not allowed to exist gives the services themselves different meaning and function. The new law is not limited to breaking the absoluteness of the scientific definition of mental illness, thus suggesting its relativity to other factors, but rather tends to question (and hence raise consciousness through the contradictions that are thereby opened up) the function of the asylum as a cover for the operation perpetuated by the system of production that has been able to exclude, through laws and sciences most adapted to this exclusion, whatever hampered its functioning.

Madness and Need

Reason includes and excludes madness, determining the sectors, modes, and times when it can speak up, hence neutralizing it. In this way, a certain legitimacy is assumed whereby madness speaks in an authorized language, whether or not it is understandable according to the canons of the *écoute*. But can there exist a rule for expressing needs and desires? Or is not the very existence of the rule an imposition and a form of violence that can only produce a violent means of manifesting these needs and desires? Where does human subjectivity lie within this rule, if mandatory modes, times and places exist for its expression? What are the consequences of this insistence on lending a voice? What happens when those who speak up and express their needs in their own language rather than in one distorted by the words of others are not heard?

The problem of madness is always the relationship between the individual and the organization. It is a problem of the space—physical and psychological—that the individual finds within the group. In a formal sense, the rationality upon which our culture is founded emphasizes the individual and his or her freedom, as does the society and organization of labor which produce them. In fact, rationality is structured on the expropriation of the individual, and the reduction of the expropriated mass to a serialized ensemble of individuals. Similarly, although it has recognized unreason as part of human nature, this rationality limits itself to absorbing it. In this way, unreason is diverted and directed to sectors created to keep it under its tutelage. This is what caused Nietszche to say: "That is the task of the Enlightenment: to make princes and statesmen unmistakably aware that everything they do is sheer falsehood."[9]

But before reason had separated out unreason, how was madness expressed? Can we not presume that just as with the historical evolution of the phenomenon, madness emerged from and was nourished by an undifferentiated world of unmet needs, and that it is the nonresponse to these needs that translated into the importance from which is derived what we call madness? Before madness had been individuated from bourgeois rationality as illness, its voice was confused with indigency, and deliquency—an indistinct totality of needs which were responded to by shattering the globality of the demand, essentially represented by misery.

The same process could also repeat itself in every individual history. People are born with a nature against which they must struggle, appropriating themselves and also producing a culture that will tend towards altering their nature. Defined by the world of needs and desires that come from the body, and by a subjectivity that wishes to be expressed, they find themselves encountering other bodies and subjectivities that must be organized. The response to these needs is entrusted to the organization that represents the group and that must allow it to live and its members to coexist. If the organization represents the whole group, individual space for one's own needs and their satisfaction will be limited by the needs of others. The problem of limits is a human problem, one that is summed up in the relationship of the person to the nature that must be tamed and exploited. But if the organization protects the interests of one group (a class) at the expense of another, if the survival of this group is based on the domination of the other, if the logic of the exploitation of nature is based on the exploitation of people, there is no human limit. For everything is involved in the inhumanity of organization—an inhumanity from which not even the protected class will be saved, because to perpetuate itself this organizational logic can only produce inhuman values.

Misery has many faces: that of hunger and indigency, and that of the total impoverishment of human existence. Bourgeois rationality has preserved the former in the pockets necessary for maintaining the equilibrium of the economic logic upon which it is founded; but it has produced the latter from within itself. It is in this generalized world of economic and psychological misery that needs are expressed in a confused and undifferentiated way. These include needs that arise from the urgency of life, from a body that does not accept mutilation and mortification, from a subjectivity that does not wish to be repressed and raped, and that finds the space it has been conceded too narrow. Rules, prohibitions, taboos, and repression; divisions of class, race, color, sex, and role; expression, tyranny, humiliation, organized and permanent violence—these are what constitute the world of the norm. No rule defends human existence, but every rule is made for its domination and manipulation. The dominated cannot identify with this norm because it is made to destroy them; but neither can those who belong to the dominating group, for they risk dulling and destroying their humanity.

From this indistinct panorama of needs (the concrete misery of the lower classes and the pauperization of the individuals from the protected class), some voices can be raised, crying out the anguish, furor, anger about the split and the fragmentation or weeping for their own impotence. It is then they will be given a voice, to silence them with the definition of an illness that will always be treated, so that it does not reveal from whence it comes.

But there is a moment when all of this is expressed in the form of demands that await responses, when everything could be simple or almost so, because human hope still cements and unites the globality of the demand. But it is this demand that remains unanswered and is broken up into as many rivulets as there are technical responses already prepared by the rationality of power. The misery of the oppressed classes, and the pauperization and belittlement of those who are subordinated to an economic logic that determines every one of their needs and desires, comprise the mute demand that bourgeois rationality prohibits them from formulating, imposing upon these needs the language of illness that makes them become other than what they are. And if this demand can not be expressed in organized, finalized forms of struggle, it can flow into forms of irrational, uncontrollable behavior, and expressions of the uncontainable aspect of suffering and the impossibility of finding different ways of communicating it. But when the label of illness is superimposed upon these, their voices are altered, their concrete reality replaced by the symbol.

When all of this has happened, someone will still take the trouble to reconstruct symbolically the knots of suffering, to rediscover the moment of rupture. Or someone—perhaps coarser, to conform to the coarseness of the client—will simply say it has to do with a "paranoid delusion" or "depressive episode" and will lock him in an asylum. When all has happened, it is difficult to reconstruct the parts of that unanswered need, to piece together those demands so as to reformulate them. The hope that could cement them will have disappeared because it was frustrated for too long. First the person is killed or prevented from living. Then science—psychiatry and the social sciences—become concerned, lamentably, with the reactions of impotence and despair, or of the apathy, refusal, and a-sociability that follow, until the person dies by asphyxiation. It is to that world of needs that responses must be made, passing through also the fragmentation of the social sciences that have contributed to disguising the game, preventing the understanding of where problems are born.

There are always false prophets. But in the case of psychiatry it is the prophecy itself that is false. With the schema of definitions and classification of behaviors, with its repressive violence, with the misunderstanding of suffering, it prevents any real understanding of its relationship to reality and of the possibility of expression that people find or do not find in it. Continuing to accept psychiatry and the definition of mental illness means accepting the dehumanized world in which we live as the only human world, natural, unmodifiable, which people face unarmed. If it is like this, we will continue to relieve symptoms, make diagnoses, administer treatments and cures, and invent new therapeutic techniques. But all the while we will remain aware that the problem is elsewhere. Because "not existence but knowledge is without hope, for in the pictoral or mathematical symbols it appropriates and perpetuates existence as a schema."[10]

Part Five ANTI-INSTITUTIONAL POLITICS AND REFORM: ON PSYCHIATRY AND LAW

Introduction

Anne M. Lovell

No alternative psychiatry groups have ever achieved the level of success that the Italian anti-institutional movement reached in the 1970s. Not only were exclusion, marginality, and psychiatric repression brought to national attention, the movement succeeded in passing a law that actually transformed the judicial definitions of mental illness, dangerousness, and internment.

But implementing the reforms of the Law 180 required the movement to shed many vestiges of post-'68 radicalism, the "Jacobinism" Basaglia was accused of and which he addresses in the second selection. Democratic psychiatry had always encompassed a heterogeneity of stances. But with the Law 180 enacted, the alternative psychiatry movement shifted away from an often conflictual relationship with parties, administrators, and bureaucracies, to one of participation in carrying out new policies and reforms. Such a change in strategy could be dangerous, threatening to substitute for a radical context a planned program controlled by administrative hierarchies. It could also dampen the spirit of the movement, minimizing the gains of the past fifteen years, distorting the meaning of its values and model experiences, as befalls many grass-roots movements. This awareness of the double-edged nature of the Law 180 runs like an undercurrent through the two selections in this section.

"Problems of Law and Psychiatry" provides a historical and comparative framework for the law. Picking up from the earlier piece, "Madness/Delirium", Basaglia elaborates upon psychiatry's gradual incorporation of judicial sanctions for controlling part of what is disruptive, dangerous to the social equilibrium, and unproductive. By the turn of this century, European legislation governing asylums and commitment procedures had accomplished this. Law, not medicine, had come to define the domain and boundaries of psychiatry, emphasizing the *social* aspect of medicine and attributing primary importance to the asylum (which was, after all, not so structurally different from the prison).

In Basaglia's analysis of post-World War II developments, chronicity emerges as a social construction, the overproduction of illness. Corresponding to this period of economic expansion is a flowering of notions and techniques for rehabilitating unproductive individuals; i.e. "chronics." Yet in the United States and Europe, a major cause of social chronicity—the asylum—remained untouched by community psychiatry reforms, which merely modified the relationship between judicial norms and the psychiatric system.

Ultimately, the attack on chronicity failed. Not only did outpatient facilities and services produce a new, "soft" form of chronicity, whose bearers are dependent on not one total institution, but they also produced a series of social and mental health services that perpetuate their marginality ad infinitum.[1] Community psychiatry, despite its emphasis on efficiency and efficacy, also failed to address the social and welfare needs of "chronic" patients, old and new. Nevertheless, Italy in the seventies had yet to target chronic patients. The 1968 "Mariotti Law," which established voluntary commitment, and community mental health centers, remained untried.

By gradually eliminating public mental hospitals, the Law 180 quickly bypasses its predecessors in other countries. In contrast, the France *secteur* model retains the mental hospital as one of the essential components of each catchment area.[2] And while American community mental health centers grew during deinstitutionalization, they essentially short-circuited the mental hospital, by serving a new rapidly expanding acute population while ignoring the increasing number of discharged patients.

The asylum as a major "sick-producing" institution is confronted in Article F (See Appendix) of the Law 180 which explicitly prohibits the construction of new mental hospitals and the creation of new or use of existing mental health departments or units in general hospitals (except the 15-bed diagnostic and treatment unit), neurological or neuropsychiatric departments. Article

8 requires that the status of public, long-stay patients be reexamined within three months of the law's enactment and that the names of those in need of further compulsory treatment be sent to the mayors of their respective towns of residence. Furthermore, by emphasizing a network of services outside the hospital system, the law assumes that long-stay patients should have access to the same resources as any other disadvantaged group. Unfortunately, these services are not spelled out, as both advocates and detractors of the Law 180 have pointed out.

Not surprisingly, the law incorporates some of the major principles antipsychiatry and patients' rights groups have long advocated in other countries. The principle of the "least restrictive alternative," elaborated in judicial decisions pertaining to patients' rights lawsuits in the United States, is expressed by one of the three criteria for compulsory treatment, that "there are not the conditions and the circumstances for taking immediate and timely health care measures outside the hospital." The right to treatment is also established in the place of judicial sanctions—for example, confinement—based on dangerousness. Patients retain their civil rights.

Yet two aspects of the law have met criticism from antipsychiatry groups outside Italy.[3] First, it does retain some form of compulsory treatment, which was a result of the compromise the law represents. The Italian response to those who would push either more legislated guarantees or, at the other extreme, no state intervention, is that with an adequate network of services compulsory treatment can be avoided. And while the reasons for demanding hospitalization are often complex and culturally determined to some extent,[4] one explanation for possible increase in cases of compulsory treatment (*Trattamenti Sanitari Obbligatori*), since 1980 is probably the lack of services available to patients outside of the diagnostic and treatment unit.

Second, the Law attributes responsibility to the state for responding to individuals suffering from psychic distress. Elsewhere, in contrast, many branches of antipsychiatry refused to work within a state-run system (see the "Dialogue with R.D. Laing in Part Three); others, such as the French groups, either operated at a totally symbolic level (e.g., the radical Lacaniens), or challenged only the most repressive aspects of state power (e.g. in-

270 ANTI-INSTITUTIONAL POLITICS AND REFORM

voluntary commitment as manifested through psychiatry).[5] The Italians, however, are apprehensive about allowing psychiatrists to abdicate responsibility for people experiencing psychological difficulties; such neglect was common after the Law 180 was passed (see Franca Ongaro Basaglia's preface to this book).

Nowhere does Basaglia express the dilemma faced by anti-institutional workers on the dawn of the new law as well as in the last selection, "Critical Psychiatry after the Law 180." The knowledge gained over fifteen years could balance the sudden loss of identity and common reference points—the model experiences such as Trieste and Arrezzo, no longer needing to fight against institutional psychiatry. And yet, without the definitions and social space of the old institutional psychiatry, practitioners are left with a world to construct. This is the moment to seize: when one stands, with few cultural tools at one's disposal, before a type of suffering heretofore not seen. It is the behavior of people no longer identified or identifiable with the institution.

Basaglia's description brings to mind certain parallels with the situation after deinstitutionalization in the United States. In the United States, mental health workers suddenly faced a void in their knowledge when confronted with each new, noninstitutionalized group—the youth who had "fallen through the cracks" of a system that used hopitals less and less (the so-called young chronics), those among the homeless who manifested psychiatric problems that went untreated, the older ex-patients who were no longer in a captive situation. In both cases, a moment exists in which there are no clear institutional schemas to fall back on, to define the problem. The difference in the Italian situation is that with the Law 180 there is no institutional apparatus, because the last station—the mental hospital—is prohibited. The only possibility left is a new network of social and health services, a new social space still to be invented.

7. Problems of Law and Psychiatry: The Italian Experience

The Task and Definition of Psychiatry and the Norms Governing Its Conduct

The debate on the definition of madness, the classification of lunatics, psychiatry as a science, and its institutions was already almost a century old when, at the beginning of the nineteenth century, in industrialized countries, the first laws on the subject of psychiatric treatment appeared. The story, however, dates back to the far-reaching social changes brought about at the dawn of the industrialized era when the structuring and organizing of production on a national scale concentrated and deposited the reserves of required manpower in the suburbs and outskirts of the larger industrial cities.

Madness, thus, slowly began to take on its various shapes in that vast and varied social terrain which makes up both a nation's wealth (because the mad are one source of reserve manpower) and its poverty (because of the misery and wretchedness of their living conditions.) The task of the productive organizations is to force this wretchedness to fit into preordained structures, dictated by reason, to rationalize and order it so that it produces the wealth required by the new society.

"Unreason" in wretchedness becomes, therefore, a "social problem," since the social organization as a whole has to take on responsibility for it and provide for it or, at least, bend it to its will so that it does not become a disruptive element of the producing system. Misery, as unreason, must therefore be channelled

With Maria Grazia Gianichedda.

into a social order which identifies itself with the orderly production of wealth. Each of these terms is defined negatively: the former is the possession of nothing save one's own bodily existence (as a source of manpower) while the latter is the absence of reason, the irrational, all that which refuses to comply with the rules of rational thought and, moreover, disturb its equilibrium. Misery is redeemed through work and ordered where production itself takes place; in return, identity and basic rights are guaranteed to those who adhere to and benefit from the social contract. Unreason, disqualified from the outset, must be deliberately cut off from the institution of rationality and separated from centres of production in places devised for that purpose. It may only return to form part of the social order if transformed by science and confined within the latter's institutions. "Sickness" becomes its rational definition and the asylum the place wherein it is confined and ordered.

From the vast and variegated world of misery, emerge then, within it, zones which are productive and therefore, rational or sane. At the opposite pole, we have all that which is unproductive, disqualified as such from the outset and relegated to that social area where science discovers, identifies, and classifies deviation as sickness and, in time, deviations from sicknesses. The rationalizing action of the state's institutions justifies their emergence within the social fabric, safeguarding the freedom of action of those integrated in the producing society by organizing the lives of those who are excluded from it.

Medicine, entrusted with the treatment of everything that has been set within the sphere of illness, conceals the fundamental contradiction between the separation of the productive and the unproductive which then becomes opposition between sane and sick. The failure to produce, which medicine must remedy, is symbolized by and concentrated in the body which is to become the object of its practices. The sickness and its physical symbol, the sick body, thus become mirror images of the techniques that medical science is gradually evolving. It is the birth of the clinic which seems to indicate that the identification of unproductive with sick has been reached, as has the integration of medicine and productive organization. What production rejects is sick and must subsequently be isolated and cared for by its institutions. In that enormous laboratory which is the clinic, illnesses are observed, classified, selected, and saved or condemned according to whether they comply with the rationality of the techniques which medical science has devised.

The contradiction reemerges when deviation from the psychic norm (madness) falls, as sickness, within medicine's sphere or competence. The new discipline, however, gradually taking shape along the same lines as the medical disciplines which are its model, is unable with its tools alone to control that pathology of relationship which is its real and specific task. Judicial sanctions then become its logical and basic complement. The concept of "dangerous to the community," which strictly belongs to the legal field, is justified and rationalized in medical categories or rather, the medical model is forced into the same forms as the judicial sanctions. The basic contradiction of psychiatry, thus, takes shape from the very outset—hovering between care of the sick and protection of the community, between medicine and law and order.

Together, those themes of the protection of the lunatic and the protection of the community from the excesses which lunacy may commit, are the two poles around which the debate on psychiatry's function takes place and which determine the relevant decisions in the organizational and legislative sector. They are interwoven in England in the dream of the Enlightenment of an ordered society producing wealth for mankind; in France, they are closely bound up with the great libertarian principles of the Revolution and, later, in Italy, they are constantly absorbed in the enormity of the "social question." Around these themes are set both the framework of principles, fixed by the first legislation on the subject, defining the criteria of the so-called "danger to the community" and the aims and methods of its treatment.

We see, therefore, clearly defined, on one hand the criteria for the identification of everything which, disqualified as unproductive, is a serious menace to community life and, on the other, the norms which justify this definition and plan ways of treating it with the inevitable corollary of separation and control.

If, in the medical field, the original compromise between science and productive organizations evolves with the former yielding to the exigencies of the latter, though still maintaining its autonomy as a specifically medical science in the definition and treatment of the object of its concerns (the body which is unproductive is sick), psychiatric knowledge finds, set out in the definition according to accepted norms, both its social functions and the form which the latter will take. In other words, the law not only clearly defines the limits within which the tasks and institutions of the new science will have to move, but goes so far as to identify its object: the sickness itself and the symptoms accompanying its outbreak. The idea of possible danger to the community is, at the same time, the justification for legal sanctions and the great category of diagnoses from which others stem and subsequently take shape. In fact, significant variations either in treatment techniques or in the administration of the institutions will be brought about by the proliferation and variety of these new categories until the first stages of the crisis of the old laws, i.e., after World War II.

Thus, legal actions loom permanently over the whole realm of psychiatric knowledge contaminating it to its very depths. The outlines of the body to be treated, clearly identified in medicine within the physical limits of the *soma*, on which the very nature and autonomy of medical science is based, become blurred as far as psychiatry is concerned and can even expand and be identified with the whole social fabric—the social body. That which psychiatry defines as sick is, in fact, that which the social setup defines as dangerous for its equilibrium, according to its changing requirements. Health and recovery are therefore, in psychiatry, the health and recovery of the social body. The individual sick body becomes a mere germ, a source of infection and an agent of contagion to be identified, isolated, and sterilized within the social vacuum of the asylum.

The interrelationship fostered by medical science between the individual body and the social structure, between the needs of the former and the way the latter functions, enabled a certain permeability between the productive and the unproductive, on which medicine, in fact, based its own functions. The chance of restoring the single body to the social organization, once it has been healed and enabled to form part of the productive apparatus, and/or when the latter presented an opening in which to insert it, has always been one of medicine's fundamental roles, unleashing, so to speak, its therapeutic qualities. In the case of psychiatry, the necessity of keeping the patient in custody, defined by the law as condition and form of the treatment, is in fact, identified by the asylum with the treatment itself and has frozen the contradiction between the individual body and the social fabric and made them irreconcilable opponents.

The productive body able to carry out useful and, therefore, socially relevant functions, the body as potential labour force to be revalued and restored to health, is withdrawn from the sphere of the development of psychiatric knowledge. On the other hand, the body which is the object of psychiatry's concerns only takes on its significance inasmuch as it is a "content of the asylum," after its removal from the general social context has blunted its potentially dangerous qualities. In this sense, the techniques used in treatment are to be identified with the organization and methods of the asylum itself, while illness and recovery are only the degree to which the individual yields to his integration into the organization of the institutions or stubbornly refuses to do so. Within its four walls, the insignificance of the inmate becomes definitive; he is reduced to a mere object, an image of the asylum itself, and only in this sense, has he become productive, though not of wealth but at least of social order.

It is precisely this production of social order which becomes the principle upon which the founding of the asylum and the conquering of madness are based. Madness is only conquered as a social problem, however, and this system will, for at least a century, until substantial modifications of the productive organization emerge, tend to preclude—unlike medicine—any possibility of the individual being restored to health. What can, however, be integrated into normal social life and form part of its rational set-up is the asylum itself, as the container within which madness is confined, which is the real object of psychiatric science's concerns and the driving force behind the development of its knowledge.

Within its four walls, the pulse of history ceases to beat, the social identity of the individual therein contained is suppressed, and the process of total identification of the individual with his psychic deviations takes place. The conditions of his life may be offered as proof of his innate inferiority, and his culture disregarded as the mere expression of his irrational deviation. The silence which thus sets in, in the asylum, becomes both typical of it and the guarantee that, from it, no messages will reach the outside world. The only possible message, clear from the very existence of those four walls, is the threat of sanctions to illustrate the abnormality of all that for which the mentality of a producing society has no room.

The asylum and the organization are not, however, only to be seen in the light of such negative productivity. The asylum is also an extraordinary observatory of behaviour patterns and the huge experimental laboratory where the lack of individual life (i.e., lack of productive and rational life) is the excuse for the failure to apply ethical principles to the same extent as in medicine and, moreover, justifies the withholding, temporary or permanent, of individual rights to a greater extent than in the prison system.

The criteria according to which psychiatry's norms are applied, have, throughout its history, always been particularly strict and careful not to allow any practices or ideologies, masquerading as therapeutic, to cast doubt on the fundamental identity of treatment and custody, on the sickness-sanctions symdrome, and to channel them along its own lines or brand them as dangerously political. On the other hand, as far as the safeguarding of the individual's rights laid down by the law and entrusted to the relevant bodies is concerned, ample scope has always been available when approved by the responsible authorities. In fact, the more severely and explicitly the law defines the sphere of competence and the organizational methods of the asylum (for example, the Italian legislation of 1904 and [1959] British legislation, at the other end of the scale), the more seriously are considered the slightest infringements of custody norms, and the less seriously any oversights in treatment.

The governing norms have, therefore, contributed, to a considerable extent, to forcing the development of psychiatric knowledge into certain channels, nearer to those of the state's judiciary apparatus than those of medicine. As is the case with the judiciary apparatus, it is the danger represented by deviant behaviour which is the real object of psychiatry's attention. Moreover, justice and psychiatry have the principles of sanction and separation in common, as well as a great deal of their institutional organization. Similarly, the system of norms sets up, in psychiatry's field too, a vast network of rules governing all the stages of the activity of the expert official: how to identify the disease (ascertaining the existence of criteria determining the danger to society), immediate sanction against it (generally restraint), and subsequent restriction of personal liberty (internment). The doctor/warden himself is responsible for the severity of the application of the above, to the extent that he may be cited as accessory should failure to confine the lunatic give rise to deviant behaviour. Treatment centers must, therefore, be up to the job and hence even physically resemble prisons. In the majority of European countries, this analogy is taken to extremes when the supervision of the functioning psychiatric institutions becomes the task of the Ministry of the Interior, which is responsible for law and order.

The scope for psychiatry to develop its medical side has, in all European countries, always been strictly limited by these principles and within these organizational rules, though to a varying extent. Such scope is, however, in theory provided for by the laws of the individual countries which entrust psychiatry with a clear role involving treatment, albeit in custody. Psychiatry's task, in its interventions, must become, in practice, that of harmonizing its strictly medical with its penal functions.

The debate on the various ways of treating madness, which explicitly have to lead to the convergence of medical techniques with judicial norms, is punctuated by many attempts to enable the medical model (as the therapeutic aim of the doctor's intervention) to prevail within the prison-like structure. The resulting tension, which is often accompanied by claims for greater autonomy on the part of psychiatrists as a professional body, who are also animated by the desire for a scientific enrichment of this hitherto dimly-outlined brance of science, manages to find room for practical action where the law is less rigid and the network of institutions more complex and widely distributed. Therefore, for almost a century and a half of psychiatry's history, the contrast between norms and techniques has evolved differently in the various countries, giving rise to Connoly's nonrestraint system in England, and on the other hand, the programs of Cerletti in Italy,[1] and Simmon in Germany, at the opposite ends of a hypothetical scale of coincidence between judicial norms and psychiatric technique. However, throughout Europe, the asylum continues to be the cor-

nerstone of the whole psychiatric structure. The knowledge and
culture developing around it, sanctioned by laws remaining largely
unchanged, are its cumbersome ideological and organizational
heritage. All those projected reforms envisaging its integration into
richer and more complex organizational and normative systems
have clashed with this heritage and hardly ever prevailed.

The New Psychiatric Order

The crisis of the asylum, as psychiatry's only organizational
model, rises to the surface in the three great victorious countries:
England, France, and the United States, immediately after World
War II. The process of redefinition and reorganization of psychiatry in each of these countries develops along different lines and
at a different pace, both as far as institutional transformation and
the revision of the norms are concerned. Any generalization attempting to heap together in one single model the process of the
nationalization of medicine in England, the sectorial policy in
France, and the diffusion of welfare in the United States would
not therefore correspond to reality. It would be even less justifi-
able to identify the results of the attempts at institutional transformation in these countries, with the relevant norms subsequently
issued. Yet, the vast difference in background, producing organizational apparatuses and ideological models with their own typical, unmistakable characteristics, appear less significant when
taken in the overall context of norms or, rather, the relationship
between the revision of norms and the redefinition of psychiatry
as a branch of learning and as an institution. Against this backdrop, some constants, though not in comparable normative contexts, can be traced. They emerge from the definition of norms
and in fact the new psychiatric order resulting from the crisis of
the asylum both as practice and as ideology, hinges on them to
this very day.

The automatic way in which, in the asylum, the diagnosis of illness means the prognosis of its chronic nature, followed in
turn by permanent confinement, has, for more than a century, in-
sured control over inclusion in or exclusion from the labor market
of those social classes which have been isolated and relegated to

the margins of the productive organization. The irrevocable nature of this exclusion from the world, sanctioned by the asylum, clashes at this point with the expanding economy and, hence, with the demand for new sources of labor and the rehabilitation, where possible, of the unfit. The overproduction of chronic sickness, thus, takes on the guise of waste of productive forces hoarded and administered within an institution. It is this sentence to loss of liberty which hinders recovery and integration into the productive world. The two mechanisms, part though not the whole of the asylum model, present themselves at this stage as the problem to be solved before psychiatry's functional efficiency can be restored or its ends achieved. They are, moreover, the focal points of psychiatrists' reforming impulses, reforming of the law, and organizational planning.

The point where the asylum and the productive organization clash, therefore, is where the aforementioned mechanisms insure that the two institutions shall be insulated one from the other, where the sanction is automatic and confinement irrevocable. The perceived effects of this friction emerge as ideological inconsistency and the inefficient running of the asylum; the one takes the form of a general suspicion of individual rights just at a moment in history when they are being stressed, while the other threatens the productive organization as it hinders the absorption of new sources of labor and the fruitful use of what has already been integrated.

The welding together of these discrepancies is a prerequisite of the renaissance of psychiatry. It is to be achieved by means of an organic relationship, ideological and organizational, between the restoration of the social body (control of its productive equilibrium) and the restoration of the individual body (defending its labor potential).

The object of these attempts to reform is, therefore, the asylum as an organization with its set of strict rules regulating internal organization and with its norms governing contacts with the outside world. Other features of the asylum, even though they have been dealt with at the ideological level, have not been included in the scope of reforming action. Doubts are cast neither on the identification of madness with illness nor on the necessity of particular, separate treatment, but rather on the efficiency of custody as the only means of treatment and on the general extension of judicial sanctions to all those inmates of the institution who are diagnosed as representing a threat to the community. The contours of the relationship between the institution and its contents (the individual suffering), between the request for treatment and the need behind it, become blurred, because the institution mechanically defines in terms of illness any sort of need which is presented. As neither the individual suffering nor its real meaning are perceptible outside the asylum, or before the latter's doors have closed behind him, total identification between the inmate and the structure around him sets in. Thereafter the crisis begins and criticism follows; both are centered on the form of the institution as, on the one hand, treatment's aim and technique and, on the other hand, the limited purport of the sickness. Only when the institution is no longer responsible for producing wide-ranging chronicity, will it be possible to realize that mental illness is not always chronic and will experience show that the rules of everyday living may actually be reacquired in an altered institutional context. Only when the institution is no longer compelled to imprison whoever falls within its grasp, will it be possible to discover that not all cases are dangerous, that not all kind of illness are dangerous to the same extent, and that even the issuing of sanctions may, under different treatment conditions, be graduated in both intensity and time.

The experiences of the tranformation of institutions which took place in France and the Anglo-Saxon countries are the great laboratory where the internal structure of the asylum set-up is analyzed in its single components and thoroughly rethought. Segregation is replaced by an emphasis on socialization under the supervision of a technician who constructs a network of sheltered relationships aiming at the recreation, within the institution, of models and living conditions resembling as closely as possible those of real life. Thus, social awareness filters through the walls into the asylum on the one hand as a search for increased contacts and democracy in social relationships, and on the other, finds its way out into the microsocial context where the illness originated. The course of these experiences, though rich in critical stimuli and practical suggestion, confines itself to the model of the institutional management of the illness as its field of study and makes no attempt to define or determine its own specific goals. Even where, for example in some post-war American sociological studies, the great processes relegating to the institution specific social classes and not others *are* described, even where (as the English experience shows) a relationship between the productive world and the management of the institution *does* emerge, or (in France) the connection between the existence of existential problems and social alienation is established, they only suggest new areas where the expert may intervene or new treatment techniques be applied.

All experiences of alternative management of institutions have, therefore, been circumscribed with the specific and separate field of psychiatry. They affect the transformation of both norms and organizational services through the practical application of certain ways of conceiving the asylum model and through the indication of organizational patterns leading to a continuous relationship between the institution and its catchment area. The old norms governing compulsory admission to the institution (the rigidly socialized sanction) are accompanied, though neither replaced nor modified, by regulations facilitating voluntary or informal admission. It is, though, still the doctor who decides which type of admission is suitable for the patient to be admitted, with varying degrees of urgency and permanency, to one of the range of available institutions. Individual rights, which these regulations contribute to guaranteeing, are enhanced therefore inside the institution itself and entrusted to the doctor as a strictly medical problem. So, as far as the norms are concerned, the declaration of principles becomes, in practice, a recommendation to the doctor to ensure that sanction and disorder are each accorded due weight. Yet, while the experiences of alternative management have been aimed at reducing sanctions and eliminating segregation, in practice, psychiatrists still operate within the limits of the old ideology, reaffirming its basic worth and only slightly mitigating its rigidity (for example, the very limited application of voluntary and informal admission).

Though being able to graduate sanctions in time and place has limited effects as far as the definition of the illness of the individual patient is concerned, it does allow the fixed nature of the institutional organization to be perceptibly modified. The enclosed world of the asylum is surrounded and integrated, though neither replaced nor reduced, by a complex network of institutions which in England lead to psychiatry being absorbed by medicine and social welfare, in France the establishment of a therapeutic link between the institution and its catchment area, and in the United States the integration of psychiatry and medicine into the welfare system. The latest transformations in this field since World War II appear to be macroscopic; we have seen the proliferation of a network of services and the training of a host of technicians which has apparently shifted the asylum away from the center towards the outskirts of the network. These transformations appear to have conquered the chronic nature of the illness in that the ratio between new arrivals and permanent inmates has been considerably increased. They appear, too, to have eliminated the dangerous nature of the disease which, while it is still liable to break out, may yet be controlled in the proper places and in a suitable way. The sanctions are thus divided up into their various components, present, at varying intensities, at different levels of the circuit. They then coalesce in the classic form of confinement in the strictest and most rigid spots of the whole circuit which are, of course, the asylum and the criminal asylum. These institutions survive, virtually unchanged, as the centers into which, as a result of a gradual and automatic process, are discharged those forms of illness which are least responsive to the new method of control and most resistant to the services offered. The sanctions become less apparent, enabling new treatment techniques to be invented, which mitigate its presence in the asylum and, outside, permit new selective criteria for the various forms of treatment to be found.

The organization of psychiatry as a widespread network of institutions has led to the polarization of sanctions around one particular spot, which, in the interplay of responsibilities, both guarantees and pollutes the functioning of the whole sector. The problem of rehabilitation and chronicity is transformed and recycled along the same lines. The practice of confinement for short periods and the subsequent rapid turnover in the services avoids or at least reduces the perpetuation of chronicity in the typical forms the asylum presents, such as permanent confinement with no hope of ever emerging. Irreversible forms of the disease thus sur-

vive in only a limited number of patients (the aged and the severely handicapped) and chronicity, seen as total dependence on
the services is attenuated in that it takes the form of regular sessions. Around the services themselves, we find the polarization of
"soft" chronicity which maintains contact with the social fabric
by means of unstable or part-time jobs and the socialization of the
patients' own world. Both are controlled and supported by resorting to the services where the psychiatrist's supervision permits different types of treatment and contact that corresponds to this
chronic individual. In other words, a composite area of diversified
social groups has formed around the services. These groups have
in common their dependency on the institution which is resorted
to either permanently or periodically. A complex social area thus
arises containing within itself contradictions and posing a series of
problems recalling the origins of psychiatry as a branch of learning and a distinctive organization. As resorting to the services is
automatically qualified as illness, the status of the sick person per-
ilously widens; all the more so where the norms establishing this
condition have remained unchanged since the time when the definition of illness referred to a specific group of cases or was clearly
differentiated according to the social class to which the individual
case belonged. Accordingly, psychiatry can no longer cope with
too wide and varied a range of demands and conditions which, in
the absence of alternatives, tend to flow automatically into the
psychiatric services.

It is in this sense and with these dimensions that the
problem of the norms governing psychiatry's conduct reemerges.
The evolution of the organizational model of the asylum into the
diffusion of psychiatric institutions has been based on a minimum
of legislative changes which, though not altering the structure or
meaning of the old nineteenth-century norms, still forms the
framework of a complex organizational set-up involving successive series of planning attempts. The network of services has
deeply modified the features of the illness and its requirements as
well as the specific field in which psychiatry operates involving
certain social groups and institutions which, in various ways, fall
within it. The contradiction which thus emerges through the problem of the norms regards the definition of the illness as the criteria
whereby psychiatry's particular field is identified with and/or dis-

tinguished from those of medicine, welfare, and the law. So, we witness the reemergence of old ambiguities still present in the laws and sociologically recognizable today in the survival of the asylum on too broad a scale and in the disorderly proliferation of medical and welfare apparatuses around it. The way in which psychiatry operates today has led to its boundaries becoming less distinct, yet they are still outlined by old-fashioned judicial sanctions. The network of institutions psychiatry administers has become more rigid and contaminated by the presence of the asylum, the place where inmates are gathered together and sanctions and segregation thrive. It is no accident that these contradictions tend to become clearly defined within the field of the norms. It is this field that reveals and legitimates those categories that have hitherto inspired the ideology and practices of psychiatrists as a professional body and overflowed into the social context with the increasing availability of experts. The crisis requires a complete rethinking of the whole function of psychiatry within the social framework. It demands that a series of laws face up to this crisis fairly and squarely. This crisis and the ensuing process of reflection were nurtured by groups of technicians, consumer groups, and political movements and have already swept over the greater part of the Western world.

The Italian Experience

The situation in Italy, too, has mobilized around these same issues, albeit in different ways and at a different pace than other European countries. Moreover, Italy's institutions have been only marginally affected by the changes which have characterized more highly-developed industrialized countries since the war. The first attempt at legal reform (Law No. 431) dates back to 1968 and, as with other European countries, supplements the old 1904 norms on asylums and lunatics with rulings concerning voluntary admission to psychiatric hospitals and enabling involuntary commitment to be transformed into voluntary, at the psychiatrist's discretion. This measure and the administrative directives aimed at the setting up of a community network of services—mental health centers—complementing psychiatric hospitals, are to be

seen in the same light as the other intervention hitherto examined. They do not affect the basic nature of the judicial sanctions
(the patient, if his admission is compulsory, continues to be defined as a danger to himself and others, and a public disgrace) but
they do aim at setting up mechanisms able to correct the severity
of the application of sanctions and do outline psychiatry as a service belonging to the field of general health through fostering
those territorial services which draw their inspiration from French
models of sectorial organization.

Rather than because of the flimsiness of these directives,
the reasons why the microreform has had such limited effects on a
national scale, lie in the discrepancies between the vastness of the
problems to which the institutional transformations evolving
since the 1960s have given rise and the overall intransigence of a
system of institutions wholly based on the various asylums which
sprang up at the beginning of the century and were run by a type
of psychiatry (medicine's step-sister) still based on antiquated
nineteenth-century positivist ideas and cut off from the regular
flow of international information. In a context characterized by
opposing and extreme positions, the intervention of the state has
been of limited significance at a normative level and has led to a
minimum of planning at an administrative one. It has not even
led to those widespread changes which have taken place in other
European countries since the 1950s but which have not lived up
to expectations (for example, the resorting to informal admission
has been extremely limited in England and there has been no generalized development of French sectorial organization).

In Italy the situation has been characterized by further
polarization: experiments of alternative management of the institutions have been able to exploit the new directives to render the
asylum obsolete and to plan an alternative system of services,
whereas the majority of psychiatric hospitals continue to be based
on the concept of the asylum as a prison-like institution cut off
from its surroundings. Hence, within the professional body of psychiatrists have formed two schools of thought: one advocating
strict application of the old asylum-psychiatry, and the other questioning the whole nature of psychiatry and its scope, as well as the
role and limits of its experts' authority. This schism has led advocates of alternative management to move in the direction of a po-

litical collaboration with those social forces struggling to affirm their rights (namely the students and workers in 1968 and 1969) than towards theoretical models of reform, hardly viable in any case considering the ingrained resistance to change on the part of the state and its apparatus.

In Italy, this type of process, with characteristics of its own compared with other European countries, has seen the function of psychiatry itself dragged into the crisis of the asylum model, with a whole host of other issues and conflicts not of a specifically psychiatric nature. In other words, the effects of the crisis in psychiatry have only been able to make themselves felt in the apparatus of the state, indirectly, through social areas and political movements which, despite furthering certain interests with undoubted connections with psychiatry, as far as function and apparatus are concerned, did not originally set out with specific psychiatric concerns. The process of redefinition of psychiatry, which is still going on, began, therefore, less as a plan of reform of the management model than as a social process rising from the base of the whole social fabric around which, and particularly around its transformation experiments, coalesces a whole movement. The practical expression and extension of the latter have enabled a critical approach to the asylum as an institution and as an ideology to reach a wider audience on a cultural level. In this sense, the contradictions of the postasylum period (as an historical stage following World War II) were only felt and given form in some areas of the Italian psychiatric organization, in the shapes of various criticisms of the continued use of sanctions, the problems of chronicity, the rendering obsolete of the management of the asylum as an isolated institution, and the impulse to replace it with a network of social services. These contradictions have become interwoven with criticisms of the old norms. Thus, a series of critical studies and analyses show that there are still internal links between the old asylum set-up and the new management models. They also shed light on the ideological and practical affinities between the two models; practical indications for intervention emerge, too, and when they are translated into terms of institutional activities, they point the way to, or at least lay down the guidelines for, possible future developments.

In these terms and on this scale, the political problem of

new legal and organizational definitions of psychiatry emerged in the late 1970s. The Italian experience is in one sense unique—as far as the relationship between these developments and the institutions are concerned—and can, therefore, hardly serve as a model in other social circumstances. It does, however, provide a useful observation point from which to view the whole array of contradictions and conflicts flowing into the mainstream of psychiatric evolutions. The recently approved norms contain both the themes which have given rise to the criticism of the asylum since the war and the attempt to come to terms with the contradictions rife within the organizational systems, stemming in their turn from the need to proceed beyond the asylum as the focal point of the structure. While general post-war legal amendments have either underestimated or avoided the problem of judicial sanctions and the asylum as a structure (possibly with the best of intentions to supersede them with purely organizational means), Italian law focuses precisely on these points and redefines them.

The very terminology chosen to define the law ("voluntary and compulsory health treatment") suggests a changed approach. The law's concern is no longer the definition of the disease itself or its classifications but its treatment. It is the forms of, and reasons for, this treatment which are the objects of the law's intervention. The treatment falls into the general category of health care and covers any type of illness requiring compulsory treatment. So much so that the final provisions stress the need for one single text to cover all rulings in force as far as international prophylaxis and infectious diseases are concerned. One type of illness which falls into the category of compulsory health treatment is mental illness. As the first paragraph of Article 1 states that diagnosis and health treatment are voluntary, the approach can be seen to have radically changed compared with other laws in force. Proof has to be provided of the necessity for compulsory health treatment whereas other laws consider it either an integral part of the definition of mental illness or, as in England, inherent in a given form of disturbance ("psychopathic disorder") and characterized by abnormal aggressive or clearly irresponsible behaviour. Indeed, English law is significant in this sense in that we find it specified within one Act (Article 4, paragraphs 4 and 5, Act 29, July 1959) that a distinction must be made between dangerous behaviour due to illness and that due to other reasons. This approach shows how ambiguous this definition of dangerousness can be. It is in any case vague and lays down a general principle (the dangerousness of mental illnesses) rather than providing concrete rulings for the doctor/judge.

Italian law, on the other hand, shifts the emphasis from the behavior of the sick person to the services made available for him. The basic principle (which is, as we have seen, the principle on which psychiatric action is based, despite contradictions on an ideological plane) is that it is the services which must identify the disease and establish its gravity. Hence, compulsory health treatment's resorting to hospitalization is only justified in emergencies, in the event of the patient refusing treatment or of "circumstances not permitting prompt and effective treatment elsewhere." All of which illustrates that the problems involved in compulsory health treatment are at least twofold: on the one hand the difficulty of the patient and on the other the response of the services which only resort to the psychiatric hospital inasmuch as they have failed to arrange suitable alternative measures. Hospital treatment, then, is necessary not only in the case of dangerous behaviour as such, but also as the last resort of an inadequate territorial network of services unable to cope with the requirements of a specific case.

Before going on to discuss the particular features of the Italian laws, some general remarks prompted by an analysis of compulsory health treatment would appear to be in order. Stressing the text of a law (as in Italy) or criticising the same, as hitherto in the present work, may seem to hint at a sort of equivalence between norms and the actual situation. In this light, and with a naive approach, a definition of compulsory health treatment might appear sufficient in itself to eradicate the power of both the expert and the services and to force suffering and behaviour patterns to fix into their own organizational and ideological schemes. Quite the reverse. The discrepancy between norms and the actual situation is based on a real stratification of interests inspired by precise ideological models and structured according to social status. Only if this is kept in mind shall we come to appreciate the partiality which the norms have made their own. Stressing mental illness as a social danger or allowing the doctor to assess its dangerousness at his own discretion or even forcing it into a precise organizational framework, where its dangerousness must be proved and is in any case the reflection of the inadequacy of the technical response, all involve taking a very clear stand with reference to conflicts and interests inherent in psychiatry's field of action and that of its experts.

The Italian law is innovative, clearly not because it mitigates the identification of illness with crime, which can still be determined by the doctor, but rather inasmuch as the expert may be reprehended if his intervention oversteps the limits which the law imposes on him. The principle on which the law is based aims at safeguarding, first and foremost, the patient's right to treatment which, in turn, means the protection of the social fabric through a network of services. We can see a real shift in emphasis in the contradiction between the medical and the legal field, which thus moves out of the abstract sphere of the law into practical reality. The ambiguity of the various legal definitions becomes the practical problem of the expert who must make his decision according to the merits of each individual case, whether to assume responsibility himself for treatment of a specifically sanitary nature, or whether to defer the whole problem to judicial power. In the event of the latter choice, the law is too generic to be able to dispel any doubts as to the expert's diagnosis and he cannot be protected by it. If, therefore, the illness is no longer considered socially dangerous but rather in the same need of the services as other diseases, though on different terms, the survival of the asylum in any form as a place of confinement and segregation is totally unjustified. Psychiatric assistance is, therefore, no longer a combination of intramural and extramural treatment but is envisaged as decentralized treatment given outside any institution. The construction of new psychiatric hospitals is forbidden and local authorities are entrusted with the task of organizing replacement services and finding a new use for the old asylum premises. Mental health services and wards accommodating no more than fifteen patients on the premises of the general hospitals are envisaged to replace institutional confinement in case of admission.

The article of the law concerning the number of beds

available in the general hospitals is a particularly controversial point at the stage of the formulation of the law; it is an attempt to integrate medicine and psychiatry in a philosophy which yet declines to iron out the outstanding problems concerning a psychiatric intervention into a merely medical model. We have seen that the contradiction between institution and territory is central to psychiatry and reconciled by the new norms on the principle of spreading psychiatric services over the whole territory. It is reflected in the nature of the hospital which is the pivot of the medical organization still centered on hospital admission. That new types of conflicts do arise, is borne out by the reluctance of the general hospital to assign the necessary accommodation for psychiatry's uses. Psychiatry, given its rightful place within the general hospital, can be the organizational and cultural link between health services and the territory's social needs.

This is how the channel along which new arrivals flow into the asylum tends to be dammed up. Yet, the real superceding of the asylum as an institution can be brought about only if the problem of chronicity—of long-stay patients still confined in mental hospitals or those who periodically resort to them—is solved first. Here, too, the principle laid down by the law, i.e., planning the superceding of psychiatric hospitals at local levels, is no guarantee of its application nor does it avert the risk of purely administrative solutions. Yet, the shift in emphasis brought about by the law can totally alter the meaning of the condition of inmate; the stigma of psychiatric treatment within the asylum is transformed into the right to an alternative solution, that is, to a type of welfare treatment guaranteeing that requirements will be met in the form of income and social services and no longer by compulsory treatment and the condition of permanent invalid. This process has experienced all the institutional transformations and is now beginning to take the shape of a widespread demand for welfare and health services from various social groups such as workers, women and young people. Quite rightly, the law makes the mayor who represents the local authority at both the political and administrative level (and no longer the magistrate), the supervisor of compulsory health treatment and responsible, with others, for the functioning of the services. Hence, the problem of safeguarding society from illness and infirmity becomes a political responsibility, inasmuch as it concerns the organization of services and is no longer a pretext for isolating the sick in a form of ghetto.

On account of the whole range of social processes which the application of this law has set off, the one year since it has been in force is insufficient to enable an assessment of it to be made. The law, both because of its inherent qualities and because of the characteristics of the social terrain in which it works, creates more contradictions than it solves. We do feel that any general approach blindly identifying the efficiency of a law with its clear and frictionless application is misleading. However, the terrain of psychic disorders, into which strong cultural prejudices and stratified, vested, and class interests flow, prevents any intervention from affecting existing conditions deeply because the latter can confine itself to the purely administrative planning sphere. The contradictions to be resolved lie neither in the planning nor in the law but in the social processes to which they either give rise or prevent. The possibility of their practical application is linked less to the rationality of internal mechanisms of law and planning than to the cohesion and mobilization which their principles and solutions either favour or hinder. In this sense, the new Italian psychiatric law is an attempt to link the transformation of one sector of the state's apparatus to the growth, in terms of both awareness and organization, of the base of the social fabric, for example, local authorities, individual institutions, peripheral groupings of experts and patients, political and trade union movements, and such like. The application of this law will be possible to the extent to which a resolve to overcome historical backwardness and shortcomings (lack of services, health assistance in private hands, intransigence of the medical class, and politicians' unwillingness to commit themselves) emerges from the base and influences the organization of the state. Similarly, the same resolve on the people's part will serve to overcome their historical absence and exclusion from the management of institutions. A law may enable this to be achieved but cannot, by its very nature, guarantee that it will. Therefore, the problem remains unsolved, as these laws or series of laws belong to a type of process indicating a radically new stage in the management of madness and the definition of its social significance.

Appendix

Law N. 180, May 13, 1978
   The House of Deputies and the Senate
      of the Republic passed:
         THE PRESIDENT OF THE REPUBLIC
         promulgates
the following law:

Article 1
Voluntary and Compulsory Health Survey and Treatment

Health assessment (diagnosis) and treatment are voluntary.

In the cases mentioned in this law and in those cases explicitly foreseen by State laws, the Health Authority can order compulsory health survey and treatment with respect for the person's dignity and the civil and political rights guaranteed by the Constitution, including, in as much as possible, the right to freely choose the physician and the health care center.

Compulsory health survey and treatment at the expense of the State, public bodies or institutions, are carried out by public territorial health care centers and, when hospitalization is needed, in public or state-subsidized hospital facilities.

During the compulsory health treatment, those who are under treatment have the right to communicate with any person they think right.

Compulsory health survey and treatment mentioned in the previous paragraphs, must be associated with initiatives that will assure the consent and participation of the patient.

Compulsory health survey and treatment are ordered by a Mayor proceeding, in his capacity of local Health Authority, on a justified proposal made by a physician.

Article 2
Compulsory Health Survey and Treatment for Mental Disorder

The measures mentioned in paragraph 2 of Article 1, can be taken against those persons suffering from mental disorder.

In the cases mentioned in the previous paragraph, the proposal for compulsory health treatment can envisage hospitalization care only if mental disturbances are such as to require urgent therapeutic intervention, if these interventions are not accepted by the patient, and if there are not the conditions and the circumstances for taking immediate and timely health care measures outside the hospital.

The measure implementing compulsory health treatment in hospitalization conditions must be preceded by the ratification of the proposal mentioned in the last paragraph of Article 1, made by a public health service physician, and must be justified in accordance with the previous paragraph.

Article 3
Procedure Relative to Compulsory Health Survey and Treatment in Hospitalization Conditions for Mental Disorder

The measure, mentioned in Article 2, by which the Mayor imposes compulsory health treatment in hospitalization conditions, supplemented with the justified proposal of a physician—as mentioned in the last paragraph of Article 1—and with the confirmation—as mentioned in the last paragraph of Article 2—must be notified by a communal Messenger within 48 hours from the admission into the health center, to the tutelary judge of the same district of the communal administration.

The tutelary judge within the following 48 hours, after having made inquiries and ordered the necessary controls, issues a justified decree for the confirmation or nonconfirmation of the measure, and communicates it to the Mayor. In case of nonconfirmation, the Mayor orders the cessation of the compulsory health treatment in hospitalization conditions.

If the measure mentioned in the first paragraph of this article, is taken by the Mayor of a communal administration different from the patient's place of residence, the Mayor of the patient's domicile must be informed. If the measure mentioned in the first paragraph of this article is taken against aliens or stateless persons, the Prefect must inform the Home Office and the competent Consulates.

Should compulsory health treatment exceed 7 days or should it be further prolonged, the physician responsible for the mental health service, as mentioned in Article 6, must in due time send a justified proposal indicating the further assumable duration of the treatment itself to the Mayor who has ordered the hospitalization of the patient; and the Mayor must inform the tutelary judge, with the formalities and for the accomplishments mentioned in paragraph 1 and 2 of this Article.

The physician mentioned in the previous paragraph is obliged to inform the Mayor (either the patient is discharged or remains in the hospital) of the cessation of the conditions which require compulsory health treatment; moreover he is obliged to communicate the eventual impossibility to carry on the treatment itself. The Mayor within 48 hours from the receipt of the communication of the physician, must inform the tutelary judge.

If necessary, the tutelary judge takes the required urgent measures to preserve and administer the patient's properties.

Omission of the communications mentioned in paragraph 1, 4 and 5 of this article causes the cessation of all effects of the measure, and is considered and "omission of office deeds crime," unless there is sufficient evidence for a more serious crime.

Article 4
Publication and Modification of Compulsory Health Treatment Measure

Anyone can make a request to the Mayor for the revocation or modification of the measure enforcing or prolonging compulsory health treatment.

The Mayor decides within 10 days on the request of revocation or modification. Revocation or modification measures are put into force with the same procedure as for modified or revoked measures.

Article 5
Jurisdictional Protection

Anyone who undergoes the compulsory health treatment and anyone who has interest in it, can appeal against the measure ratified by the tutelary judge, to the Court of his jurisdiction.

Within 30 days, beginning from the expiry of the period of time as mentioned in the second paragraph of Article 3, the Mayor can appeal against the nonratification of the measure enforcing the compulsory health treatment.

In the trial held in a court of law, the parties can stand without defence counsels and can be represented by a person in possession of a mandate written at the foot of the appeal or in a separate document. The appeal can be sent to the Court by means of registered letter with a receipt notice.

The president of the Court fixes the hearing of the parties with a decree written at the foot of the appeal which is notified to the parties and to the Public Prosecutor by the Registrar.

The president of the Court, after having received the measure enforcing the compulsory health treatment and after having heard the Public Prosecutor can suspend the treatment itself even before the hearing.

The president of the Court decides on the request of suspension within 10 days.

The Court after having heard the Public Prosecutor decides in the counsel room on the basis of information and evidence requested by the Court or by the parties.

The appeals and the following proceedings are stamp-duty free. The decision of the Court is not subject to registration.

Article 6
Procedures Relative to Compulsory Health Survey and Treatment in Hospitalization Conditions for Mental Disorder

Prevention, care, and rehabilitation relative to mental illness are usually carried out by mental health service centers outside the hospital.

From the coming into force of this law, mental health treatments which require hospitalization and which are at the expense of the State or public bodies and institutions are carried out in the mental care centers mentioned in the following paragraphs, except for what is specified in Article 8.

The autonomous regional and provincial administrations of Trento and Bolzano—taking also into account the territorial ambits foreseen in paragraph 2 and 3 of Article 25 of the Decree of the President of the Republic N. 616 of July 24, 1977—single out the general hospitals in which appropriate mental health centers for diagnosis and care must be created within 60 days from the coming into force of this law.

The centers mentioned in paragraphs 2 and 3 of this article— which are regulated in accordance with the Decree of the President of the Republic No. 128 of March 28, 1969, concerning compulsory special centers in the general hospitals and which must not have more than 15 beds—with the purpose of guaranteeing the continuity of the health service for the protection of mental health, are linked to the other mental health service centers of the territory, as far as staff and functions are concerned, in a departmental organization.

The autonomous regional and provincial administrations of Trento and Bolzano single out the private medical establishments which have the compulsory requirements necessary for voluntary and compulsory health treatments in the hospital context.

As to health service needs, the provincial administrations can draw up conventions with the establishments mentioned in the previous paragraph in accordance with the following Article 7.

Article 7
Transference to Regional Administrations of the Functions Relative to Mental Hospital Services

Beginning from the coming into force of this law, the administrative functions—until now carried out by provincial administrations—concerning mental health service in hospitalization conditions, are transferred to both ordinary and special statute regional administrations, for the territories under their jurisdiction. The autonomous provincial administrations of Trento and Bolzano maintain their present competence.

Hospital health service—regulated under Articles 12 and 13 of the Decree N. 264 of July 8, 1974, afterwards modified and transformed in Law N. 386 of August 17, 1974—includes hospitalization for mental disorders. The present regulations concerning the competence of the expenditures are in force until December 31, 1978.

Beginning from the coming into force of this law, the regional administrations exercise the functions which they accomplish for the other hospitals, for mental hospitals as well.

Until the date of coming into force of the National Health Service Reform, and at any rate not further than January 1, 1979, the provincial administrations continue to perform the administrative functions relative to the management of the mental hospitals, and any other function relative to mental health and hygiene centers.

The autonomous regional and provincial administrations of Trento and Bolzano plan and coordinate the organization of mental health and hygiene centers with the other health service facilities of the territory, and carry out the gradual removal of the mental hospitals and the different utilization of the existing facilities. These initiatives cannot involve higher expenses in the provincial administration budgets.

At any rate it is forbidden to build new mental hospitals, to use the existing ones as specialized mental departments of general hospitals, to create mental departments or units in general hospitals, and to use for this purpose neurological or neuropsychiatric departments or units.

The prohibitions—mentioned in Article 6 of the Decree N. 946 of December 29, 1977, afterwards modified and transformed in Law N. 43 of February 27, 1978—are applied to mental hospitals which depend upon provincial administrations or other public bodies, or upon public welfare and charity institutions.

Personnel of public mental hospitals and mental health service centers outside the hospital are employable in mental diagnosis and care centers of general hospitals as mentioned in Article 6.

The relationships between provincial administrations, hospital administrations, and other health care and in-patient facilities are regulated by appropriate conventions, in compliance with a standard scheme, which must be approved, within 30 days from the coming into force of this law, by means of a Decree of the Ministry of Health agreed by the regional administrations and the Italian provincial administration association and after having heard, as far as personnel problems are concerned, the most representative trade unions.

The standard scheme of Convention shall also regulate the staff and functions liaisons, mentioned in paragraph 4 of Article 6, the financial relations between provincial administration and in-patients facilities and the employment, also by command, of the personnel mentioned in paragraph 8 of this article.

From January 1, 1979, during the negotiations for the renewal of the labour agreement, between the agreement, regulations will be set out for the gradual equalization between the salary and economic regulations of the personnel of public mental hospitals and mental health and hygiene service centers and the salary and economic regulations of the corresponding categories of the personnel of general hospitals.

Article 8
Patients Already Admitted in Mental Hospitals

The rules of this law are also applied to patients already admitted in mental hospitals at the time of the coming into force of this law.

The head physician responsible for the unit, within 90 days from the coming into force of this law (with single justified reports), communicates the names of the patients who, in his opinion need to continue the compulsory health treatment in the same in-patient facility, and indicates the assumable duration of the treatment itself to the Mayor of the respective places of residence. The head physician responsible for the unit is also bound to accomplish the duties mentioned in paragraph 5 of Article 3.

The mayor applies the measure of compulsory health treatment in hospitalization conditions in accordance with the regulations mentioned in the last paragraph of Article 2 and notifies it to the tutelary judge with the formalities and for the accomplishments mentioned in Article 3.

Omission of the communications mentioned in the previous paragraphs causes the cessation of all effects of the measure and is considered an "omission of office deeds crime," unless there is sufficient evidence for a more serious crime.

Taking into account paragraph 5 of Article 7 and in temporary derogation from what is established in paragraph 2 of Article 6, only those who had been admitted before the coming into force of this law and that need mental health treatment in hospitalization conditions can be admitted in the present mental hospitals, provided that they request it.

8. Critical Psychiatry
After the Law 180

When this collection of writings was published,[1] we questioned its timeliness. Indeed, it refers to a precise period, between the years 1977 and 1978, during which specific themes were recurring in the debate among the psychiatric practitioners. These concerned both the types of service organization concentrated primarily in the hospital or community, and the theoretical and practical weight of exemplary experiences that attested to a generalizable model of the "new" psychiatry. Today, with the implementation of the Mental Health Law 180 and the establishment of the National Health Service, the situation of Italian psychiatry and the issues seem radically changed. . . .

After the law had been in force for a year, the number of inpatients in psychiatric hospitals was reduced considerably, and the cases of compulsory treatment were greatly contained. A certain debate still persists regarding the quality and characteristics of the new intermediate care and [general] hospital structures that are still lacking. In the midst of many criticisms and with a deliberate emphasis on the dangers that this law brings, we are witnessing the first steps towards the diffusion of a new way of practicing psychiatry that differs from the recent past and goes far beyond the prototype of a few experiences. Yet we are not quite certain—and it is too early to know—what these necessary changes entail.

We need only reread the Mental Health Law to be convinced that what appears, in the eyes of many, to be a risky adventure, full of threats, merely inserts into the medical norm a civil

Translated by Anne M. Lovell.

and constitutional principle that should have been implicit, but was not: the recognition that all men and women, whether healthy or sick, have rights. The originality of this law lies, basically, 1) in the disappearance of the judicial concept of "dangerousness," from which was deduced the need for custody of the mentally ill, and hence for violating and repressing them; 2) in the opposition, following from the above, to the creation of new, segregative structures; 3) in the reversal of the traditional psychiatric view; for the first time, psychiatry must be prepared to confront those who suffer from psychic disturbances without protecting itself behind the screen of dangerousness and custody. In fact, where hospitalization is to be used, it is no longer the sick person who determines the type of intervention in terms of the seriousness and dangerousness of his or her illness, but rather the social organization, according to its capacity for responding or not to the needs and rights of the citizen, in sickness and in health.

The law can be easily attacked, on the one hand, by the most backward segments of this country as being risky and guaranteeing little in the way of protection for either the sick or the healthy. Yet at the same time it is a target of facile attacks by those who consider these changes and their underlying assumptions to be merely normative interventions, rationalizations committed to reinforcing the very institutions they were meant to negate. But if these changes are situated within the framework of the theoretical and practical tensions that have provoked significant struggles against the mechanisms of oppression and marginalization in the last few years, they cannot help but carry the content of these struggles to the forefront. To create a crisis, as is the actual case, in a service that, being psychiatric, is rigidly custodial, means calling into question one of our society's most significant safety valves. For this means breaking the certainty of the clear separation between health and illness, normal and abnormal, on which the social order itself is founded. If there has been a crisis, it was provoked by the clearly expressed will to negate the institutions of repression and violence, rather than to rebuild them. It is the asylum, negated in practice, destroyed, dismantled, and the rigidity of its scientific certainty and its punitive rules overturned, that has fractured its own internal logic. It avoids the ambiguities inherent when cultural models capable of filling up the void created by this crisis are simply recycled.

In Italy, then, a law that prohibits the construction of new hospitals and provides for the gradual elimination of those still in use was generated by this break, at a practical level, with the logic of perpetuating a marginal class that is implied in the very existence of the asylum. As it prevents the recent crisis from becoming absorbed by a new theory or ideology that would leave the reality unaltered while interpreting it differently, this operation is the inverse of that already achieved in other countries. There the problem was seemingly confronted by expanding services for controlling deviance into the community without effecting any change in the asylum's logic or reality. Indeed, the persistance of social marginalization, justified by the alibi of illness and treatment, can only reproduce and reaffirm the same logic in the community and the new services, at the same time reinforcing the asylum and its logic. The new Mental Health Law has produced a struggle to vindicate the existence of a subjectivity, visible in a vigorously positivistic terrain, revealing that what exists is other than unmodifiable "nature." The reality and the project of our life is what we make of it, just as what exists now was previously "produced."

Even if it is the fruit of a struggle, a law can only be the result of the rationalization of a revolt; but it can also succeed in diffusing the message of a practice, rendering it a collective legacy. Even if the fruit of a struggle, a law can provoke a levelling of the heights reached by exemplary experiences; but it can also diffuse and homogenize a discourse, creating the common bases for subsequent action. For this law allows for what has been desired more than once: the possibility of transferring the contents of a struggle from the hands of a few into those of an ever larger number of people, even if this means the slow abandonment of exemplary experiences as the practical reference point.

In this sense it has tended to modify, or at least to lessen, the heroism, romanticism, and perhaps rhetoric with which all of us—in our Jacobinism—were and are somewhat stricken. It has forced us to confront one another more carefully than was the case in the last few years, when our style also stemmed from our practical rage against the institution. This law, then, has in some ways forced alternative psychiatric practitioners to change their awareness of themselves and their work. And now it is as if a loss of the "faith" that had sustained us all these years, up through the advent of the law, now threatens us. Yet the character of the new, emerging secularization is still undefined.

Today all of us find ourselves starting from this law, caught between some things finished and others not yet defined. The people who were part of this movement have caught a glimpse of this situation; they express a concern with filling up this void, emptied of identity and lacking any of the historical dimension of our work.

Traditional psychiatry offered the worker a precise identity only as the guarantor of social control. Similarly, the process of overcoming the asylum offered the possibility of identifying with the refusal of such control. But once the latter has been accomplished, sanctioned by the law to which we are now anchored, we reduce the possibility that allows the liberating quality of a role identified with the struggle against the asylum to coexist with the often asserted need for overcoming the normalizing function implicit in every psychiatric practitioner's work.

The psychiatrist continues to be concerned with individual suffering that, however, remains instilled with a precise definition of what is the norm. The limits of the norm shift, expanding and contracting according to the necessity for and change in social values; but in the dominant logic what must be maintained is always the clear definition of the limit. The way in which suffering is expressed continues to be rigid and enclosed within the classic parameters of mental illness. For there are still the cultural conceptions according to which one determines who suffers from psychic disturbances, who is on the edge, at the point of exceeding the norm's limit, beyond which lie punishment and sanction.

Once the logic of the asylum—sanction of the abnormal world—has been broken, psychiatric practitioners find themselves disarmed before a sick person who still moves according to the old parameters of illness and who hides and defends him or herself behind them. Identification with the institution is no longer possible because the asylum has revealed its function as defender of the healthy with respect to the ill. An identification with psychiatry is no longer possible because it has revealed itself to be the instrument that permits this defense of the healthy world through the creation of a sick place. Nor is it any longer possible to identify with the role of those who struggle against the asylum, because there now exists a law that has decreed its death. But nevertheless psychiatrists continue to be concerned with a suffering which they must confront without tools, without defenses. They must grasp the world of needs from which suffering emerges, restoring it to the history from which it was banished in the very moment it was defined as an illness.

It is this lack of identity that constitutes the implicit challenge to what could be a different way of practicing psychiatry. For it is in this ideological and institutional vacuum, outside the parameters and instruments that until now have prevented us from approaching psychic disturbances, that we will now be forced to act.

Filling up this void, crowning this moment of suspension, of perplexity, of uncertainty with other exchangeable ideologies, can prevent us from embarking on an understanding outside of the cultural schemes that imprison us. It would be easy to pour into this empty space the already proven theories of interpretation that rationalize our uncertainties. Italy, always culturally "backwards" when compared to other countries, is now ready to welcome psychoanalysis, behaviorism, therapies, etc. This readiness is evidenced by the recent demands and requirements for the ideological and scientific reassurance that those theories bring. Yet elsewhere they have left intact both the process of social marginalization and the logic of the asylum that justifies it. But the focal point that the new Italian law tends to fracture, without halting the crisis engendered by these new theories, is the logic of perpetuating a marginal class. And this permits us to see directly which unmet needs and concrete frustrations feed psychic disturbances, what real impotence causes illness to explode, once we have decided to avoid seeing that which we wish to cover with metaphors. This does not mean affirming that psychic suffering originates only out of material misery (which certainly has its effect on both the origin of the disturbance and the types of responses it receives), but rather that a social misery exists which prevents us from expressing our own needs and forces us to find anomalous and tortuous paths that pass through the mediations of illness, because we are prevented from expressing it in an immediate way.

The need for a new science and a new theory is part of what gets incorrectly defined as an "ideological void" and which, in reality, is the felicitous moment when we might begin to face problems in a different way. The happy moment when, disarmed as we are, deprived of tools so that we cannot use them as an explicit defense in the face of anguish and suffering, we are forced to relate to this anguish and this suffering without automatically objectifying them with the schema of sickness, and without having at our disposal a new interpretative code that would require the ancient distance between those who understand and those who are ignorant, those who suffer and those who help. It is only in this indirect encounter, without the mediation of sickness and its interpretation, that the subjectivity of those who suffer from psychic disturbances can emerge. This subjectivity can only surface in a relationship that, having finally detached itself from the objectifying categories of positivist psychiatry (of which the asylum is its most complete expression), succeeds by refusing to enclose abnormal experience in further objectification, and by maintaining it instead in a close relationship of individual to social history.

Notes

INTRODUCTION: THE UTOPIA OF REALITY: FRANCO BASAGLIA AND THE PRACTICE OF A DEMOCRATIC PSYCHIATRY

1. Robert Castel, *L'Ordre Psychiatrique: l'Age d'Or d'Alienisme* (Paris: Les Editions de Minuit, 1976), p. 74. Translated by Anne M. Lovell. Unless otherwise indicated, all translations from the Italian are by Anne M. Lovell and Teresa Shtob.

2. David Rothman, *The Discovery of the Asylum: Social Order and Disorder in the New Republic* (Boston: Little-Brown, 1971); Joseph P. Morrissey and Howard P. Goldman, "The Ambitious Legacy: 1856–1968," in Joseph P. Morrissey, Howard Goldman, and Lorraine Klerman, eds., *The Enduring Asylum: Cycles of Institutional Reform at Worcester State Hospital* (New York: Grune and Stratton, 1980), pp. 247–278.

3. For example, Franz G. Alexander and Sheldon T. Selesnik, *The History of Psychiatry: Thought and Practice from Prehistoric Times to the Present* (New York: Harper and Row, 1966).

4. Michel Foucault, *Madness and Civilization* (New York: New American Library, 1967).

5. R. Semelaigne, cited in Kathleen Jones, "Moral Management and the Therapeutic Community." Address to the Society for the Social History of Medicine, July 3, 1971, p. 2.

6. Pinel, cited in Foucault, *Madness and Civilization*, p. 242.

7. Nancy J. Tomes, "A Generous Confidence: Thomas Story Kirkbride's Philosophy of Asylum Construction and Management," in Andrew Scull, ed., *Madhouses, Maddoctors, and Madmen: The Social History of Psychiatry in the Victorian Age* (Philadelphia: University of Pennsylvania Press, 1981), p. 138.

8. William Ll. Parry-Jones, "The Model of the Gheel Lunatic Colony and Its Influence on the Nineteenth-Century Asylum System in Britain," in Scull, ed., *Madhouses, Maddoctors, and Madmen*.

9. Franco Basaglia, "L'utopia della realta," in Basaglia, *Scritti, II, Dall'apertura del manicomio alla nuova legge sull' assistenza psichiatrica* (Turin: Einaudi, 1982).

10. Mario Tommasini, cited in Mario Tommasini and Franca Ongaro Basaglia, "Voci di Periferia, Parma 1965–1983." Manuscript, p. 16.

11. Jean-Paul Sartre, *Situations II* (Paris: Gallimard, 1948).

12. Franco Basaglia, "Le istituzioni di violenza," in Basaglia, *Scritti I, Dalla psichiatria fenomenologica all'esperienza di Gorizia* (Turin: Einaudi, 1981).

13. Basaglia, *Scritti I;* Basaglia, *Scritti II* (Turin: Einaudi, 1981, 1982).

14. Cited in Franco Basaglia, ed., *L'Istituzione Negata* (Turin: Einaudi, 1968), p. 3.

15. Americans, too, drew the parallel between Nazi concentration camps and psychiatric hospitals. A journalist whose exposé on hospitals provided cannon fodder for the reform movement in the United States wrote in 1948: "As I passed through some of

Byberry's wards, I was reminded of the pictures of the Nazi concentration camps at Belsen and Buchenwald. I entered buildings swarming with naked humans herded like cattle and treated with less concern, pervaded by a fetid odor so heavy, so nauseating, that the stench seemed to have a physical existence of its own." Albert Deutsch, *The Mentally Ill in America: A History of Their Care and Treatment from Colonial Times,* 2d. ed. (New York: Columbia University Press, 1949). However, American reformers did not, as did Basaglia, draw the connection between hospital conditions and the larger society.

16. See Basaglia, *Scritti I.*

17. Franco Basaglia, "Crisi istituzionale o crisi psichiatrica?" in Basaglia, *Scritti I,* p. 443.

18. Basaglia, *L'Istituzione Negata,* pp. 32, 33.

19. *Politique de secteur* is the community mental health policy established in France by ministerial memorandum of March 15, 1960. It establishes catchment areas of around 67,000 inhabitants, to be served by a psychiatric team and facilities for prevention, treatment and after-care. Each sector is linked to a psychiatric hospital, although the emphasis is placed on community-based psychiatry.

20. R. Burton, *Institutionalism* (Bristol: John Wright, 1959); John K. Wing, "Institutionalism in Mental Hospitals," *British Journal of Social and Clinical Psychology* (1962), vol. 1.

21. Franco Basaglia, "La distruzione dell'ospedale psichiatrico come luogo di istituzionalizzazione," in Basaglia, *Scritti I,* p. 251.

22. Franco Basaglia, "Problems of Law and Psychiatry: The Italian Experience, this volume, pp. 275–276.

23. Franco Basaglia and Franca Ongaro Basaglia, "Follia/Delirio," in Basaglia, *Scritti II.*

24. A. B. Hollingshead and F. C. Redlich, *Social Class and Mental Illness* (New York: Wiley, 1958).

25. Paolo Tranchina, *Norma e Antinorma* (Milan: Feltrinelli, 1977), p. 169.

26. Agostino Pirella, interview in Franco Basaglia, Franca Ongaro Basaglia, Agostino Pirella, and Salvatore Taverna, *La Nave Che Affonda* (Rome: Savelli, 1978), p. 40.

27. *Ibid.*

28. Basaglia, "Conversazione: A proposito della nuova legge 180," *Scritti II,* p. 481.

29. Robert Rubenstein and Harold D. Lasswell, *The Sharing of Power in a Psychiatric Hospital* (New Haven: Yale University Press, 1966); Robert N. Rappaport, *Community as Doctor: New Perspectives on the Therapeutic Community* (London: Tavistock, 1960).

30. Basaglia, "La distruzione," p. 256.

31. *Ibid.*

32. This and similar illustrations of the work at Gorizia can be found in Basaglia, ed., *L'Istituzione Negata.*

33. Basaglia, ed., *L'Istituzione Negata.*

34. Silvano Agosti, Marco Bellocchio, Sandro Petraglia, and Stefano Rulli, *Fit To Be Untied.*

35. This discussion relies on information from Antonio Buonatesta, "Mythe et Réalité de la Psychiatrie Alternative Italienne: De l'Alternative à la Réforme," Thesis, Université Catholique de Louvain, Belgium, 1981.

36. Yvonne Bonner, "La thérapie familiale et son utilisation dans un service publique en Italie," *Psychologie et Société,* no. 4, Faculté de Psychologie et des Sciences de l'Education, Universite Catholique de Louvain, Belgium, 1981.

37. Buonatesta, "Mythe et realité. . ."

38. Agostino Pirella, cited in Buonatesta, "Mythe et realité. . ." p. 38.

39. G. Micheli, *I Nuovi Catari: Centralità della Conoscenza nell'Esperienza Psichiatrica di Perugia* (Bologna: Il Mulino, 1982).

40. Michel Vandeleene, cited in Michel Legrand, "Le procéssus de transformation des institutions psychiatriques à Perouse," *Psycologie et Société,* no. 12, Faculté de Psychologie et des Sciences de l'Education, Université Catholique de Louvain, Belgium, 1983, p. 10.

41. Micheli, *I Nuovi Catari.*

42. The more psychotherapeutic tendencies are represented in the writings: Francesco Scotti and Carlo Brutti, *Quale Psichiatria?* vol. 1 (Rome: Borli, 1980) and Carlo Brutti and Francesco Scotti, *Quale Psichiatria?* vol. 2 (Rome: Borli, 1981).

43. The "encirclement strategy" involved destroying the hospital from the outside by surrounding it with a network of mental health centers that could act as a buffer between potential patients and the institution. Buonatesta, "Mythe et Realité," ch. I.

44. Giovanna Gallio, "La memoria del manicomio," in Diana Mauri, ed., *La Liberta e Terapeutica? L'Esperienza Psichiatrica di Trieste* (Milan: Feltrinelli, 1983).

45. Gallio, "La memoria," p. 22.

46. Anne M. Lovell, "Breaking the Circuit of Control: A Report on the Trieste Conference," *State and Mind,* (1978), vol. 6, no. 2.

47. Guiseppe dell'Acqua, cited in Mauri, ed., *La Liberta,* p. 266.

48. Gallio, "La Memoria."

49. Cited in Anne M. Lovell, "From Confinement to Community: The Radical Transformation of an Italian Mental Hospital," in Phil Brown, ed., *Mental Health Care and Social Policy* (Boston: Routledge and Kegan Paul, 1985), p. 381.

50. Franco Basaglia, in Basaglia et al., *La Nave Che Affonda,* pp. 31, 32.

51. Ota de Leonardis, "Il sistema sanitario, Dalla politica delle riforme alla politica delle istituzione," *Problemi del Socialismo* (Spring 1984), pp. 152–175.

52. Nevertheless, many feminists disagreed with the anti-institutional practices, because the burden of care in the community, especially if the patient lived at home, fell primarily on the shoulders of women. It was felt that many of these services should be provided by the state, not by the free labor of women. Women and madness, however, was a subject elaborated upon in conferences and meetings, though less so in publications. One exception is selections in Franca Ongaro Basaglia, *Una Voce* (Turin: Einaudi, 1980).

53. Raffaele Misiti, Augusto DeBernardi, and Carlo Gerbaldo. *La Riforma Psichiatrica. Prima Fase di Attuazione* (Rome: Il Pensiero Scientifico, 1981).

54. Buonatesta, "Mythe et Realité."

55. Sergio Piro, "Leggi sulla psichiatria e Meridione in Italia," *in Psichiatria Senza Manicomio: Epidemiologia Critica sulla Riforma,* Domenico DeSalvia and Paolo Crepet, eds. (Milan: Feltrinelli, 1982).

56. *Ibid.*

57. B. Podbersig, "Elementi di legislazione psichiatrica regionale," *Prospettive Sociali e Sanitarie* (1983), 13: 49–53.

58. Franco Basaglia, "Prefazione a Il Giardino dei Gelsi," in Basaglia, *Scritti II,* p. 469. Some discussion of the law and its implementation also exists in English-language writings. See Loren Mosher, "Italy's Revolutionary Mental Health Law: An Assessment," *American Journal of Psychiatry* (February 1982), 139: 199–203; Shulamith Ramon, *"Psichiatria Democratica:* A Study of an Italian Community Mental Health Service," *International Journal of Health Services* (1983), 13: 307–324; Mario Tobino, "Psychiatry in Italy Since the Promulgation of Law 180, *International Journal of Mental Health* 14 (1985) 1–2: 125–138; Richard Mollica, ed., "The Unfinished Revolution in Italian Psychiatry: An Inter-

national Perspective," special issue of *The International Journal of Mental Health*, (1985), vol. 14, nos. 1–2.

59. Yasmine Ergas,"Allargamento della cittadinanza e governo dei conflitto: Le politiche sociali negli anni settanta in Italia," *State e Mercato* (December 1982), 6:429–454.

60. Lovell, "From Confinement to Community," p. 374.

61. Andrew Scull, *Decarceration: Community Treatment and the Deviant* (New Brunswick, N.J.: Rutgers University Press, 1977).

62. *Ibid.*, p. 144.

63. Howard H. Goldman and Joseph P. Morrissey, "The Alchemy of Mental Health Policy: Homelessness and the Fourth Cycle of Reform," *American Journal of Public Health* (1985), 75:727.

64. Scull, *Decarceration*,

65. For example, Ellen L. Bassuk and Samuel Gerson, "Deinstitutionalization and Mental Health Services," *Scientific American* (February 1978), 238:46–53.

66. H. Richard Lamb, ed., *The Homeless Mentally Ill: A Task Force Report of the American Psychiatric Association* (Washington D.C.: American Psychiatric Press, 1985).

67. Goldman and Morrissey, "The Alchemy," p. 728.

68. Robert Castel, Francoise Castel, and Anne Lovell, *The Psychiatric Society* (New York: Columbia University Press, 1982).

69. Stanley P. Hoffman, *Who Are the Homeless? A Study of Randomly Selected Men Who Use the New York City Shelters* (New York: New York State Office of Mental Health, 1982); C. Brown, S. MacFarlane, R. Paredes and L. Stark, *The Homeless of Phoenix: Who Are They?* (Phoenix, AZ: Phoenix South Community Health Center, 1983); and Dee Roth, Jerry Bean and Nancy Luet et al., *Homelessness in Ohio: A Study of People in Need* (Ohio: Ohio Department of Mental Health, 1985).

70. Sue E. Estroff, "Medicalizing the Margins: On Being Disgraced, Disordered, and Deserving," *Psychosocial Rehabilitation Journal* (1985), 85:35.

71. Nancy Scheper-Hughes, "Dilemmas in Deinstitutionalization," *Journal of Operational Psychiatry* (1981), 12:90–99; Sue E. Estroff, *Making It Crazy* (Berkeley: University of California Press, 1981).

72. Estroff, *Making It Crazy.*

73. Scheper-Hughes, "Dilemmas in Deinstitutionalization," p. 94.

74. Steven P. Segal and Jim Baumohl, "The Community Living Room," *Social Casework* (February 1985), p. 112.

75. *Ibid.*

76. Michel Foucault, *Mental Illness and Psychology* (New York: Harper and Row, 1976), p. 80.

77. Susan Sontag, *Illness as Metaphor* (New York: Random House, 1979), p. 1.

78. Giuseppe Bruno-Bossio, personal communication.

PART ONE: DESTROYING THE MENTAL HOSPITAL

1. A. R. Favazza, "Editor's Comments," *Journal of Operational Psychiatry* (1981), vol. 12, no. 2 (cover).

2. David J. Rothman, "Decarcerating Prisoners and Patients," *Civil Liberties Review* (1973), 1(1):8–30.

3. H. Richard Lamb, ed., *The Homeless Mentally Ill* (Washington, D.C.: American Psychiatric Association, 1984).

4. Leona Bachrach, "The Effects of Deinstitutionalization on General Hospital Psychiatry," *Hospital and Community Psychiatry* (1981), 32(11):786–790. Also, Leona Bachrach and H. R. Lamb, "Conceptual Issues in the Evaluation of the Deinsti-

tutionalization Movement," In G. J.. Stahler and W. R. Tash, eds., *Innovative Approaches to Mental Health Evaluation* (New York: Academic Press, 1982).

5. Richard F. Mollica, "From Asylum to Community: The Threatened Disintegration of Public Psychiatry," *New England Journal of Medicine* (1983), 308:367–373.

6. Kathleen Jones, "Address to the National Association for Mental Health," Annual Conference, March 1, 1973, England.

7. David Rothman, "Decarcerating Prisoners and Patients."

8. Lee Coleman, *The Reign of Error* (Boston: Beacon Press, 1984).

9. Franco Basaglia, *L'Istituzione Negata* (Turin: Einaudi, 1967).

10. Erving Goffman, *Asylums* (Garden City, N.Y.: Doubleday, 1961).

11. See: T. Van Putten, E. Crumpton, and C. Yale, "Drug Refusal and the Wish to be Crazy," *Archives of General Psychiatry* (1976),33:1443–1446; D. A. Treffert, "Dying With Your Rights On," paper presented at the 127th Annual Meeting of the American Psychiatric Association, Detroit, Michigan, May 6–10, 1974; Stephen Rachlin, "With Liberty and Psychosis For All," *Psychiatric Quarterly* (1974), 48:1–9; T. Gutheil, "Editorial: In Search of True Freedom: Drug Refusal, Involuntary Medication, and 'Rotting With Your Rights On,' " *American Journal of Psychiatry* (1980), 137:327.

12. S. Rachlin, p. 418.

13. H. C. Modlin, "Balancing Patients' Rights With the Rights of Others," *Hospital and Community Psychiatry* (1974), 25:474–475.

14. Rogers V. Okin, U.S. District Court, District of Massachusetts, CA 75-1610-T. Order and judgement by D.J. Tauro, October 29, 1979.

15. Peter Breggin, *Psychiatric Drugs: Hazards to the Brain, p. 268* (New York: Springer, 1983).

1. INSTITUTIONS OF VIOLENCE

1. Erving Goffman, *Asylums* (Garden City, N.Y.: Doubleday, 1961).

2. Community mental health has the advantage of providing a more extensive and convenient form of prevention. However, if it it not accompanied by the simultaneous destruction of the psychiatric hospital as a closed, coercive, and institutionalizing space, then it will be discredited. The asylum will continue to exist as a threat to the patient, whose only salvation would be to escape. Prevention, through an efficient mental health service, would certainly stop many patients from entering the asylum, thus avoiding the danger and risks of hospitalization, given the current condition of our psychiatric hospitals. But the principle of preventive community mental health services continues to operate in a climate where there is fear of the hospital: it would be the extreme step taken when all other measures have failed. The creation of so-called open wards will not resolve the problem either. This would maintain, within hospital, the privilege of those fortunate enough to have medical coverage, while the so-called closed wards would still contain those involuntarily committed.

3. The first excerpt is taken from "La Distruzione dell'ospedale psichiatrico," *Annali di Neurologia e Psichiatria,* Lis, f.l, 1965. The others are taken from internal documents written by the Gorizia *equipe* during the various phases of the movement.—ED.

4. It should be noted that the Italian for evil (*male*) is the root of the word illness (*malattia*).—ED.

5. John Conolly (1794–1866) abolished restraints at the Hanwell Asylum in England. His teachings that restraining a patient was more harmful than neglecting him were influential throughout England and, later, in Russia. Once the restraints were removed, the attitudes of asylum personnel also changed and violence toward patients became the

exception rather than the rule. The climate of the asylum changed and two-thirds of the patients were discharged. Among many of Basaglia's co-workers, Conolly represented the birth of an awareness that psychiatry is both a social problem and a scientific one. Conolly advocated for a "state" form of psychiatric care and for university courses in this discipline. See A. Pirella and D. Casagrande, "John Conolly, *dalla filantropia alla psichiatria sociale*" in F. Basaglia, ed., *Che Cos'e la Psichiatria?* (Parma: Administrazione Provinciale di Parma, 1967).—ED.

6. The English example is the most representative in terms of this issue. Psychiatry no longer has a subordinate status in the National Health Service, but mental patients are considered like any other patients and thus part of the general medical system. While we are in agreement with the general approach, it raises some questions because integration into the system can mean an avoidance of the problem of mental illness and creates the illusion that one of the greatest contradictions of our reality has been eliminated. Some psychiatric institutions run the risk of suppressing contradictions by creating a pleasant communal regression. For example, unless there is true community control, Maxwell Jones' "living-learning situation" or his "sensitivity training" end up as methods of nonproblematic integration. When they are used as techniques to resolve social conflicts, applicable as well to healthy workers in industrial settings, they can easily become ideological solutions that do not take real contradictions into account, similar to Lewin's concept of "resolving social conflict." The English approach is exciting, nonetheless, because it does give the patient an active role in his or her self-construction, but it is unacceptable when this self-making tends toward integration. Since the organization of the hospital in which we work starts from similar assumptions, we are well aware of the risks we can easily encounter. The meaning of the patient's role and her self-making are to found in struggle and in conflict, not in integration. See F. O. Basaglia and F. Basaglia, G. F. Minguzzi. "Exclusion, Programmation, et Integration," *Recherches* (1967), no. 5.

7. Cited by Jurij Davydov, *Il lavoro e la liberta,* (Turin: Einaudi, 1966).

PART TWO: DEVIANCE, "TOLERANCE," AND MARGINALITY

1. See, for example: Thomas J. Scheff, *Being Mentally Ill* (Chicago: Aldine, 1966); Edwin Lemert, "Paranoia and the Dynamics of Exclusion" from the volume *Human Deviance, Social Problems, and Social Control* (Englewood Cliffs: Prentice Hall, 1967).

2. Jurgen Ruesch, "Social Disability: the Problem of Misfits in Society," paper presented at the Congress entitled, "Towards a Healthy Community," organized by the World Federation for Mental Health and Social Psychiatry, Edinburgh, 1969.

3. Scheff, T. *Being Mentally Ill.* See especially part one.

3. THE DISEASE AND ITS DOUBLE AND THE DEVIANT MAJORITY

1. In bourgeois democracies, the state manages to keep the forces of opposition under control, which enables them to manipulate the situation. Tolerance of antagonistic forces is directly proportional to the strength and certainty of control.

2. Compare the techniques used by psychoanalysis and social psychiatry, both of which started out as responses to practical needs, but which later became tools of manipulation by reifying the original dynamic.

3. When it is said that the more deviants there are, the less deviant they will be, the only logical consequence would be for them to change the definition of the norm and its boundaries. But since the norm is defined in terms of productivity, the increase in the number of deviants has not caused a change in its definition. We might say that deviants have been assimilated at different levels as new subjects and objects of production, consumption and control.

4. F. and F. Basaglia, "L'utopia della realta," in L. Forti, ed., *L'altra pazzia* (Milan: Feltrinelli, 1975).

5. Consider the origins of the English community psychiatry movement after World War II. In the postwar economy, England needed manpower, and it was then that the first psychiatric institutions were established for the rehabilitation of mental patients because the country needed them for production.

6. This ferment arises from real needs, both because the public begins to see that it has a nonexistent service which has only a custodial function and because the paraprofessional staff perceives the possibility of a more human, less degrading job than being the jailer of innocent prisoners. Even though it is still fragmentary and isolated, this pressure from below is beginning to force governmental agencies to take positions and formulate programs. Nonetheless, these programs are limited in nature because they are drawn up by politicians. In general it is a matter of preelectoral projects which are rarely carried out; they are planned as long-term initiatives with no experimental stages to clarify the appropriate approach to take. It is far easier to formulate far-reaching programs than to plan experimental programs and study their effect on a given reality. Thus we can see the true political concerns of these social programs—the imposition of new laws and dogmas means that no practical solutions are found for the demands being made, and a new theoretical structure is created which once again hides the lack of action.

7. We are still at a stage of capitalist development in which the ideology of diversity is indispensable for the maintenance of order.

8. The classification does not even justify itself by saying there is no internal conflict in psychopathic behavior, which would make the negative judgment of all his behavior more convincing.

9. J. Ruesch, "Social Disability: The Problem of Misfits in Society." Paper presented at the Conference of the World Federation for Mental Health and Social Psychiatry, "Towards a Healthy Community," Edinburgh, Scotland, September 3–5, 1969.

10. How can you define 65 percent of the population, which has no alternative to nonwork, as the "world of leisure?"

11. Talcott Parsons, *The Social System* (New York: Free Press, 1951), p. 522.

12. Antonin Artaud, *The Theatre and Its Double,* Mary Caroline Richards, tr. (New York: Grove Press, 1958), p. 7.

13. As regards these two new disciplines: for polemology, we refer the reader to the arguments of F. Fornari, who is considered the most authoritative exponent in Italy. For thanatology, we are not aware of any Italian contributions and we therefore quote from a relevant item in the authoritative French newspaper, *Le Monde,* April 2, 1970, p. 15:

"A New Discipline: Thanatology

"The changes in our society, particularly the fact that the population is increasingly concentrated in large cities, forces our attention to problems involving death, funerals, and exhumation, and to find reasonable solutions to them.

"Towards this end, philosophers, clergymen, doctors, mayors, hospital directors, urban planners, etc. have established interdisciplinary ties in order to study everything that relates to death.

"Created in 1966, the French Thanatology Society plans to study these different aspects. Up to now, the Society has concentrated most of its work on suicide, euthanasia, the death penalty, organ transplants, and the problems of death and urban ecology. On many occasions, its officials have noted the inadequate hygiene generally found as regards death, on the usefulness of thanataproxy (the preservation of corpses), and of "athenia" and "funeraria" (establishments which would be hygienically equipped to receive the dead and their families in the period between death and burial).

"Other studies that are to be undertaken soon are on the scientific use of autopsies, and the changes needed in cemetaries, funerals, and cremations. (M. A. R.)"

14. As published in *The Dialectic of Liberation*, David Cooper, ed., (Hammondsworth: Penguin, 1968).

15. This is clear from how certain groups of intellectuals use an esoteric language, and how intellectualism itself becomes a weapon of domination over the class that they think they are liberating. Is there a difference between a political, revolutionary esoteric language and this technical, professional language which is the scientific expression of an ideology serving the dominant class? The incomprehensibility of the language creates and maintains distance from the class they hope to unite with, and it maintains their domination as well.

4. LETTER FROM AMERICA

1. Basaglia would define therapy as a change not adjustment.—Trans.

2. Basaglia uses this word transitively, much the way *Exist* is used by Laing and Cooper in *Reason and Violence.—Trans.*

PART THREE: PRACTICING KNOWLEDGE: REFLECTIONS ON THE ROLE OF INTELLECTUALS

1. Antonio Gramsci, *Selections from the Prison Notebooks,* Quentin Hoare and Geoffrey Nowell Smith, trs. (New York: International Publishers, 1971), ch. 1.

2. Serge Mallet, *La nouvelle classe ouvrière* (Paris: 1963).

3. "Technicians and the Capitalist Division of Labor," *Il Manifesto* (October–November 1969), no. 5/6; French translation published in *Les Temps Modernes* (April 1970), p. 285.

4. *Ibid.* An abridged English-language version appeared in *Socialist Revolution,* (May–June 1972), 2(3): 65–84,

5. See, for example, C. Boggs, "The Italian Left: A New Political Synthesis," *Socialist Revolution* (May–June 1972), 2(3): 91–113.

6. P. Sedgewick, *Psychopolitics* (New York: Harper and Row, 1981), part 2.

7. Discussed in A. Scull, *Decarceration: Community Treatment and the Deviant—A Radical View,* (Englewood Cliff, N.J.: Prentice-Hall, 1977), p. 71.

8. American Federation of State, County, and Municipal Employees, *Out of Their Beds and Into the Streets* (Washington D. C.: AFSCME, 1975).

9. M. El-Kaim, ed., *Reseau Alternative à La Psychiatrie* (Paris: Dix/Dix-Huit, 1977). Differences between the French and Italian unions' relationships to the antipsychiatric and anti-institutional movements are discussed in this book. They are beyond the scope of this introduction.

10. D. Mauri, ed., *La Libertà e Terapeutica?* (Milano: Feltrinelli, 1983). All other information about Trieste is taken from this book, unless otherwise indicated.

11. Report from the Nurses of Trieste Psychiatric Zone IIa., *in Il Circuito del Controllo: Dal Manicomio al Decentramento Psichiatrico,* E. Battiston, M. Costantino, F. Faoro, C. Piccardo, and M. Reali, eds. (Trieste: Cooperative Libraria-Centro Culturale "Via Gambini", 1980); pp. 111–113.

12. See, for example, the comments by the C.G.I.L. to the first convention of Psyichiatria Democratica in *La Pratica della Follia,* Atti del 1° Convegno Nazionale di Psichiatria Democratica (Venice: Critica delle Instituzioni, 1975).

13. S. Piro and M. Risso, "La Formazione degli Operatori di Salute Mentale," in *La Practica della Follia*, pp. 263–275.

14. This seemingly paradoxical position actually reflects an understanding of the complexities of psychiatric treatment, especially the thin, poorly defined line between providing much-needed treatment and applying a chemical strait-jacket. Aware of the power inherent in knowledge, the nurses wanted technical information. Yet they refused to carry out potentially oppressive decisions the doctors had freed themselves of by delegating to them. At other times the Trieste nurses' control over deciding upon the type and amount of medication was interpreted as a form of autonomy (see Mauri, ed., *La Liberata*, p. 152). Nurses elsewhere demanded a say in how psychiatric funding should be spent (R. Manfredi, "Per Una Reale Unita Fra Operatori Sanitarie Classe Operaia," (On Behalf of 76 Psychiatric Nurses in Ravenna), in *La Pratica della Follia*, p. 201.

15. See especially the first volume of collected works by F. Basaglia (*Scritti I: 1953–1968*, Turin: Einaudi, 1982), and R. D. Laing and D. Cooper, *Reason and Violence* (New York: Partheon Books, 1971).

16. Mauri, ed., *La Liberta*; G. dell'Acqua, *Non Ho L'Arma che Uccide II Leone. Storie del Manicomio di Triestre* (Trieste: Cooperative Libraria-Centro Culturale "Via Gambini," 1980).

5. PEACETIME CRIMES: TECHNICIANS OF PRACTICAL KNOWLEDGE

1. Antonio Gramsci, *Selections from the Prison Notebooks of Antonio Gramsci*, Q. Hoare and G. N. Smith, eds. (New York: International Publishers, 1971), p. 12.

2. The Resistance refers to the Italian anti-Fascist and anti-German opposition, which gained widespread support after the armistice of September 8, 1943. It included an active and armed movement and the passive resistance of a large part of the Italian population.—ED.

3. Basaglia is using the term as defined by Gramsci, for whom functionaries are members of the middle and upper echelons of bureaucracy. See Gramsci *Selections*, p. 13. —ED.

4. See Franco Basaglia and Franca Ongaro Basaglia, "Preface," in Maxwell Jones, *Ideologia e Pratica della Psichiatria Sociale* (Milan: Etas Kompass, 1970).

5. F. A. Tambroni, a Christian Democrat (DC) and government Minister from 1953 to 1960, became President of the government council in March 1960. During that time, he gave tacit consent to attempts by neo-Fascist forces, including the Movimento Sociale Italiano (MSI) Party to determine the direction of Italy's policies. This was finally met by public protests, resulting in the deaths of several demonstrators and in Tambroni's resignation.—ED.

6. M. Langer and A. Bouleo, "Algo mas sovre tortura," *Questionamos*, No. 2, Granica editor, Collecion Izquierda Freudiana, n.d.

7. The "kiss of death," an expression quoted by Eleanor Roosevelt and told to Yugoslavian historian Vladimir Dedijer during the U.S. General Assembly of 1948, refers to a concept of manipulation. She described it as a "dangerous technique" used in the Anglo-Saxon countries to destroy nonconformists by suffocating them with praise, "the kiss of death," thus diverting them from their original objectives. (V. Dedijer, "Notes on Historiography as an Instrument of Identification with the Aggressor," in Franco Basaglia and Franca Ongaro Basaglia, eds., *Crimini di pace: Ricerche sugli intelletuali e sui tecnici come addetti all' oppressione.* (Turin: Einaudi, 1975)—ED.

8. The concept of "negative worker" was used by Rene Lorau, a sociologist and

major representative of the French movement of *analyse institutionelle,* which grew out of both the May Events in 1968 and the earlier institutional psychotherapy. Institutional analysis used symbolic actions within institutions to expose their true functions. Rather than identifying with the dominant class which delegated power to them, the "negative worker" (e.g., a doctor) sided with the "deviant" (e.g., the patient who refuses treatment), who acted in ways that were dysfunctional to the institution's goals. See René Lorau, "Negative Workers, Unite!," in Basaglia and Ongaro Basaglia, *Crimini di Pace*—ED.

9. Franco Basaglia, "L'Utopia della realta," in Basaglia, *Scritti II,* (Turin: Einaudi, 1982).

10. See Franco Basaglia, "Illness and its Double," in this volume.

11. Naturally, this discussion applies to every other institution in our social system.

12. At the Psychiatric Hospital of Gorizia, we brought about changes in the logic of the asylum that led to the development of an anti-institutional movement that shifted psychiatric problems from a purely technical context to a social and political one. This experience has been written about in Franco Basaglia, ed., *Che Cos'è La Psichiatria?* (Parma: Amministrazione Provinciale, 1967); and in Franco Basaglia, ed., *L'Istituzione Negata* (Turin: Einaudi, 1968). (See also the first two selections in this volume.—ED.) Our intent was to increase public knowledge of and involvement in health and psychiatric issues.

13. By "opening" the asylum, the Basaglias refer to the process of eliminating all forms of confinement and restraint within the institution, e.g., locked wards.—ED.

14. To understand the process that led to the suppression of Basaglia's anti-institutional work at Gorizia, see Part 1. During this period in 1972, Basaglia was already director of the Psychiatric Hospital of Trieste. However, several of his original team members had stayed on and recruited other mental health workers to Gorizia.—ED.

15. Until this mental health law of 1968, voluntary hospitalization was nonexistent. The Law of 1904, which established the equivalent of state hospitals in every Italian Province, required patients to be committed involuntarily.—ED.

16. Statement released on October 20, 1972, by Domenico Casagrande, then director of the Psychiatric Hospital at Gorizia.

17. Letter from Franco Basaglia sent to the President of the Provincial Administration on October 23, 1972.

18. Letter sent on November 20, 1972, to the patients at the Psychiatric Hospital of Gorizia from the resigning doctors and staff, who had participated in the transformation of the hospital.

19. M.S.I. (Movimento Sociale Italiano), or Italian neo-Fascist party.—ED.

20. Letter sent on November 20, 1972, to the President of the Provincial Administration of Gorizia by Franco Basaglia, then member of the nominating committee to select a new director for the hospital.

21. The Thirteenth Arrondissement, a mental health center so named for its location in one of Paris' administrative districts, is considered the model of the French version of community mental health, the *politique de secteur.* Founded in 1954, it quickly developed a vast array of services for children and adults that included day hospitals, sheltered workshops, etc. Unlike most French community mental health services, however, it has semi-private status and no psychiatric hospital attached to it.—ED.

22. The G.I.P. (Groupe d'information des prisons) was founded in 1970–71 by a group of leftist French intellectuals, notably Michel Foucault, Jacques Donzelot, Daniel Defert, and the editor, Jean-Marie Domenach. At first exerting pressure on authorities to obtain political prisoner status for activists imprisoned during the May Events, the G.I.P.

quickly quickly moved to an exposure of the disciplinary and violent nature of prisons. —ED.

23. Journal founded at the end of World War II by Sartre, Simone de Beauvoir, and Maurice Merleau-Ponty.—ED.

24. See Part Five for discussions of the law.

25. In particular, those at Gorizia, Parma, Trieste, Arrezzo, Perugia.—ED.

26. We are referring to the creation of the organization, Democratic Psychiatry (in 1974).

27. Right-wing violence was used by the Christian-Democratic governments from 1969 to 1974 as a means of controlling the actions of the strong social movements. The series of terrorist acts ranged from attacks on leftist demonstrations and injuries and assassinations of individual militants to the bombing of numerous trains and of the Bologna train station in 1980, where 84 persons died. In 1974, the M.S.I. (neo-Fascist party) increased the percentage of its votes from 4.5 to 8.7 percent, partly through "red scare" tactics. (Alberto Melucci, "New Movements, Terrorism, and the Political System. Reflections on the Italian Case," *Socialist Review* (March–April 1981), 56:97–135.—ED.

28. Antonio Gramsci, *Quaderni del Carcere: Gli Intelletuali el'Organizzazione della Cultura* (Turin: Einaudi, 1955).

29. See David Cooper, *The Death of the Family* (London: Penguin, 1971) and *Psychiatry and Anti-Psychiatry* (New York: Ballantine, 1967). By the late seventies, Cooper considered what he meant by antipsychiatry to be closer to Basaglia's work.—ED.

30. See Ivan Illich, *Medical Nemesis* (New York: Pantheon, 1976).

31. See parts one and two of this volume. See also, Erving Goffman, *Asylums* (Garden City, N.Y.: Doubleday, 1961).—ED.

32. See, for example, Robert Castel, Francoise Castel, and Anne Lovell, *The Psychiatric Society* (New York: Columbia University Press, 1982), and Robert Castel, *La Gestion des Risques* (Paris: Editions de Minuit, 1981) for elaboration of these points.—ED.

33. Stanley Cohen, "Uno scenario per il sistema carcerario futuro," in Franco Basaglia and Franca Ongaro Basaglia, eds., *Crimini di pace,* pp. 441–470.

34. General Jacques Massu, *La vrai bataille d'Alger,* (Paris: Plon, 1971).

PART FOUR: ON THE NATURE OF MADNESS

1. Franco Basaglia, "Conference Brasiliane," Foglie d'Informazione, March 1984, p. 8.

2. *Enciclopaedia Einaudi,* vol. 6, (Turin: Einaudi, 1979).

3. Franco Basaglia, "Esposizione Riassuntivo," *Scritti I* (Turin: Einaudi, 1981), p. xxviii.

4. Michel Foucault, *Madness and Civilization: A History of Insanity in the Age of Reason.* Richard Howard, tr. (New York: Vintage Books, 1965).

5. Max Horkheimer and Theodor W. Adorno. *Dialectic of Enlightenment.* John Cumming, tr. (New York: Herder and Herder, 1972).

6. Franca Ongaro Basaglia, "Premessa," in Basaglia, *Scritti I,* p. ix.

7. See for example essays written between 1953 and 1966 and collected in Basaglia, *Scritti I.*

8. The Trieste group often conceptualized their work in the terms of this theory, whose major proponent was the Hungarian scholar and disciple of Georg Lukacs, Agnes Heller. See her *Theory of Need in Marx* (New York: St. Martin Press, 1976).

For example, one community mental health center stated that: "The hypothesis of our center tends to create a discussion around radical needs, which are the needs for

316   FOUR: ON THE NATURE OF MADNESS

community, for authentic interpersonal relationships, for structuring one's own identity and corporal image. With the concept of radical, we are indicating needs that cannot be met in the social market, which objectify themselves in exchanges not defined in an alienated way. (In the long run, even the need for a home can become radical in a certain historical and economic context)."

9. Edgardo Battiston and Mario Reale, "Esperienze di trasformatione: Dall'ospedale al Centro" (Trieste: Cooperative Libraria Centro Culturale Via Gambini, 1977), p. 10.

10. Basaglia, "Conferenze Brasiliane," p. 32.

11. During the years of Basaglia's anti-institutional work, few psychiatrists who trained with him and other democratic psychiatrists returned to teach in the universities. The lessons from their alternative practices have not been incorporated into university training, creating the problem of passing on knowledge.

6. MADNESS/DELIRIUM

Epigraph: Max Horkheimer and Theodor W. Adorno, *Dialectic of Enlightenment*. John Cumming, tr. (New York: Herder and Herder, 1972).

1. M. Foucault, *Madness and Civilization: A History of Insanity in the Age of Reason*, translated from the French by Richard Howard (New York: Vintage Books, 1965), p. xi.

2. Translator's Note: The term "delirium" has been retained here in the place of "delusion." In Italian, *delirio* refers to both the confused mental condition that results from an organic base, such as fever, that produces hallucinations and delusions, and to a belief held without factual evidence (delusion). Basaglia and Basaglia also use "delirium" in a historical sense. In this chapter, "delusion" will be used only when "delirium" is clearly awkward or misleading.

4. *Follis* is the root of the root of the Italian word for madness, *follia.—Trans.*

5. Nietzsche, cited in Horkheimer and Adorno, *Dialectic of Enlightenment*.

6. T. R. Malthus, *An Essay on the Principle of Population* (London: Johnson, 1978).

7. Translators' Note: D. Diderot and M. d'Alembert, *Enciclopédie ou Dictionnaire Raisonné des Sciences, des Arts, et des Metiers*. Vol. X, 2nd Edition. (Geneva: Pettet, 1777–1779), p. 609.

8. Translator's Note: *Enciclopedia Italiana Trecciani*. Vol. 12 (Milano: Rizzoli, 1931), p. 540.

9. F. Nietzche, cited in Horkheimer and Adorno, *Dialectic of Enlightenment*.

10. M. Horkheimer and T.W. Adorno, *Dialectic of Enlightenment*, translated from the German by John Cumming (New York: Herder and Herder, 1972), pp. 27–28.

PART FIVE: ANTI-INSTITUTIONAL POLITICS AND REFORM: ON PSYCHIATRY AND LAW

1. The concept of social chronicity in a North American context is nicely illustrated in Sue E. Estroff, *Making It Crazy* (Berkeley: University of California Press, 1981). For Italian discussions see Diana Mauri, ed., *La Libertà è Terapeutica? L'Esperienza Psichiatrica di Trieste* (Milan: Feltrinelli, 1983).

2. The *secteur* model is discussed in Robert Castel, *La Gestion des Risques: de l'Anti-Psychiatrie à l'Apres-Analyse* (Paris: Les Editions de Minuit, 1981). The community mental health movement in the United States is discussed in Robert Castel, Françoise Castel, and Anne Lovell, *The Psychiatric Society*. (New York: Columbia University Press, 1982). See also Phil Brown, *The Transfer of Care* (Boston: Routledge and Kegan Paul, 1984).

3. By the 1980s, many anti-psychiatry groups were shifting positions. The concern with treatment and the reality of mental illness is reflected in the late Peter Sedgewick's writings, especially *Psychopolitics* (New York: Harper and Row, 1981). The range of critical positions are analyzed in David Ingleby, ed., *Critical Psychiatry: The Politics of Mental Health* (New York: Pantheon, 1980). Although many of the groups in the United States have folded (for example, the *Radical Therapy* journal collective, in its many metamorphoses, from *Rough Times* to *State and Mind*), in California, Network Against Psychiatric Assault (NAPA) helped defeat electroconvulsive therapy legislation in Berkeley. In Europe, many anti-psychiatry groups, such as Le Cheval Bleu in France and the Réseau, Alternatives to Psychiatry affiliate in Belgium, have focused attention on the Italian law, under the leadership of the Trieste group and Franco Rotelli, Basaglia's successor as director.

4. It has been suggested that where the cultural expectation that the public mental hospital is the valid form of treatment for psychiatric problems does *not* exist, such as in two Southern Italian cities that never established the asylums required by the 1904 law, use of community-based alternatives as the choice for psychiatric care is more easily accomplished. See Sergio Piro, "Leggi sulla Psichiatria e Meridione d'Italia," in Domenico Desalvia and Paolo Crepet, eds., *Psichiatria Senza Manicomio: Epidemiologia Critica Sulla Riforma,* (Milan: Feltrinelli, 1982). The site of an area and the nature of the relationships between its doctors and elected officials may also affect frequency of commitments, under "the 180." One psychiatrist provides the following illustration of what might happen when the mayor calls a doctor about a person in crisis:

" 'Listen, doctor, is compulsory hospitalization really necessary for Mr. So-and-so? We don't like to sign the ordinances, either. Can't you figure out another way [to handle him]?' " Every now and then this sort of telephone call takes place, usually when the patient is from a township or the area is small and the policeman who is supposed to go pick up the patient was playing cards with him the night before. These are the small, very profound positive changes provoked by the 180 in areas where it has been worked on honestly." Leo Nahon, "La Legge Negata," *SE: Scienza Esperienza,* April 1984, p. 8. A contrasting example is provided from a rural area in the rice-growing region of Italy. There, day-to-day work takes place in individual rice fields. The inhabitants, who live in isolated houses rather than villages, as in southern Italy, are not used to managing social problems together. Since the 180 was passed, families have used the Diagnosis and Cure Units heavily for their members in psychological distress. Dr. Orlando Erlicher, personal communication, April 1984.

5. The radical currents of Jacques Lacan's psychoanalysis and other anti-psychiatry groups that focus on the symbolic realm are discussed in Sherry Turkle, *Psychoanalytic Politics: Freud's French Revolution* (New York: Basic Books, 1978). Castel contends that after the May events of 1968, most psychiatric practitioners used the momentum engendered for reform to implement already-existing plans for social programs, particularly the community mental health policy (*politique de secteur*) which had been decreed in 1960 (Castel, *La Gestion des Risques*).

7. PROBLEMS OF LAW AND PSYCHIATRY: THE ITALIAN EXPERIENCE

1. Conolly's nonrestraining system is discussed in note 5, editor's Introduction to chapter 1. Ugo Cerletti (1877–1963), an Italian neurologist, developed and perfected electroconvulsive therapy in the late thirties.

8. CRITICAL PSYCHOLOGY AFTER THE LAW 180

1. Basaglia is referring to Ernesto Venturini, ed., *Il Giardino dei Gelsi,* (Turin: Einaudi, 1979), a collection of interviews with psychiatrists working in community settings. This selection was originally published as a preface to the second edition of that book.—ED.